THE ENCYCLOPEDIA OF

CHILDREN'S HEALTH AND WELLNESS

Volume II

Carol Turkington
and
Albert Tzeel, M.D., F.A.A.P.

☑®
Facts On File, Inc.

The Encyclopedia of Children's Health and Wellness

Facts On File, Inc.
132 West 31st Street
New York NY 10001

Library of Congress Cataloging-in-Publication Data

Turkington, Carol.
The encyclopedia of children's health and wellness / Carol Turkington ; foreword by Albert Tzeel
p. cm.
Includes bibliographical references and index.
ISBN 0-8160-4821-5 (hc. ; alk. paper)
1. Pediatrics—Encyclopedias. 2. Children—Diseases—Encyclopedias. I. Title.
[DNLM: 1. Pediatrics—Encyclopedias—English. WS 13 T939e2004]
RJ45.T9465 2004
618.92—dc22   2004043251

Facts On File books are available at special discounts when purchased in bulk quantities for businesses, associations, institutions, or sales promotions. Please call our Special Sales Department in New York at (212) 967-8800 or (800) 322-8755.

You can find Facts On File on the World Wide Web at http://www.factsonfile.com

Text and cover design by Cathy Rincon

Printed in the United States of America

VB Hermitage 10 9 8 7 6 5 4 3 2 1

This book is printed on acid-free paper.

CONTENTS

ENTRIES M–Z

mainstreaming The placement of disabled students in the regular education classroom. Mainstreaming was introduced in the 1970s as a result of Public Law 94-142, which mandated that special needs children be placed in the least restrictive environment. Until the approval of P.L. 94-142 in 1975, most special needs children (from mildly to severely disabled), were educated in self-contained settings.

The philosophy of mainstreaming disabled children into the regular classroom comes from the idea that since most individuals will be "mainstreamed" into society, the integration of regular and special needs students should begin at an early age. It was also believed that school resources could be used more efficiently if special needs students were placed in the regular classroom. Mainstreaming also required regular educators to share the responsibility for disabled students with special educators. Conversely, mainstreaming benefits regular education students by increasing their understanding and tolerance of students with differences.

Studies of mainstreaming over the past two decades indicate that the practice is defined differently depending on the school and school district. In most school systems, mainstreaming involves placing a special needs student in the regular classroom setting for one subject area or a portion of the day depending on what is best for the student. According to research, mainstreaming can be a valid alternative to self-contained classrooms, but it is not an appropriate practice for all special needs students. A delicate balance must be struck between the student's need, teacher training, attitudes toward mainstreaming, and cost factors.

Most students with learning disabilities are educated in the regular classroom while receiving support services. Although parents sometimes worry that their children's needs will not be met in a regular classroom setting, mainstreaming does not mean that special education students are "dumped" into classes indiscriminately. Rather, students are placed in a regular classroom with support services so they can perform adequately. The concept of mainstreaming is a response to the fact that students can benefit from regular classroom placement if they get additional assistance at the same time. Forms of assistance might be an aide, modification of instruction, more instruction time, and communication with the regular classroom teacher.

Parents of nondisabled children often complain that the disabled child might disrupt the class or take up too much of the teacher's time. Both are legitimate concerns, and if any child is so disruptive that it interferes with the functioning of the class, then intervention is necessary.

Considerable time, energy, and planning go into every successful mainstreaming experience. Parents must be advocates for their children and provide input about the type and amount of mainstreaming that takes place, and they need to forge positive relationships with school personnel. This should be done during the development and implementation of the individualized education program (IEP).

Mainstreaming works best when:

- Parents and teachers work together.

- Specific mainstreaming experiences are recorded in the child's education plan.

- Special education teachers meet with regular classroom teachers in the mainstreamed setting.

- Mainstream teachers get information on the special education student's strengths and needs, and teaching techniques considered helpful for the student's particular learning disability.

- Mainstream teachers have time to consult with special education teachers to discuss student progress.

- Regular students are given information that enables them to better understand students with special needs.

malaria   An infectious disease caused by a parasitic protozoan within the red blood cells, now believed to be one of the major reemerging infections of the world. It is so serious that every 30 seconds somewhere in the world, a child dies of the disease.

Malaria is one of the oldest known infections described in detail by Hippocrates in the fifth century B.C. The incidence of the disease peaked in 1875 in this country, but it is estimated that more than 600,000 cases were reported in 1914. By 1934 the number of cases dropped to 125,556, and by the 1950s experts concluded that malaria had been eliminated in the United States through the efforts of mosquito spraying, removing breeding sites, accurate assessment, and focused control. It was still understood that international travel could reintroduce the disease into this country.

Since 1957 nearly all cases diagnosed in the United States have been acquired by mosquito transmission in areas where malaria is known to exist. About half the cases occur among native U.S. citizens, and half occur in foreign-born people. Environmental changes, the spread of drug resistance, and increased air travel could lead to the reemergence of malaria as a serious public health problem in the United States, according to the U.S. Centers for Disease Control and Prevention. Recent outbreaks of other mosquito-transmitted diseases in densely populated areas of New Jersey, New York, Texas, and Michigan are evidence that the risk exists.

The parasite that causes malaria has become resistant to the usual antimalarial drugs. Only 10 percent of the world's population was at risk of catching this disease in 1960, but today that number has grown to 40 percent. The number of deaths worldwide is very high, up to 2.4 million a year.

Most of the deaths occur in children under age five in Africa.

Cause

Malaria is caused by four different species of the *Plasmodium* parasite transmitted by the *Anopheles* mosquito. The deadliest parasite causing the sometimes-fatal version of malaria is *Plasmodium falciparum;* others are *P. vivas, P. malariae,* and *P. ovale.*

Parasites in the blood of an infected child are taken into the stomach of the mosquito as it feeds; when the mosquito bites a person, parasites are injected into the person's bloodstream, migrating to the liver and other organs. After an incubation period, parasites return to the blood and invade the red blood cells. At this point, symptoms appear. Rapid multiplication of the parasites destroys the red cells and releases more parasites capable of infecting other cells. This leads to the shivering, fever, and sweating that are the hallmarks of the disease.

The mature parasites remain in the blood and do not reinvade the liver, although a few may remain behind in the liver in a dormant state. These can be released months or years later, causing a relapse of malaria in people who thought they were cured.

Symptoms

Symptoms vary and may appear from eight to 12 days after a bite (falciparum malaria) to as many as 30 days for other types. Early signs may mimic the flu, with fever, chills, headache, muscle aches, and malaise. As each new batch of parasites is released, symptoms of shivering and fever reappear. The interval between fever attacks is different in different types of malaria.

In the most serious form of malaria (falciparum malaria), red blood cells become sticky, blocking and damaging the small blood vessels to the brain, kidney, and lungs. Patients with this variety can die within several days without antibiotics. Irreversible complications can appear suddenly. Malaria is more severe in children; more than 10 percent of untreated children will die.

Anyone who becomes ill with chills and fever after being in an area where malaria is endemic must see a doctor immediately. Delaying treatment of falciparum malaria can be fatal.

Diagnosis

Because malaria is often misdiagnosed by North American doctors, travelers to malaria-ridden areas must be tested with a specific blood test, which requires direct microscopic exam of the red blood cells to look for the parasite. Antibody tests are not always helpful, because many people have antibodies from past infections.

Treatment

Malaria can be treated effectively in the early stages, but delaying treatment can have serious consequences. Effective drugs include mefloquine, quinine, chloroquine, quinacrine, and atovaquone, chloroguanide. More recently, scientists in China discovered a drug called artemether that appears to be as effective as quinine in preventing malarial deaths. The need for a different drug is imperative, since the parasite is becoming resistant to quinine and chloroquine.

There are side effects with both the standard and the newer treatments. Quinine increases the risk of low blood sugar and abscesses at the injection site. Patients treated with artemether are slower to come out of a malaria-induced coma and more likely to have convulsions. Other animal studies suggest brain stem damage is related to high doses of artemether.

Falciparum malaria requires hospitalization, with intravenous fluids, red blood cell transfusions, kidney dialysis, and assistance in breathing.

Prevention

The World Health Organization has been trying to eradicate malaria for the past 30 years by killing mosquitoes that carry the parasite, but as the mosquitoes and parasites become resistant to insecticides, prevention now aims at avoiding bites and taking preventive drugs such as mefloquine or lariam.

Malaria often can be prevented by using antimalarial drugs and personal protection measures against mosquito bites. While the risk of malaria is slight in the United States, people traveling to high-risk areas should take precautions. The risk for tourists who stay in air-conditioned hotels on tourist trips in urban or resort areas is lower than for backpackers, missionaries, and Peace Corps volunteers. Decisions on whether to use antimalarial drugs depends on the traveler's itinerary and duration of travel. Researchers are studying possible vaccines, but the parasite's complex life cycle inside its human host makes vaccination difficult.

malnutrition For proper function, the body must have the correct amount of food, including glucose, vitamins, minerals, and other essential chemicals. For example, the fuel the brain uses is glucose, which is produced from eating carbohydrates or other foods that can be converted to glucose. To grow new connections or add myelin, a fatty sheath to axons, the brain must manufacture the right proteins and fats. It does this by digesting proteins and fats in food and using the resulting amino acids and fatty acids to make the new brain proteins and fats. Without the correct amount and balance of particular building blocks, the brain will not work properly. Too little or too much of the necessary nutrient can affect the nervous system.

Vitamin and mineral deficiencies can be caused by:

- starvation
- poor diet
- poor absorption of vitamins and minerals
- damage to the digestive system
- infection
- alcoholism

The brain of a human fetus grows rapidly from the 10th to 18th week of pregnancy, so it is important for the mother to eat nutritious foods during this time.

The brain also grows rapidly just before and for about two years after birth. Malnutrition during these periods of rapid brain growth may have devastating effects on the nervous system and can affect not only neurons but also glial cell development and growth, which can affect myelin development. Babies born to mothers who had poor diets may have some form of mental retardation or behavioral problems, and children who do not eat well in their first few years of life may develop problems later. Often the effects of malnutrition and environmental problems, such as emotional and physical abuse, can combine to create behavioral problems. Therefore, the exact causes of behavioral disorders are difficult to determine.

Some effects of malnutrition can be repaired by a proper diet, so not all of the effects of poor diets are permanent. Researchers believe that the timing of malnutrition is an important factor in determining whether problems will occur. This means that missing out on a particular nutrient at the time when a part of the brain is growing and needs that nutrient will cause a specific problem there.

Scientists have just begun to understand how changes in particular nutrients alter the brain and how these neural changes then affect intelligence, mood, and the way people act. Experiments that investigate this nutrition-brain-behavior interaction, particularly those that study the effects of malnutrition, are difficult for several reasons. First, there is a link between poor nutrition and environmental factors, so that changes in behavior may not be due to poor nutrition only but to factors such as education, social, or family problems.

Because it is hard to alter only one substance in the human diet, it can be difficult to determine if a particular vitamin or mineral has a certain effect on behavior. For ethical reasons, experiments in which a person is not allowed to eat a particular nutrient cannot be done, so much of the data come from animal experiments. Studies in humans are generally limited to examining the effects of famine and starvation, situations where many nutrients are missing.

Children respond to different diets in different ways. In other words, there is a large individual variation in the body's response and need for different nutrients. A change in diet may have a placebo effect. The placebo effect occurs because a person thinks something will have an effect. In other words, if a person thinks a change in diet will affect behavior, it may actually affect behavior even if the nutrients are not causing the change. Therefore, experiments must have a placebo control and be performed in a double-blind manner where neither the experimental subject nor the experimenter knows who has received an altered diet.

manic depression   See BIPOLAR DISORDER.

Mantoux test   See TUBERCULIN TEST.

March of Dimes Birth Defects Foundation   A nonprofit organization originally established to conquer polio that since 1958 has been funding research and innovative programs to save babies from birth defects, premature birth, and low birth weight.

The March of Dimes was founded in January 1938, when President Franklin D. Roosevelt, himself a polio victim and alarmed by decades of worsening polio epidemics, established the National Foundation for Infantile Paralysis. At the time, comedian Eddie Cantor coined the phrase "March of Dimes" (playing on the popular newsreel feature "The March of Time"), appealing to radio listeners all over the country to send their dimes directly to the White House. The campaign was extremely successful, and over the next 17 years, the National Foundation focused on funding research to develop a vaccine against polio.

In 1948, with funding provided by the March of Dimes, Dr. Jonas Salk was able to grow the three known types of polio virus in his lab and eventually to develop an experimental killed-virus vaccine. In the summer of 1952 Dr. Salk tested the vaccine on children who had already recovered from polio. Following vaccination, the level of polio antibodies in their blood increased. The next step was to try it on volunteers who had not had polio—including himself, his wife, and their children. The volunteers all produced antibodies; none got sick. By 1954 nationwide testing of the vaccine inoculated nearly two million schoolchildren. Statistics showed that the Salk vaccine was 80 percent to 90 percent effective in preventing polio.

In the next four years 450 million doses of the vaccine were administered, and it became a standard fixture among childhood immunizations. Later, in 1962, an oral polio vaccine, developed by Dr. Albert Sabin, with funding from the March of Dimes, was licensed.

With the virtual elimination of polio as a childhood epidemic, the National Foundation officially changed its name to the March of Dimes in 1979.

Marfan syndrome   A genetic disorder of the connective tissue that affects many organ systems, including the skeleton, lungs, eyes, heart, and blood vessels. The condition affects both boys and girls of all races and ethnic groups and affects at least 200,000 people in the United States.

Symptoms

The most serious problems associated with Marfan syndrome involve the heart. The two parts of the mitral valve may move backward when the heart contracts (mitral valve prolapse), which can lead to mitral valve leaks or irregular heart rhythm. In addition, the main artery carrying blood away from the heart is often wider and more delicate in these patients. This progressive widening can lead to leaks or tears in the artery, which may require surgical repair.

Skeletal problems are common in Marfan syndrome, including curvature of the spine (SCOLIO-SIS), abnormally shaped chest, loose joints, and disproportionate growth (many patients will be quite tall). Children with Marfan syndrome are often nearsighted, and about half have a dislocated ocular lens.

Cause

A single abnormal gene causes Marfan syndrome, usually inherited from a parent who is also affected, but one-fourth of the cases involve a spontaneous mutation. Marfan syndrome is autosomal dominant, which means that any child of someone with the condition has a 50-50 chance of inheriting it.

Diagnosis

Marfan syndrome is hard to diagnose because there is no lab test for the condition, and symptoms vary a great deal. Most affected children do not have all of the possible signs and complications of the syndrome. A complete physical exam that focuses on the systems affected by the disorder may include a complete family history, an echocardiogram of the heart, a slit-lamp eye examination by an ophthalmologist, and a skeletal examination by an orthopedist.

Lab tests may eventually be possible, since scientists have discovered the chromosome, gene, and component of connective tissue (fibrillin) in which the mutation for the Marfan syndrome is located. It is hoped that as scientists better understand fibrillin, earlier and more accurate diagnosis of Marfan syndrome will be possible.

Treatment

There is no cure for the disorder yet, but careful medical management can greatly improve the prognosis and lengthen the life span. Treatment usually includes:

- *Echocardiogram* This annual test can monitor the size and function of the heart and aorta.
- *Eye exams* After the initial diagnosis with a slit-lamp to detect lens dislocation, periodic follow-ups with an ophthalmologist are required.
- *Drugs* Beta-blocker medications may be prescribed to lower blood pressure and ease stress on the aorta.
- *Antibiotics* These drugs may be prescribed prior to dental or genitourinary procedures to lower the risk of infection in people who experience mitral valve prolapse or who have artificial heart valves. (For contact information, see Appendix I.)

marijuana The world's most commonly used hallucinogenic drug that is derived from a plant *(Cannabis sativa)* containing delta-9 tetrahydrocannabinol (THC). Marijuana is usually smoked like a cigarette, but it also can be cooked into baked goods such as brownies or cookies, or brewed like a tea. THC is also contained in hashish, which is the resin from the plant. Hashish is usually smoked in a pipe. Other names for marijuana include grass, reefer, pot, and weed.

THC acts on cannabinoid receptors, which are found on brain cells in many places throughout the brain. These cells are found in areas involved in memory (the hippocampus), concentration (cerebral cortex), perception (sensory portions of the cerebral cortex), and movement (the cerebellum). When THC activates cannabinoid receptors, it interferes with the normal functioning of these brain areas.

In low to medium doses, marijuana causes relaxation, reduced coordination, low blood pressure, sleepiness, disruption in attention, and an altered sense of time and space. In high doses, it can cause hallucinations, delusions, impaired memory, and disorientation. The effects of marijuana begin within one to 10 minutes and can last from three to four hours.

Scientists have known for a long time that THC interacted with cannabinoid receptors in the brain, but they did not know why the brain would have such receptors. In 1992 scientists discovered anandamide, the brain's own THC, but they are not yet sure what the function of this chemical might be in a normal brain. Experts do not agree about whether marijuana can produce addiction and whether it causes long-term mental problems. While there have been no documented cases of fatal overdoses produced by marijuana, there is a high level of tar and other chemicals in marijuana cigarettes; smoking the drug causes similar health problems to cigarette smoking. There is a bigger risk of lung problems and lung cancer later in life due to marijuana cigarette smoking.

mastoiditis An infection of the prominent bone behind the ear (mastoid bone) usually as a result of an EAR INFECTION. Mastoiditis usually affects children and can sometimes lead to HEARING PROBLEMS. This disease has become uncommon since the widespread use of antibiotics to control ear infections.

Cause
The disease occurs when infection spreads from the middle ear to a cavity in the mastoid bone, and from there to a honeycomb of air cells in the bone itself.

Symptoms
Severe EARACHE, headache, and fatigue. Swelling behind the ear is often enough to actually push the external ear out of position. Other symptoms may include fever, creamy discharge from the ear, and progressive hearing loss.

Complications
The infection may spread to inside the skull, causing MENINGITIS, brain abscess, or a blood clot in veins inside the brain. Alternatively, the infection may spread outward, affecting the facial nerve and causing a facial paralysis.

Diagnosis
Mastoiditis can be identified from a physical exam. Early diagnosis is essential because of the potential serious complications.

Treatment
This infection is not easy to treat and often requires intravenous antibiotics for several days. If the infection persists, an operation called a mastoidectomy may be required. In this procedure, the surgeon makes an incision behind the ear to open up the mastoid bone and remove the infected air cells. A drainage tube is left in place and removed several days after the operation.

Maternal and Child Health Bureau Federal department that provides national leadership in working with states, communities, public and private partners, and families to strengthen maternal and child health. The Children's Bureau was established in 1912; by 1935 the U.S. Congress enacted Title V of the Social Security Act, which authorized the Maternal and Child Health Services programs and provided a foundation and structure for assuring the health of American mothers and children.

The bureau administers seven major programs with a budget of $872.4 million:

- The Maternal and Child Health Services Block Grant
- The Healthy Start initiative
- Emergency Medical Services for Children Program
- The Abstinence Education Program
- Traumatic Brain Injury
- Universal Newborn Hearing Screening
- Poison Control Centers Program

The bureau is part of the Health Resources and Services Administration of the U.S. Department of Health and Human Services. (For contact information, see Appendix I.)

mathematics disorder A disorder in which mathematical ability, as measured by standardized tests, is substantially below what is expected given the child's chronological age, intelligence, and education level. The disorder significantly interferes with academic achievement and with activities of daily living that require mathematical ability.

measles   A childhood viral illness causing a widespread red rash and fever considered to be the most contagious disease in the world. One infected person in a crowded room is able to transmit the illness to almost every unvaccinated person in the room. The medical name for measles is "rubeola," and it is sometimes called "red measles" to distinguish it from the much milder disease known as rubella (GERMAN MEASLES). While measles was once commonly found throughout the world and was not normally considered to be dangerous, complications can be fatal.

In populations that have never been exposed to it, measles can be a killer; 800 children died of measles during an epidemic in the Charlestown area of Boston in 1772. It is so remarkably virulent that in 1951, a single person with measles landed in Greenland and within six weeks, all but five of the 4,300 never-before-exposed Greenland natives came down with the disease.

Although measles has been known to be a viral disease since 1911, it was not until 1954 that two Harvard researchers isolated the actual measles virus in the lab. When a vaccine was finally licensed in 1963, experts thought the disease would be eradicated by 1982. When this did not occur, the target date was revised to 1990. But instead of disappearing, measles cases began to rise again from only 1,500 cases in 1983 to 28,000 cases in 1990 in the United States. Half of those reported cases occurred in children under age five. Because many high schools and colleges experienced measles outbreaks in the late 1980s and early 1990s, most schools now require older students to be re-immunized.

Since 1991 measles cases have again been decreasing; there were 963 cases in 1994 and just 301 in 1995 (the lowest number for a single year since the disease became reportable in 1912). However, it is still a killer in developing countries, where more than one million deaths a year are recorded, especially among malnourished children with impaired immunity.

One case of measles confers lifelong immunity; the vaccine also confers lifelong immunity after two doses; anyone who received two doses of vaccine during childhood will not get measles.

Cause
The measles virus is spread by airborne droplets from nasal secretions. The incubation period is between nine and 11 days, and the patient is infectious from shortly after the beginning of this period until up to a week after symptoms have developed. Infants under six months of age rarely contract measles because they still harbor some immunity from their mothers.

The virus survives best in low humidity; it can survive in the air for several hours. It is so infectious that it is capable of traveling down a hall on air currents and into other rooms where healthy people are located, infecting them. It is also possible to contract the disease from touching bedding or towels touched by an infected person, or by directly touching secretions from a person's nose, mouth, eyes, or cough. The patient is most infectious right before the rash beings.

A milder form of the disease can occur among those who do not develop adequate immunity from just one dose of vaccine, who were immunized too early, or who had received an older, less effective variety of the vaccine. As their immunity wears off, these people become susceptible to measles.

Symptoms
About 10 days after the virus enters the body, symptoms of a high fever (up to 105°F) and general sick feeling begin. This is followed the next day by red, sore eyes, a stuffy nose, and cough. On the second day of fever, a rash of tiny white dots on a red base appears inside the mouth. After three or four days, a bright red splotchy rash will begin on the head and neck, spreading down to cover the entire body. The spots may be so numerous that they appear together as a large, reddened area. The rash begins to fade within three days and will disappear by six days. The fever will begin to drop on the second day of the rash, and the runny nose and sore eyes also lessen as the fever falls. The cough, however, may last for up to two weeks. Everyone with measles feels terrible, but babies and young children usually fare the worst, feeling much sicker than they would with a cold, the flu, or CHICKEN POX.

A physician should be called immediately if any of the following signs appear:

- vomiting

- dehydration

- wheezing or breathing problems (this may be a sign that the virus has spread to the lungs, causing measles PNEUMONIA)

- fever for more than four days after the rash appears

- unusual drowsiness, fussiness, or stiff neck (signs of measles ENCEPHALITIS) caused by the spread of the virus into the brain

- ear pain or pulling at the ear

Diagnosis

Physicians can diagnose measles from symptoms alone, although blood tests that check for antibodies to the virus are available.

Treatment

There is no cure for measles. Symptoms are treated with fluids and acetaminophen. Antibiotics will not affect the virus but may be needed to treat secondary infection. Patients need to rest in a darkened room because their eyes are sensitive to light.

Complications

Infants and those with serious health problems may become severely ill with measles and die. Infants are the most likely patients to have complications, including secondary ear and chest infections that usually occur as the fever returns after the rash appears. There also may be diarrhea, vomiting, and abdominal pain. Measles pneumonia in children may trigger serious breathing problems.

About one in every 1,000 patients goes on to develop encephalitis with headache, drowsiness, and vomiting, beginning seven to 10 days after the rash starts. This may be followed by seizures and coma, leading to mental retardation or death. (Febrile seizures are common with measles, however, and do not necessarily indicate the presence of encephalitis.)

Measles during pregnancy can cause fetal death in about one-fifth of all cases, but there is no evidence that measles causes birth defects.

Prevention

In the United States, children are routinely vaccinated first at age 12 months and again at age four or older with an injection usually combined with mumps and rubella that produces immunity in 97 percent of patients. Side effects of the vaccine are reported to be mild, including low fever, slight cold, and a rash about a week after the shot. The vaccine was first licensed for use in 1963 and is very effective; only one injection produces long-lasting protection.

The vaccine should not be given to infants under age one, or to those with a family history of epilepsy or who have had seizures before. In these children, simultaneous injection of measles-specific immunoglobulin, which contains antibodies against the virus, should be given.

A booster is recommended to be given at age four to six years, or at 10 to 12 years, to protect 95 percent of those who may have failed to become immune after their first vaccine dose.

Schools require evidence of measles immunity upon enrollment. Any children immunized before their first birthday should be re-immunized.

measles-mumps-rubella vaccine   See MMR VACCINE.

medical history   Every child's medical history should be written down in case of illness or accident that requires emergency care. In these situations, paramedics and emergency room doctors may have many questions about the child's medical history, and it is much easier to recall written information in the middle of a life-or-death emergency. Every second counts during an emergency, and having an up-to-date health record may help a doctor make quicker decisions.

Parents should keep a detailed medical record for each child in a safe place at home, one in each family car, and another in briefcase or purse. The child's day-care center and babysitters also should have a copy.

The medical history record should include the following items.

Allergies

This can help reveal a cause for problems like seizures or difficulty breathing. Record any known allergies to medications (list each specific name), insect stings and bites, food, and other substances. Note if the child has asthma and uses inhalers.

Medications

Some drugs just do not mix, so paramedics need to know all medications a child takes. This should include the name of medication, dose, and dosing schedule for each drug.

Illnesses or Chronic Conditions

Any chronic condition (such as asthma or diabetes) can affect emergency tests or treatments. For added protection, these children should wear an identifying bracelet tag.

Hospitalizations

All hospitalization dates for the child should be listed, along with any surgeries performed.

Immunizations

The medical history should include an updated record of all the child's immunizations, especially when the last tetanus shot was given. Information about any reactions after immunization (seizures, high fever, and so on) should be included.

Height and Weight

Because it is important to know a child's height and weight when calculating medication doses, this information should be kept updated constantly.

medication, giving Parents are often called upon to administer medication to their children at home. When obtaining a prescription or buying over-the-counter medicine, parents should know the child's exact weight. Most over-the-counter medicines list a chart on the bottle or package that outlines how much medicine should be given, according to weight.

When giving medicine to a child, the parent should use a measuring spoon or the plastic calibrated cup that comes with the medicine, but not a kitchen teaspoon.

Medicine for children is of a different concentration than infant's preparations. They should never be mixed or substituted one for the other.

Many medicines in suspension should be refrigerated; all should be shaken well before administration.

Parents should always call the pediatrician if they are not sure of the dose, even if the pharmacist has provided written instructions. Parents should also immediately call either the pharmacist or pediatrician if they have any doubts about the medication. Parents should check the name on the pill with the prescription and check the dosage to make sure it seems correct. They should always read the label twice and never give medicine in the dark.

Even if the child is getting better, all of the prescribed medicine must be used. This is especially important with antibiotics. Failure to use all the medication can lead to relapse or another illness.

meningitis Any infection or inflammation of the membranes covering the brain and spinal cord, caused by either bacteria, virus, or fungi. Bacterial meningitis is by far the most serious type of meningitis, but most of the time the infectious agent is a virus.

Before 1992 most patients under age five were infected with *Haemophilus influenzae*. Today this type of meningitis has almost disappeared in children younger than five because of an effective vaccine. Pneumococcal meningitis (caused by *Streptococcus pneumoniae*) and meningococcal meningitis (caused by *Neisseria meningitidis*) are now the most common and serious types of bacterial meningitis.

Bacterial Meningitis

More than two-thirds of all people who get bacterial meningitis are under age five, and before 1992 most of them would have been infected with *Haemophilus influenzae* type B (Hib). This illness has nothing to do with influenza, however, despite the name of the bacterium. Because of an effective vaccine, HIB meningitis has practically disappeared among young children in the United States.

The dread of bacterial meningitis, no matter which bacterium is responsible, is not just on its reputation as a killer but also on the real possibility of lingering neurological complications. These lingering deficits, which occur in between 20 percent and 30 percent of those surviving bacterial meningitis, can be especially devastating in infants and children. The deficits can include persistent hearing loss, mental retardation, and recurrent convulsions.

Cause   Today the most common causes of bacterial meningitis are pneumococcal meningitis caused by *Streptococcus pneumoniae*, meningococcal meningitis caused by *Neisseria meningitidis,* and *Listeria* in babies two months of age and younger.

Meningococcal meningitis affects about 3,000 Americans a year; about half are younger than two, and two-thirds are younger than 20. The highest-risk populations are babies between four months and 12 months of age, and young adults living together in close proximity (such as in a college dormitory). Patients can become infected by inhaling the bacteria, but most patients develop only very mild upper respiratory symptoms. More serious cases occur when the bacteria enter the bloodstream. Up to 30 percent of healthy people have this bacteria in their throats without having symptoms. In North America this type of meningitis usually occurs in isolated cases, usually in February and March (and least often in September).

Pneumococcal meningitis is the second most common type of bacterial meningitis, which kills one out of every five people who contract it. Children under age two are among the most easily infected. This type of meningitis occurs sporadically during the cold and flu season but not in epidemics. This bacteria is also responsible for EAR INFECTION, PNEUMONIA, and SINUSITIS. There are more than 80 types of *N. meningitidis.*

Symptoms   Classic signs of meningitis include sudden high fever (between 100°F and 106°F), with chills, vomiting, stiff neck, seizures, and intense headache in the front of the head. The neck will hurt if the child tries to touch the chin to the chest. There may be muscle spasms or leg pains, and bright lights may irritate the eyes.

All types of bacterial meningitis can appear suddenly or gradually in children. The less-common gradual type is harder to diagnose because symptoms are similar to other mild childhood illnesses: cold symptoms, fever, lethargy, vomiting, appetite loss. A sudden attack is easier to diagnose, although it may indicate a more serious case.

Abnormal behavior also may announce the onset of meningitis, including aggressiveness, irritability, agitation, delirium, or screaming. This is followed by lethargy and stupor or coma.

Babies between the ages of three months and two years may have fever, vomiting, irritability, seizures, and a high-pitched cry. The baby may become rigid, and the soft spot on the front of the baby's head may bulge.

Sometimes the illness may be preceded by a cold or an ear infection. Any sudden change in consciousness or any unusual behavior in a young child may be a sign of meningitis.

Diagnosis   A spinal tap must be done to diagnose meningitis. The normally clear fluid is analyzed for the presence of bacteria and other evidence of infection. Bacteria will grow in the fluid within 48 hours; rapid tests on urine or blood can give results in a few hours and are most helpful in determining what type of bacteria are causing the infection. However, since the disease can progress so quickly, treatment with intravenous antibiotics is usually started even before test results are available.

Treatment   Without treatment, most children would die from meningitis; with antibiotics, 95 percent recover. Current antibiotics used to treat bacterial meningitis include cephalosporins (especially cefotaxime and ceftriaxone) and various types of penicillin. At least one week of treatment is required.

Viral Meningitis

Viral meningitis is a fairly common and less severe version that is rarely fatal, although infections involving arbovirus, herpesviruses, or polio may be more severe.

Causes   Viral meningitis is usually caused by an enterovirus, a type of virus that infects only humans and is spread by the fecal-oral route. Enteroviruses live in human intestines; the two most common are ECHOVIRUSES and COXSACKIEVIRUS. The virus is spread by direct contact with infected feces, or nose or throat secretions. Most children are carriers without symptoms; the virus spreads most easily among young children in a group. Viral meningitis usually strikes young children in the summer and early fall. Scientists do not know why so few children who are exposed to the disease come down with symptoms; those who are well fed, well rested, and healthy are less likely to become infected.

Symptoms Symptoms usually appear quite suddenly, with a high fever, severe headache, nausea and vomiting, and stiff neck. There may be sensitivity to light and noise, sore throat, or eye infections. There also may be accompanying neurological problems, such as blurred vision. Most people recover completely within two weeks, although there may be muscle weakness, tiredness, headache, muscle spasms, insomnia, or personality changes such as an inability to concentrate for months afterward. These are rarely permanent.

Diagnosis Viral meningitis can be diagnosed by a spinal tap.

Treatment There is no cure for viral meningitis; eventually the immune system will develop antibodies to destroy the virus. Hospitalization with intravenous fluids and painkillers may be necessary for the severe headache, dehydration, nausea, and vomiting. Patients should drink clear fluids, eat a bland diet, and get plenty of rest. A few weeks after recovery, children's hearing should be tested.

Complications Increased pressure on the brain from a buildup of fluid in the meninges is a serious complication. Some infants who have meningitis early in life experience delayed language development. Patients with a weakened immune system may have chronic infections with enterovirus.

Prevention A vaccine to prevent meningitis due to *S. pneumoniae* is not effective in children under two years of age but is recommended for all persons over 65 years of age and younger persons with certain chronic medical problems.

meningoencephalitis An inflammation of both the brain and the meninges, usually caused by a bacterial infection.

menstruation The reproductive cycle that begins when an ovary releases an egg. At the same time, estrogen is released, stimulating the lining of the uterus to thicken with blood. If an egg is not fertilized, progesterone levels drop and blood vessels constrict, the uterine lining sheds, and the menstrual flow begins. This cycle repeats itself about every 28 days until interrupted by pregnancy or ended by menopause.

Normally, menstruation begins at some point between the ages of 11 and 13, although a delay through age 17 is still considered to be normal. A girl who is older than 17 and has never had a menstrual period should see a doctor. Lack of weight gain, stress, or hormone irregularities all can contribute to a delayed period.

mental health Good mental health allows children to think clearly, develop socially, and learn new skills. Mental health can be fostered by making sure a child has some good friends and receives encouraging words from adults. All this is important in helping children develop self-confidence, high self-esteem, and a healthy emotional outlook on life. In order to develop good mental health, a child needs:

• unconditional love

• self-confidence and high self-esteem

• the opportunity to play with other children

• encouraging teachers

• supportive caretakers

• safe surroundings

• guidance and discipline

Unconditional Love

For optimum mental health, a child should find love, security, and acceptance at home among the family. Children need to understand that their parents' love does not depend on accomplishments, and mistakes should be expected and accepted.

Self-Confidence

A child becomes more confident in a family that expresses unconditional love and affection. Children should be praised and encouraged so that they develop a desire to explore and learn about their surroundings. Parents who actively participate in children's activities help build their self-confidence and self-esteem.

Parents should not hide failures from their children, because it is important for them to know that everyone makes mistakes.

Encouragement

Encouragement helps children strive to do their best and enjoy the process of achievement. Trying new activities teaches children about teamwork, self-esteem, and new skills.

Playtime

Playtime is as important to a child's development as food and good care, because play teaches children to be creative, to learn problem-solving skills, and to have self-control. Running and exercise help children be physically and mentally healthy. By playing with others, children discover their strengths and weaknesses, develop a sense of belonging, and learn how to get along with others. Parents can be playmates, too; playing a board game or coloring with a child gives parents a great opportunity to share ideas and spend time together in a relaxed setting. This also helps teach children that winning is not as important as being involved and enjoying the activity. One of the most important questions to ask children is "Did you have fun?" not "Did you win?"

Guidance and Discipline

Parents should provide appropriate guidance and discipline because children need the opportunity to explore and develop new skills and independence. At the same time, they need to learn that certain behavior is unacceptable, and that they are responsible for the consequences of their actions.

Parents should be fair and consistent, being firm, kind, and realistic. Nagging, threats, and bribery should be avoided.

When to Seek Help

Caregivers are usually the first to notice if a child has problems with emotions or behavior. If a problem is suspected, parents should consult a pediatrician or mental health professional. The following signs may indicate the need for professional assistance or evaluation:

- decline in school performance
- poor grades despite strong efforts
- worry or anxiety
- repeated refusal to go to school or take part in normal activities

- hyperactivity or fidgeting
- persistent nightmares
- persistent disobedience or aggression
- frequent temper tantrums
- depression, sadness, or irritability

See also MENTAL ILLNESS.

mental illness   Mental health problems affect one in every five children and adolescents at any given time, and an estimated two-thirds of all young people with mental health problems are not getting the help they need. Estimates of the number of children who have mental disorders range from 7.7 million to 12.8 million.

If a child is having an emotional or behavioral problem, it is important to intervene as quickly as possible; often, a good therapist can recognize a problem and treat it effectively. Child and family psychologists are specifically trained to work with young children and teenagers. A child's pediatrician should first examine the child if there is a suspicion of depression or other emotional problems, because a doctor should rule out medical problems as a possible cause of symptoms.

Preschoolers could benefit from seeing a therapist if there is a significant delay in achieving developmental milestones (walking, language, and toilet training). Emotional difficulty in older children may well appear as problems at school, because behavior that may be tolerated at home may be recognized as inappropriate in a school setting. Although "normal" behavior varies depending on a child's age and maturity level, some of the signs that your child may be experiencing stress include:

- developmental delays
- behavioral problems (anger, acting out, or eating disorders)
- significant drop in grades, especially in a child formerly doing well
- prolonged or inappropriate sadness or depression
- social withdrawal or isolation
- decreased interest in previously enjoyed activities

- overly aggressive behavior
- appetite changes (particularly in adolescents)
- insomnia or fatigue
- school absenteeism or tardiness
- mood swings
- excessive physical complaints (especially headaches or stomachaches)

Finding a Therapist

Child psychologists, social workers, and child psychiatrists all diagnose and treat mental health disorders in youngsters. It is important to find a well-qualified, experienced therapist with whom your child can relate well, who seems friendly, warm, and approachable. Because the right therapist-client match is so important, it may require visits to several counselors before a final choice is made. A therapist who works with children should have a license and a professional degree in psychology, social work, or psychiatry.

A psychiatrist (M.D. or D.O.) is a medical doctor with advanced training and experience in mental illness and pharmacology. They are the only mental health providers who can prescribe medications. Clinical psychologists (Ph.D., Psy.D., or Ed.D.) are therapists with a doctorate that includes advanced training in the practice of psychology and psychotherapy. Many specialize in treating children and adolescents and their families. A clinical social worker (L.C.S.W., A.C.S.W., L.I.C.S.W., or C.S.W.) has a master's degree and specializes in clinical social work; an L.C.S.W. (licensed clinical social worker) is licensed by the state (accredited clinical social workers—A.C.S.W.—may also be accredited to work in more than one state). An L.I.C.S.W. is a licensed clinical social worker, which is a similar accreditation to the A.C.S.W., which means that these social workers can work in any state. A C.S.W. is a clinical social worker who is not yet licensed to practice.

Types of Therapy

There are many types of psychotherapy that may be most appropriate for a particular problem and a particular child and family. Therapists will often spend a portion of each session with the parents alone, with the child alone, and with the family together. Strategies include:

Individual therapy With this type of therapy, a therapist works one-on-one with a child on problems such as depression, social difficulties, or worry.

Family therapy With this technique, counseling sessions are scheduled with some or all family members as a way of improving communication skills. Family therapy can be helpful in many cases, especially if family members are having problems getting along. Treatment focuses on problem-solving techniques and can help parents reestablish their roles as authority figures.

Cognitive behavioral therapy This type of approach is often helpful with children over age 12 who are depressed, anxious, or having problems coping with stress. Cognitive behavioral therapy attempts to identify and alter maladaptive ways of thinking, restructuring negative thoughts into more positive ways of thinking.

Stress management If stress seems to trigger or worsen your child's condition, this type of therapy may help him learn ways to recognize stress and how to deal with it. Stress management may include relaxation training, a method that teaches children how to relax so they can better cope with stress. With this approach, children are encouraged to take responsibility for their own care, which can make them feel more in control of their situation.

Preparing a Child for Counseling

Parents should be honest with their child about a therapy session and why she or the family will be going, emphasizing that this type of doctor talks with children and families to help solve problems. Young children may need to be reassured that a visit to a therapist does not involve shots or physicals. Older children may need to be reassured that anything they say to the therapist is confidential and cannot be shared with anyone, including parents, without their permission (unless they indicate that are considering suicide or hurting someone).

mental retardation Below-average intellectual functioning abilities as determined by intelligence quotient (IQ) testing, and low adaptive functioning at home or in a work environment. An individual is considered to have mental retardation if IQ is below 70-75, there are significant limitations in two or more adaptive skill areas, and the condition is present from childhood.

Between 6.2 million and 7.5 million people have mental retardation, which is 10 times more common than CEREBRAL PALSY and 28 times more prevalent than neural tube defects such as SPINA BIFIDA. Mental retardation cuts across the lines of racial, ethnic, educational, social, and economic backgrounds, so that one out of 10 American families is directly affected by mental retardation.

The effects of mental retardation vary considerably among people, just as the range of abilities varies considerably among people who do not have mental retardation. About 87 percent will be mildly affected and will be only a little slower than average in learning new information and skills. As children, their mental retardation is not easy to see and may not be identified until school age. The remaining 13 percent of people with mental retardation (those with IQs under 50) will have serious limits in function. However, with early intervention, a good education, and appropriate supports as an adult, all can lead satisfying lives in the community.

People with mental retardation may have trouble communicating, interacting with others, and being independent. There may also be concerns with regard to understanding health and safety issues. Not all skills are necessarily impaired, and children with mental retardation may learn to function independently in many areas. However, education programs, providing skilled assistance and ongoing support, are necessary for determining appropriate living and work environments.

Symptoms

Most parents tend to notice a problem within the first year or two of life. While all children develop different skills at different times, significant lags in several areas of development are an early warning sign. Children with mental retardation tend to reach developmental milestones later than youngsters of normal intelligence. They may not learn to sit, crawl, or walk until well after their second birthdays. Speech is likewise delayed, and some severely retarded children never learn to talk at all.

Cause

Mental retardation can be caused by any condition that impairs development of the brain before birth, during birth, or in the childhood years. Several hundred causes have been discovered, but about a third of the time the reason remains unknown. The three most common known causes of mental retardation are DOWN SYNDROME, FETAL ALCOHOL SYNDROME, and FRAGILE X SYNDROME.

Genetic conditions These conditions are caused by abnormal genes or from other disorders of the genes caused during pregnancy by infections, overexposure to X rays, and other factors. More than 500 genetic diseases are associated with mental retardation, such as:

- *PKU (PHENYLKETONURIA)* A single gene disorder caused by a defective enzyme
- *Down syndrome* A chromosomal disorder that happens sporadically, caused by too many chromosomes, or by a change in structure of a chromosome
- *Fragile X syndrome* A single gene disorder located on the X chromosome that is the leading inherited cause of mental retardation

Prenatal problems Using alcohol, drugs, or smoking during pregnancy can cause mental retardation. Other risks include malnutrition, certain environmental contaminants, and illnesses of the mother during pregnancy, such as TOXOPLASMOSIS, CYTOMEGALOVIRUS, GERMAN MEASLES, and SYPHILIS. Pregnant women who are infected with HIV and HERPES may pass the virus to their child, leading to future neurological damage.

Problems at birth Although any unusual stress during birth may injure the infant's brain, prematurity and low birth weight are more likely to predict serious problems than any other conditions.

Problems after birth Childhood diseases such as WHOOPING COUGH, CHICKEN POX, MEASLES, and HIB disease (which may lead to MENINGITIS and ENCEPHALITIS) can damage the brain, as can accidents such as a blow to the head or near drowning. Lead, mercury, and other environmental toxins can cause irreparable damage to the brain and nervous system.

Socioeconomic Children in poor families may become mentally retarded because of malnutrition, disease-producing conditions, inadequate medical care, and environmental health hazards. Also, children in disadvantaged areas may be deprived of many common cultural and day-to-day experiences provided to other youngsters. Research suggests that such under-stimulation can result in irreversible damage and can serve as a cause of mental retardation.

Diagnosis

Mental retardation is diagnosed primarily on the basis of intelligence testing, but affected children often demonstrate other brain problems such as attention deficits, movement problems, and perceptual difficulties. Dexterity and coordination also may be limited. If the child's doctor suspects a problem, parents may be referred to a psychologist or other mental health expert, who can administer a number of special tests, including standardized intelligence tests and a standardized adaptive skills test. Next, an expert should describe the child's strengths and weaknesses in intellectual and adaptive behavior skills, emotions, physical health, and environment. These skills can be assessed by formal testing, observations, interviews, and interacting with the child in daily life.

Intelligence testing alone is only one measure of functioning ability, however. A child with limits in intellectual functioning who does not have limits in adaptive skill areas may not be diagnosed as having mental retardation. "Adaptive skill areas" are those daily living skills needed to live, work, and play in the community and include communication, self-care, home living, social skills, leisure, health and safety, self-direction, functional academics (reading, writing, basic math), community use, and work. Adaptive skills are assessed in the child's typical environment.

Careful assessment is important because many children have been misdiagnosed with mental retardation, particularly at a young age, and are later diagnosed with profound learning disabilities but with average or above average intelligence.

Types of Mental Retardation

Individuals with mental retardation are not a homogenous group but have widely differing lev-els of functioning. While the term *mental retardation* still exists as a clinical diagnosis, experts today prefer terms such as *developmental disability,* which some believe does not carry the same negative connotations. In the past, those who were retarded were traditionally divided by IQ scores into *educable, trainable,* and *custodial;* today, the more commonly used terms include mild, moderate, severe, or profound categories, based on the level of functioning and IQ.

Mild retardation This classification is used to specify an individual whose IQ test scores lie between 55 and 68 or 69, and it corresponds to an educators' label of "educable retarded." The individual is capable of learning basic academic subjects. Many people with mild retardation are able to live and work independently.

Moderate retardation Children who are moderately retarded have an IQ test score between 40 and 55; the term corresponds to the earlier label of "trainable retarded." These children can usually learn basic school and job skills and often achieve coached job goals and live with limited assistance.

Severe and profound mental retardation This classification applies to children with IQ scores below 25. These children are the most seriously impaired of the mentally retarded, often characterized by physical and sensory impairment as well as mental retardation. They can sometimes achieve supported job goals, but more typically they function in sheltered employment. They generally require significant assistance with daily living skills.

Treatment

Many public and private agencies that specialize in developmental disabilities can help children with mental retardation. Although there is no cure for this condition, retarded children can be taught and supported so that they can live rewarding, happy lives.

Every state is required by law to offer early intervention programs beginning at birth for children with mental retardation, and public schools must offer special education beginning at age three.

Prevention

It is possible to prevent some forms of mental retardation. During the past 30 years, significant advances in research have prevented many cases of mental retardation. For example, every year in the United States, about 250 cases of mental retardation due to PKU are prevented by newborn screening and dietary treatment. Newborn screening and thyroid hormone replacement therapy prevent 1,000 cases of mental retardation due to congenital hypothyroidism, and more than 1,000 cases of mental retardation from Rh disease and severe jaundice are prevented by using anti-Rh immune globulin to prevent Rh disease. The HIB vaccine prevents another 5,000 cases of mental retardation caused by HIB diseases, and 4,000 cases of mental retardation due to measles encephalitis can be prevented because of the measles vaccine. Countless numbers of cases of mental retardation caused by rubella during pregnancy are prevented thanks to the rubella vaccine.

Removing lead from the environment reduces brain damage in children, and child safety seats and bicycle helmets reduce head trauma. Early intervention programs with high-risk infants and children have shown remarkable results in reducing the predicted incidence of subnormal intellectual functioning.

Finally, early prenatal care and preventive measures before and during pregnancy increase a woman's chances of preventing mental retardation. Pediatric AIDS is being reduced by AZT treatment of the mother during pregnancy, and dietary supplementation with folic acid reduces the risk of neural tube defects. Research continues on new ways to prevent mental retardation, including research on the development and function of the nervous system, a wide variety of fetal treatments, and gene therapy to correct the abnormality produced by defective genes.

methylphenidate   See RITALIN.

middle ear barotrauma   A type of EARACHE related to abnormal pressure changes in the air space behind the eardrum (the middle ear) that usually occurs during an airplane flight. Even in a pressurized aircraft cabin, there is a decrease in the cabin air pressure as the plane climbs; as the plane descends, the air pressure increases again. It is during descent when children are most likely to experience the discomfort of middle ear barotrauma.

When a plane descends and the pressure in the cabin increases, the air pressure in the middle ear must be equalized; if it is not, the increased cabin air pressure pushes on the eardrum and causes pain. Normally the eustachian tube will open to equalize pressure, which is what happens when a child yawns or swallows, causing the "popping" sensation in the ear. In children, however, the relatively smaller eustachian tube may not function effectively and pain is the result.

There are several ways to help a child more effectively equalize the air pressure in the ears. Because airplane air is dry, this thickens nasal mucus, making it harder for the eustachian tube to open. A glass of a noncaffeinated beverage (water is best) for every hour of air travel will help overcome the drying effect. Careful use of nasal decongestant sprays before takeoff and before descent will also help open the ear and nasal passages. Medications that include antihistamines should be avoided unless the child has allergies, because they can actually worsen the problem by thickening secretions. An older child may benefit from chewing gum or sucking on hard candy. A bottle works well for infants, but the child should be upright while drinking. Children with ear tubes do not have to worry about ear pain, because the tubes ensure that pressure equalization happens automatically.

middle ear infection   See EAR INFECTION.

miliaria   A common disorder of the sweat glands that often occurs during hot, humid weather and is believed to result from blocked sweat ducts, so that sweat leaks into the skin. The three types of miliaria are classified according to the level at which obstruction of the sweat duct occurs:

• *miliaria crystallina*   In this case, ductal obstruction is least severe, producing tiny, fragile, clear blisters.

• *miliaria rubra* (PRICKLY HEAT)   In this case, obstruction occurs deeper within the epidermis, causing extremely itchy erythematous papules.

• *miliaria profunda*   Ductal obstruction is at the dermal-epidermal junction, leaking sweat into the papillary dermis and producing subtle flesh-colored papules.

Miliaria occurs in individuals of all races, although some studies have shown that Asians, who produce less sweat than whites, are less likely to develop miliaria rubra. Miliaria crystallina and miliaria rubra can occur at any age but are most common in infancy. Miliaria profunda is more common in adulthood.

Cause

High heat and humidity that triggers excess sweating is the primary cause for the development of miliaria. Binding the skin with clothing or bandages can further contribute to pooling of sweat on the skin surface and overhydration of the top layer of the epidermis. If hot, humid conditions persist, the individual will continue to produce excessive sweat but will be unable to secrete the sweat onto the skin surface due to the blocked ducts. This leads to leakage of sweat en route to the skin surface, either in the dermis or in the epidermis. When the point of leakage is in the top layer of the epidermis or just below (as in miliaria crystallina), there is little inflammation. In miliaria rubra, however, leakage of sweat into the subcorneal layers produces blisters. In miliaria profunda, escape of sweat into the papillary dermis leads to white or red papules that usually do not itch.

Normal skin bacteria, such as *Staphylococcus epidermidis,* are thought to play a role in the development of miliaria. Patients with miliaria have three times as many bacteria as healthy people.

Symptoms

Miliaria crystallina is a common condition that is seen in infants, with a peak at one week of age, and in individuals with fever or who have recently moved to a hot, humid climate. *Miliaria rubra* is also common in infants who have moved to a tropical environment, occurring in up to 30 percent of people exposed to such conditions. *Miliaria profunda* is more rare, only seen in a minority of those who have had repeated bouts of miliaria rubra.

Miliaria crystallina is usually quite mild and gets better without complications over a period of days, although it may recur if hot, humid conditions persist. *Miliaria rubra* also tends to improve sponta-neously when patients are removed to a cooler environment. Unlike patients with miliaria crystallina, however, those with miliaria rubra tend to have a lot of itching and stinging. They develop a lack of sweat in affected sites that may last weeks and, if generalized, may lead to heat exhaustion. Secondary infection is another possible complication of miliaria rubra, either as IMPETIGO or as multiple discrete abscesses known as periporitis staphylogenes.

Miliaria profunda is itself a complication of repeated episodes of miliaria rubra. The lesions of miliaria profunda do not cause symptoms, but patients may develop compensatory facial excess sweating, and a widespread inability to sweat elsewhere resulting from eccrine duct rupture; this is known as tropical anhidrotic asthenia and predisposes patients to heat exhaustion during exertion in warm climates.

Treatment

There is no reason to treat miliaria crystallina, as this condition is will go away on its own and does not cause unpleasant symptoms. However, miliaria rubra can be very uncomfortable and miliaria profunda may lead to heat exhaustion, so treatment of these two conditions is necessary.

Prevention and treatment of miliaria consist primarily of controlling heat and humidity so that the patient is not stimulated to sweat. This may mean treating a fever, reducing tight clothing, limiting activity, providing air conditioning, or (as a last resort) moving the patient to a cooler climate.

Topical treatments may include lotions containing calamine, boric acid, or menthol, cool wet-to-dry compresses, frequent showering with soap (although some doctors discourage excess soap), topical corticosteroids, and topical antibiotics. Topical application of anhydrous lanolin has resulted in dramatic improvement in patients with miliaria profunda. Anhydrous lanolin is believed to prevent ductal blockage, allowing sweat to flow to the skin surface. Calamine lotion provides cooling relief.

It may be possible to prevent miliaria by using oral antibiotics. Patients have also been treated with oral retinoids, vitamin A, and vitamin C with variable success. However, there have been no controlled studies to demonstrate the effectiveness of any of these treatments.

Since increased exertion leads to sweating, which greatly worsens miliaria, patients should limit activity (especially in hot weather) until the miliaria is cured. Patients with miliaria profunda are at particularly high risk for heat exhaustion during exertion in hot weather, since they have trouble dissipating heat via evaporation of sweat.

minimal brain dysfunction (MBD) A general term used to describe a young child who shows behavioral, cognitive, and affective signs of brain injury. The term is usually used for cases in which the pattern of thought and action would typically be caused by organic abnormality, but none is apparent.

Historically, minimal brain dysfunction (MBD) was the term used to define and classify learning and behavioral difficulties now classified under the category of ATTENTION DEFICIT HYPERACTIVITY DISORDER. It generally includes HYPERACTIVITY, impulsivity, and any of a number of learning and language disabilities such as DYSLEXIA and problems with math.

The term is often used as though there were an identifiable MBD syndrome, a collection of fairly specific disorders that could be taken as hallmarks of some underlying neurological cause. Although the issue is far from settled, experts believe that the evidence to support a single MBD syndrome is largely unconvincing.

minimum competency testing An assessment that tries to establish the minimum level of achievement. At least 36 states now require some type of minimum competency, which may be tied in with the ability to graduate.

There is a great deal of controversy about minimum competency tests. Critics worry that the blame for a poor school program may be shifted to the students. While the goal of minimum competency testing is to improve overall achievement, critics worry that the tests will in fact depress some students' achievement levels. There is also concern about the impact of such tests on minority achievement.

Students with identified LEARNING DISABILITIES can waive the tests, although some schools suggest that these students take the tests anyway in the freshman year. If the student fails the entire test, he could then take it again with modifications as stipulated in his individual education plan. Students with learning disabilities as a senior can waive the tests.

missing children Child abduction and serial homicide are considered two of the most serious violent crime problems facing the United States today, according to the Federal Bureau of Investigation Child Abduction and Serial Killer Unit. Every year 114,600 children are victims of attempted nonfamily abduction, and between 3,200 and 4,600 are actually abducted by nonfamily members. More than 300 children are victims of "stereotypical abduction," in which the child is gone overnight, killed, transported more than 50 miles, or is ransomed. Many of these abducted children have been assault victims, and more than 100 have been murdered; others are considered long-term missing.

Every year 139,100 children are classified as "lost, injured or otherwise missing." (Many times a child is listed in this category when there is no proof of an abduction, but many of these are victims of exploitation, violent crimes, or homicide.)

Children of all ages are abducted, but most are girls between the ages of 11 and 14 years; boys between the ages of six and nine years old are in the next highest category.

Two-thirds of short-term abductions involve sexual assault, and most children are abducted from the street. More than 85 percent of short-term nonfamily abductions involve force, and more than 75 percent involve a weapon. The number of short-term abductions is considered to be an underestimate because of police reporting methods and lack of reporting on the part of victims.

Pictures are one of the most effective tools in recovering missing children, and with the growth of the Internet and advances in computer technology, the search for missing children has been revolutionized. The first few hours immediately after a child's disappearance are the most important, since every hour, day, and week that a child is missing lessens the likelihood of the child's safe recovery. Distributing a child's picture rapidly can be the difference between a fast recovery and a prolonged search. Computer imaging, broadcast faxing, e-mail, and the World Wide Web have replaced sketches, black-

and-white posters, and mail service. As of 1996, almost every state has developed an AMBER ALERT plan—a voluntary partnership between police agencies and broadcasters to disseminate an urgent bulletin in the most serious child-abduction cases so that entire communities can help search for abducted children. Law enforcement and broadcasters use the Emergency Alert System (formerly called the Emergency Broadcast System) to air a description of the missing child and suspected abductor. This is the same concept used to warn about severe weather. (See also NATIONAL CENTER FOR MISSING AND EXPLOITED CHILDREN.)

mixed receptive-expressive language disorder
A language disability causing problems in both understanding and expressing language. The condition was formerly called *developmental receptive language disorder.* Today it is generally understood that receptive language deficits do not occur all by themselves but appear together with problems expressing language as well.

Three to five percent of all children have both receptive and expressive language disorder. The cause of this disorder is unknown, but problems with receptive skills begins before the age of four. Difficulty understanding and using language can cause problems with social interaction and make it difficult to function independently as an adult.

Symptoms
There are a number of symptoms that indicate this condition, including problems in:

- language comprehension
- language expression
- articulation
- recalling early visual or auditory memories

Diagnosis
Parents who are concerned about their child's acquisition of language should have the child tested, since early intervention offers the best possible outcome. Standardized receptive and expressive language tests can be given to any child suspected of having this disorder. An audiogram should also be given to rule out the possibility of deafness.

Treatment
Speech and language therapy are the best way to treat this type of language disorder. Psychotherapy is also recommended for children because of the possibility of emotional or behavioral problems.

MMR vaccine   A vaccine designed to prevent MEASLES, MUMPS, and GERMAN MEASLES (rubella) that is given to all American infants at about 15 months of age. This live attenuated virus provides complete protection to more than 95 percent of those who receive it. MMR is not effective, however, when given to a child earlier than 12 months of age, because the baby often has maternal antibodies that will interfere with the vaccine's action.

The MMR vaccine has greatly reduced the number of cases of measles, mumps, and rubella each year, including serious side effects (death from measles, brain infection from mumps, and birth defects and mental retardation from rubella in pregnant women). Fewer than one child in one million who get this vaccine has a serious allergic reaction or other severe problem. A survey of 50 years' worth of data (more than 2,000 studies from around the world) found that there was not enough evidence to support a suspected link between the vaccine and an increased risk for autism or bowel disease in children.

A first dose is usually given at 12 to 15 months, followed by a booster at age four to six. Older children who missed these vaccines should have one dose of MMR. Children with a high fever or a severe allergy to neomycin should not be given the vaccine.

mole   An area of brown pigment in the skin that may either be raised or flat. Certain types of moles can eventually become malignant. A mole that is asymmetrical, that has uneven borders, that changes color or is made up of more than one color, or that has a diameter larger than 6 mm could be a malignant lesion and should be checked by a physician. (See also BIRTHMARKS; MONGOLIAN SPOTS; PORT-WINE STAINS.)

Mongolian spots   A congenital blue-black pigmented area on the skin usually found on the lower back or buttocks. The spot, which may appear alone or in a group, may be mistaken for a bruise. It is most common in Asian or African American children and is caused by a concentration of pigment-producing cells deep within the skin. The spots usually disappear by age three or four. (See also BIRTHMARKS; PORT-WINE STAINS.)

moniliasis   See THRUSH.

monkeypox   A milder relative of SMALLPOX that appeared in the United States for the first time when at least a dozen people had contact in 2003 with infected pet prairie dogs. Monkeypox was reported in humans for the first time in 1970, and until the recent outbreak in the United States, it was a disease never before seen in the Western Hemisphere. Rarely fatal, it causes pus-filled blisters, rashes, chills, and fever.

Cases of monkeypox first appeared in sick prairie dogs sold by a Milwaukee, Wisconsin, animal distributor who had obtained the animals, along with an ill Gambian giant rat, from an Illinois animal distributor. All patients reported contact with either a sick prairie dog or rabbit one to three weeks before the illness began.

Symptoms

Monkeypox in humans produces a vesicular and pustular rash similar to that of smallpox. The incubation period from exposure to fever onset is about 12 days, and the typical illness with fever, headache, muscle ache, and rash lasts from two to four weeks. The rash, which appears as raised, acne-like bumps, appears within a few days and goes through several stages before crusting and falling off.

No one has died of monkeypox in the United States, but at least 33 patients contracted the disease; 14 patients with symptoms were hospitalized, including a child in Indiana with a confirmed case who also has encephalitis.

Illness in the animals has included fever, cough, swollen, reddened eyes, and swollen glands followed by a rash and hair loss, although not all of these signs have been present in all animals. Some prairie dogs died and others recovered. The sick rabbit associated with one human case had prior contact with an ill prairie dog at a veterinary clinic. The prairie dogs appeared to have infected people through bites or when people rubbed their eyes or noses after touching discharges from the animals.

Cause

The virus that causes monkeypox is usually transmitted to humans through a bite by an infected animal, or by direct contact with the animal's lesions, body fluids, or blood. Although person-to-person transmission is extremely rare, monkeypox can be spread through direct contact with the body fluids of an infected person or with objects (such as bedding or clothing) that have become contaminated. One Wisconsin resident who apparently caught monkeypox from the prairie dog had "minimal" contact with the infected animal but slept in the same room as the caged animal.

Treatment

The human mortality rate from monkeypox in Africa has ranged from one percent to 10 percent, but the virus may be less lethal in the United States because people typically are better nourished and medical technology is more advanced.

The federal government has recommended smallpox shots for people exposed to monkeypox. The vaccine can prevent the disease up to two weeks after exposure to the virus and is most effective in the first four days, but some health officials are wary because the vaccine in rare cases can cause serious and even fatal side effects.

Prevention

The spread of monkeypox to humans can be prevented. The Centers for Disease Control and Prevention and the U.S. Food and Drug Administration (FDA) have prohibited the importation and sale of rodents from Africa, including Gambian giant pouched rats, dormice, striped mice, brush-tailed porcupines, tree squirrels, and rope squirrels.

mononucleosis   An acute herpesvirus infection caused by the Epstein-Barr (EBV) virus and characterized by sore throat, fever, swollen lymph glands, and bruising. Transmitted in saliva, young people are most often infected. In childhood the disease is often mild; the older the patient, the more severe the symptoms are likely to be. Infection confers permanent immunity.

Cause

The disease is usually transmitted by droplets of EB virus, but it is not highly contagious.

Symptoms

From four to six weeks after infection, classic mononucleosis begins gradually with symptoms of sore throat, fatigue, swollen lymph glands, and occasional bruising. Although the symptoms usually disappear after about a month, the virus remains dormant in the throat and blood for the rest of the child's life. Periodically, the virus can reactivate and be found in saliva, although it does not usually cause symptoms.

Sometimes the disease can start abruptly with a high fever and severe, swollen throat similar to a strep throat. Rarely, about 10 percent of patients have a third type, which causes a low persistent fever, nausea and vomiting, and stomach problems.

About half of all mononucleosis patients have an enlarged spleen, and a few have an enlarged liver or mild jaundice. A rash also can be seen in some cases.

Diagnosis

Symptoms of fever, sore throat, and swollen glands are used to diagnose the disease. Blood tests and blood counts are needed for confirmation. The mono spot is a rapid antibody test that looks for a specific reaction in the blood of infected patients. However, it is not helpful in children under age three. Liver function tests may reveal abnormal liver function.

Treatment

There is no specific treatment for the disease other than symptom management. No antiviral or antibiotic drugs are available. Some doctors prescribe steroids to reduce the tonsil inflammation if a patient cannot swallow. Enforced bed rest may prevent injury to the swollen spleen. Painkillers and saline gargles may help the sore throat.

Complications

In addition to a swollen spleen or liver inflammation, heart problems or involvement of the central nervous system may occur. However, this disease is almost never fatal. If the spleen ruptures, immediate surgery and blood transfusions will be necessary.

About half the time, a patient will also have a strep throat, which requires antibiotic treatment. Occasionally, patients will have such intense swelling of the lymphatic system of the throat that they require hospitalization for intravenous fluids to prevent dehydration. In some cases, Epstein Barr virus has been associated with Burkitts lymphoma.

mosquito bites Mosquitoes are found throughout the world. Mosquito bites may cause swelling and itching for several days; the main problem of these bites is the infections that may be transmitted in the insect's saliva.

Treatment

Because mosquito bites can transmit disease, they should be washed with soap and water followed by an antiseptic. To control itching, a nonprescription antihistamine, calamine lotion, anesthetic gel, or an ice pack may be used. Alternatively, a paste of salt and water, or baking soda and water, can be applied to the bite to control itching.

Prevention

Insect repellents may help to prevent mosquito bites. Although many consumers swore by the ability of Avon's Skin-So-Soft bath oil to repel mosquitoes, research by the U.S. military and Avon itself found it is not as effective as DEET. However, given the persistence of the myth, the company now markets a bug repellent that includes Skin-So-Soft.

DEET (diethyltoluamide) is an insect repellent that is sprayed on the skin to repel mosquitoes. Although in low concentrations DEET is considered to be nontoxic, the U.S. Environmental Protection Agency (EPA) prohibits child safety claims on product labels because data on DEET do not support product label claims of child safety. However, the Centers for Disease Control notes that it is acceptable to use DEET on children over age two.

motion sickness   Symptoms of nausea, vomiting, and headache triggered by motion during travel by road, water, or air. Experts believe that symptoms start in a part of the ear responsible for balance and spatial orientation. It may be that when too much visual information during motion floods the inner ear, signals are relayed to the brain which in turn trigger motion sickness signals.

Prevention

Oral medications (such as Dramamine or bonamine), or medicated patches worn behind the ear, can prevent motion sickness. However, a doctor should be consulted before these products are used on children. Once symptoms develop, these medications do not usually work.

When traveling by boat, children are less likely to experience a problem if they remain above deck where the horizon can be seen. To prevent a problem when traveling by car, parents should:

- give the child a small carbohydrate snack before starting the trip (an empty stomach increases the risk of a problem)
- allow the child to sit high enough to see the road
- have the child either look straight out in front of the car, or focus on the horizon
- be sure the car is well ventilated

motor skills   A wide range of capabilities involved in movement, such as the use of muscles and muscle groups with appropriate timing and sequencing, the ability to recall the muscular steps used to perform a task in the past, and the use of feedback from the senses to regulate muscular responses and activities.

multiple intelligences   Recent advances in cognitive science, developmental psychology, and neuroscience suggest that each person's level of intelligence, as it has been traditionally considered, is actually made up of a number of faculties that can work individually or together with other abilities. Harvard professor Howard Gardner originally identified eight such types of intelligences, including verbal/linguistic, logical/mathematical, visual/spatial, musical/rhythmic, body/kinesthetic, inter-

personal, intrapersonal, and naturalistic. Each of these eight types represents abilities within a specific area of human functioning.

Gardner believed that the forms of intelligence that are measured by most intelligence tests correspond to verbal/linguistic, logical/mathematical, and visual/spatial intelligences, meaning that traditional measures of intelligence overlook or fail to recognize abilities and gifts in other areas.

Although not based on research, Gardner's theories have become increasingly influential. However, standard measures of intelligence continue to focus on verbal and nonverbal reasoning measures that depend heavily on linguistic, logical, and visual-spatial abilities, and the common understanding of intelligence continues to be mostly closely linked to verbal capabilities.

Many school narrowly focus on linguistic and mathematical intelligences, This means that children with LEARNING DISABILITIES may have other talents that are not valued in academic settings. The theory of multiple intelligences emphasizes the need to acknowledge and cultivate different kinds of thinking and different abilities.

Musical Intelligence

The ability to perform and compose music have been scientifically pinpointed in certain areas of the brain. Each child has a different musical ability, and some are totally amusical yet continue to have very normal and successful lives. Although musical intelligence may not seem as obvious a form of intellect as mathematical or logical ability, from a neurological point of view the ability to perform and comprehend musically appears to function independently from other forms of intelligence.

Bodily Kinesthetic

One of the most controversial of Gardner's intelligences is the idea of body kinesthetic intelligence. In Gardner's theory, each person possesses a certain control of movements, balance, agility, and grace. For some extraordinary athletes, strength in bodily kinesthetic intelligence appeared even before they began formal training. Super athletes all seem to have a natural sense of how their bodies should act and react in a demanding physical situation.

However some people, argue that physical control does not constitute a designation as a form of intelligence; Gardner insists that bodily kinesthetic ability does indeed deserve such a recognition.

Logical/Mathematical

The most easily understood cognitive faculty is logical/mathematical intelligence—the ability to mentally process logical problems and equations, the type most often found on multiple-choice standardized tests. Logical/mathematical intelligence often does not require verbal articulation. Individuals who have good logical/mathematical abilities are able to process logical questions at an unusually rapid rate.

Before the advent of the theory of multiple intelligences, logical/mathematical intelligence was considered a pseudonym for intelligence itself. Although the theory of multiple intelligences agrees that logical/mathematical intelligence is indeed a key section of the intellect, it is by no means the only one that should be developed.

Linguistic

Every child possesses the ability to use language; although some can master only basic levels of communication, others learn many languages easily. For years researchers have recognized the connection between language and the brain. They know that damage to one portion of the brain will affect the ability to express clear grammatical sentences, although a person's understanding of vocabulary and syntax remains intact. As Gardner notes, even young children and deaf individuals will begin to develop their own unique language if they are not offered an alternative. A person's ability to construct and comprehend language may vary, but as a cognitive trait it is still universal.

Spatial

Spatial intelligence involves the ability to comprehend shapes and images in three dimensions. Whether trying to put together a puzzle or create a sculpture, children use their spatial intelligence to interpret what they may or may not physically see. Advances in neuroscience have now provided researchers with clear-cut proof of the role of spatial intelligence in the right hemisphere of the brain. In rare instances, for example, certain brain injuries can cause people to lose the ability to rec-

ognize their closest relatives. Though they may see the other person perfectly well, they are unable to comprehend who they see.

And yet a blind person may feel a shape and identify it with ease, although they are unable to see it. Because most people use spatial intelligence in conjunction with sight, its existence as an autonomous cognitive trait may not seem obvious, but recent research suggests that it is an independent portion of the intellect.

Interpersonal

Humans are social animals who thrive when involved with others. This ability to interact with others, understand them, and interpret their behavior is called interpersonal intelligence. According to Gardner, children's interpersonal intelligence allows them to notice the moods, temperaments, motivations, and intentions of others.

From a psychological and neurological point of view, the connection between interpersonal intelligence and the brain has been explored for generations; if the frontal lobe is damaged, that person's personality and ability to interact well with others is destroyed. Interpersonal intelligence allows children to affect others by understanding others; without it, an individual loses the ability to exist socially.

Intrapersonal

Related to interpersonal intelligence, intrapersonal intelligence is the cognitive ability to understand and sense the "self." Intrapersonal intelligence allows children to tap into internal feelings and thoughts. A strong intrapersonal intelligence can lead to self-esteem, self-enhancement, and a strength of character that can be used to solve internal problems. On the other hand, a weak intrapersonal intelligence (such as that autistic children) prevents a person from recognizing himself as separate from the surrounding environment. Intrapersonal intelligence often is not recognized from the outside unless it is expressed in some form, such as rage or joy.

Naturalist

Recently added to the original list of seven multiple intelligences, naturalist intelligence is a person's ability to identify and classify patterns in nature. During prehistory, hunter-gatherers would rely on naturalist intelligence to identify which plants or animals were edible and which were not. Today naturalist intelligence may be seen in the way humans relate to the surroundings. People who are sensitive to changes in weather patterns or are adept at distinguishing nuances between large numbers of similar objects may be expressing naturalist intelligence abilities.

multiple sclerosis A neurological disease causing unpredictable bouts of paralysis, numbness, and vision loss, once thought to strike only adults but now acknowledged to occur in children. Multiple sclerosis (MS) affects about 350,000 American adults, but experts estimate that as many as 20,000 children in the United States also have the disease yet remain undiagnosed. New medical evidence suggests that the number of pediatric patients is rising, probably because more doctors are considering the diagnosis when they see a child suffering from telltale symptoms such as a sudden visual problem.

When a childhood diagnosis is made, doctors, parents, and children are faced with a number of unanswered questions. Researchers do not know whether the drugs used to treat adults will work for children. They do not know how quickly the disease will progress.

Cause

Multiple sclerosis occurs when the body's immune cells turn and mistakenly attack the thick sheath (myelin) covering the nerve fibers of the brain and spinal cord. When the myelin is destroyed, the underlying nerve can be damaged, triggering a range of symptoms such as tremors or slurred speech.

Some adults with MS have attacks that can last several days to a week and then fully recover; others may not get another attack for a year or even a decade. Others will get several attacks spaced out over a year. A small number of people with MS get steadily worse with each attack. No one knows what will happen to children with the disease.

Diagnosis

The lack of knowledge about pediatric MS means that many children may not get a diagnosis right away. Only a few doctors at urban centers in the United States and Canada specialize in pediatric MS.

Although most children with MS have very mild cases, a small group of children have very aggressive symptoms. Instead of one or two attacks a year, these children must deal with five or more. No one knows whether these children will go on to suffer from progressively worsening disease.

Treatment

The drugs that have fueled a revolution among adults with MS have not been tested in children, and there is no proof that these drugs will work the same way for young children as they do in adults. Experts hope that these drugs, especially if started early, will stave off the worst consequences of the disease.

Researchers worry that repeated attacks can leave a child with memory and learning problems. One study found that about 30 percent of the children tested had trouble with cognitive skills, such as remembering information for a test. Some adults with MS also have such deficits but often can compensate by relying on their past experience.

mumps An acute viral illness that was at one time a common childhood disease, featuring swollen and inflamed salivary glands on one or both sides of the face or under the jaw. In 1968 there were 152,000 mumps cases; today only a few thousand patients a year get mumps.

Before the mumps vaccine was developed, almost every child got mumps sometime in childhood. While the incidence of the disease is much lower today, an unimmunized child remains at high risk for getting mumps. The disease is still widely found in developing countries, which is why anyone over age one should have a vaccine before traveling abroad.

Cause

Mumps is spread by airborne droplets of the mumps virus that are expelled by an infected patient who is coughing, sneezing, or talking. The virus invades and multiplies in the parotid gland.

Symptoms

The disease will appear two to three weeks after exposure, beginning with mild discomfort in the area just inside the angle of the jaw. Many infected children have no symptoms. In more serious cases, however, the child complains of pain and has difficulty chewing; the glands on one or both sides become painful and tender. Fever, headache, and swallowing problems may follow, but the fever falls after two to three days and the swelling fades within 10 days. When only one side is affected, the second gland often swells as the first one subsides.

Diagnosis

Mumps is usually diagnosed from symptoms; it can be confirmed by culturing the virus from saliva or urine, or by measuring antibodies to mumps virus in the blood. The skin test for mumps is considered unreliable and is no longer available.

Treatment

While there is no treatment, a patient may be given painkillers and plenty of fluids. In moderate to severe cases the child may need to stay in bed. Boys with a testicular involvement may be given a stronger painkiller; corticosteroid drugs may be needed to reduce inflammation.

Complications

While mumps is normally considered to be a mild disease, sometimes it can be more serious, causing a mild inflammation of the covering of the brain and spinal cord (MENINGITIS) in about one in every 10 children with mumps. More rarely, it can cause an inflammation of the brain itself (ENCEPHALITIS), which usually improves by itself without causing permanent brain damage.

Prevention

All healthy children who have never had mumps should be immunized at about 15 months with the MMR vaccine. If in doubt, it is safe to be immunized or reimmunized against mumps. The vaccine is available by itself, in combination with measles and rubella (MMR), or with rubella alone (MR). Typically, the combination MMR vaccine is given at 15 months of age because it protects a child against all three diseases. The vaccination has been used since 1967 and is very effective. One injection produces long-lasting immunity. According to the U.S. Centers for Disease Control, in very rare cases the mumps vaccine produces a mild, brief fever, which

may occur a week or two after the vaccination. Occasionally there is some slight swelling of the throat glands. Serious reactions are extremely rare.

Anyone with a severely impaired immune system, a severe allergy to eggs, or anyone with a high fever or who has received blood products in the preceding three months, should not receive the mumps virus vaccine.

muscular dystrophy (MD) A rare group of progressive, degenerative genetic diseases that destroy a child's muscle tissue, gradually weakening and deteriorating muscles, including the heart and breathing muscles. Different types of muscular dystrophy affect different sets of muscles and result in different degrees of muscle weakness; the most common types cause a dramatic physical weakness, so that children eventually are unable to walk, sit upright, move their arms and hands, or breathe. The increasing weakness leads to serious complications that can be fatal. Other types of muscular dystrophy (MD) cause only minor physical disabilities or develop late in life, so that people have a fairly normal life.

Cause

Most types of muscular dystrophy are caused by different abnormalities in the genes that produce muscle membrane proteins. Although the genetic problem is usually inherited, sometimes it can develop spontaneously.

The genetic abnormality triggers the development of muscle membranes with missing or malformed parts, causing muscle deterioration and weakness. Some types of muscular dystrophy (including Duchenne, the most severe type) are X-linked, which means that the abnormality is carried on the X chromosome that the mother contributes. A girl receives two X chromosomes, one from each parent, whereas a boy receives a Y chromosome from his father and an X from his mother. This means that it is almost always boys who develop symptoms, because girls inherit a normal X chromosome that may cancel out the abnormal one. Girls with such an affected X chromosome carry the MD gene but have no symptoms; however, they have a 50-50 chance of passing the condition to their sons (or carrier status to their daughters).

Symptoms

Many children with muscular dystrophy have had a normal pattern of early development, but eventually symptoms begin to appear. Symptoms can first appear during early childhood or late in adult life, depending on the type of muscular dystrophy.

The child may trip a lot, waddle, have trouble climbing stairs, or walk on toes without touching the heel to the floor. Toddlers may develop a swayback to compensate for weakening hip muscles. Children may struggle to get up from a sitting position or have trouble pushing objects such as a wagon or a tricycle. Many children also develop enlarged calf muscles as muscle tissue is destroyed and replaced by nonmuscle tissue.

The symptoms of Becker muscular dystrophy are less severe and may start during the school years, so that children live well into adulthood. In contrast, Duchenne muscular dystrophy begins during early childhood and causes fairly rapid weakness.

Diagnosis

A doctor who suspects muscular dystrophy will take a clinical history, perform a physical exam, and measure blood levels of creatine kinase, a muscle enzyme released into the blood by deteriorating muscle fibers. If a child has a high level of this enzyme, the doctor may order a DNA test or a muscle biopsy. The DNA test checks for gene abnormalities, and the muscle biopsy reveals patterns of muscle deterioration and abnormal levels of dystrophin, a building block of muscle. These tests reveal the type of muscular dystrophy the child has.

Types of Muscular Dystrophy

There are many types of muscular dystrophy; of these Duchenne is the most common and most severe.

Duchenne   This type of MD occurs when muscle fibers develop with abnormal dystrophin. Duchenne affects about one out of every 3,300 boys, who usually begin to show symptoms between ages two and five, with rapid muscle weakness first affecting the pelvic muscles. Most children lose the ability to walk by age 12 and must use a wheelchair, eventually developing muscle weakness in shoulders, back, arms, and legs. Even-

tually the muscles involved in breathing weaken, which can be fatal. Typically, children with Duchenne MD live only to about age 20 years. Although most children have average intelligence, LEARNING DISABILITIES (especially those involving verbal learning and reading comprehension) are more common in boys with Duchenne than in other children.

Becker   This type of MD is similar to Duchenne, but it progresses more slowly. Symptoms typically begin during adolescence, although they can first appear as early as age five or as late as age 25. Muscle weakness first occurs in the pelvic muscles, affecting the ability to walk. As the disease progresses, strength in the shoulders and back is also affected. Because Becker progresses so slowly, many children with Becker have a normal life span.

Myotonic   This is the most common adult form of MD, although half of all cases are still diagnosed in patients younger than 20. Primary symptoms involve facial weakness, a very slow relaxation of muscles after contraction, and weak hand muscles. The disease may be mild or severe, but because the defective gene is dominant, even someone with mild symptoms can transmit a more serious case of it to offspring. A less common congenital form affects only a small number of infants born to mothers with myotonic dystrophy, but it has a worse prognosis.

Limb-girdle   This type of MD begins between ages five and 30, first affecting either the pelvic muscles or the shoulder and back muscles; eventually both areas are affected. The severity of muscle weakness differs from person to person, as does the rate at which muscle weakness progresses. Some people develop only mild conditions, but many others develop severe disabilities by middle age.

Facioscapulohumeral   This type of MD can begin at any age, although it typically first appears during adolescence. Because this form of muscular dystrophy tends to progress slowly, teens who are affected usually have a normal life span. Muscle weakness first develops in the face, making it hard for children to close their eyes, whistle, or puff out their cheeks. The shoulder and back muscles gradually weaken, until it is hard for patients to lift objects or raise their hands over their head. Over time, the legs and pelvic muscles also lose strength. Some people develop minor physical symptoms (such as not being able to close the eyes during sleep), while others have profound disabilities. Rarely, infants develop symptoms during the first year or two of life, resulting in expressionless faces and serious muscle weakness during early childhood.

Congenital   This type of MD is actually a group of disorders with two unique characteristics: At birth, babies have weak muscles, often causing joint contractures and deformities, and muscle biopsies show nonspecific abnormalities. Joint contractures occur when muscles attached to a joint have unequal strength; the stronger muscle pulls and bends the joint into a locked and nonfunctional position. A combination of the facial, arm and leg, pelvic, respiratory, and shoulder muscles can be weak at birth, but this muscle weakness rarely gets worse.

Some types of congenital MD affect the brain, triggering seizures and gradual but constant deterioration.

Other   There are several other types of rare muscular dystrophy, including distal, ocular, oculopharyngeal, and Emery-Dreifuss.

Treatment

Muscular dystrophy is a treatable but not curable disease, although affected children today live longer and have a better quality of life due to new treatments that improve muscle and joint function, slow muscle deterioration, and keep kids comfortable, active, and independent for a longer period of time.

A team of medical specialists will work with the family of an affected child, including a neurologist, orthopedist, pulmonologist, physical and occupational therapist, nurse practitioner, and a social worker.

Different treatments are used to care for children at different stages of the disease. A combination of physical therapy, joint bracing, and prednisone treat children in the early stage, whereas assistive technology may be used in later stages.

Physical therapy and braces   The primary treatment for early MD is passive muscle stretching to maintain muscle tone and joint movement

to reduce contractures. Leg braces also can help prevent contractures and enable children to stand and walk using weakened muscles and joints more effectively. By providing extra support in just the right places, bracing lets children do more things independently for a longer period of time.

Prednisone   This steroid medication has been shown to slow the rate of muscle deterioration in children with Duchenne muscular dystrophy, which allows children to walk longer and live more active lives. In some cases, children with Duchenne are still walking in late junior high school, when in the past they would have been in a wheelchair.

Experts do not agree about the best time to begin treating children with prednisone, but most doctors prescribe it when children are five or six or when they show a significant decline in strength. Unfortunately, prednisone commonly causes weight gain, which may strain already weak muscles. It also can cause a loss of bone density that could lead to fractures.

For unknown reasons, sometimes prednisone does not slow the rate of muscle deterioration. For this reason, doctors closely monitor a child's weight and blood pressure, trying to improve muscle strength without causing excessive weight gain.

Surgery   If joints become contracted, orthopedic surgery can help improve function.

Spinal fusion   Most children with Duchenne and Becker dystrophy develop a severe curvature of the spine because the back muscles are too weak to hold the spine straight. Some children may undergo spinal fusion to place a pair of metal rods down the length of the spine so that they can sit upright in a chair and be more comfortable. Usually, a child with muscular dystrophy is a candidate for spinal fusion when there is a 25-degree spinal curvature.

Respiratory care   Many children with muscular dystrophy develop weakened heart and respiratory muscles and sometimes develop serious respiratory infections because they cannot cough out mucus easily. Good general health care and regular vaccinations are especially important for children with muscular dystrophy to prevent these infections.

In the Future

Hope for a cure for MD is centered around gene therapy, in which normal dystrophin would be introduced into a genetically engineered virus that would then bind to afflicted muscle cells, where it would transfer normal dystrophin gene to the weakened muscles.

Muscular Dystrophy Association (MDA) A voluntary health agency dedicated to conquering neuromuscular diseases that affect more than a million Americans.

The Muscular Dystrophy Association combats neuromuscular diseases through programs of worldwide research, comprehensive medical and community services, and professional and public health education. With national headquarters in Tucson, Arizona, MDA has more than 200 offices across the country, sponsors 230 hospital-affiliated clinics, and supports nearly 400 research projects around the world. The association offers medical examinations, flu shots, support groups, MDA summer camps, and financial assistance to buy wheelchairs and leg braces.

The association supports more research on neuromuscular diseases than any other private organization in the world. MDA scientists have uncovered the genetic defects responsible for several forms of muscular dystrophy, including Charcot-Marie-Tooth disease, a form of amyotrophic lateral sclerosis (ALS, or Lou Gehrig's disease), childhood spinal muscular atrophy, and several other neuromuscular conditions.

The association was created in 1950 by a group of adults with muscular dystrophy, parents of children with muscular dystrophy, and a physician-scientist studying the disorder. Since its earliest days it has been energized by its national chairman, entertainer Jerry Lewis, who hosts an annual Labor Day telethon in support of muscular dystrophy research.

The association's programs are funded almost entirely by individual private contributors. The MDA seeks no government grants, United Way funding, or fees from those it serves. (For contact information, see Appendix I.)

mushroom poisoning Since the 1970s, the United States has seen a marked increase in mushroom poisoning due to an increase in the popularity of natural foods, the use of mushrooms as recreational hallucinogens, and the gourmet qualities of wild mushrooms. About 90 percent of the deaths due to mushroom poisoning in the United States and western Europe result from eating a type of mushroom known as the *Amanita phalloides*. Higher death rates of more than 50 percent occur in children less than 10 years of age.

Out of the more than 5,000 varieties of mushrooms found in the United States, about 100 are toxic—and most of these cause only mild stomach problems. A few, however, can cause fatal reactions. Most of the toxic symptoms are caused by the stomach irritants that lead to the vomiting and diarrhea common in mushroom poisoning. In most cases onset of symptoms is rapid, but if the onset is delayed past six to 12 hours, the more serious toxins may be suspected.

Although only an expert can tell for sure if a mushroom is poisonous by looking at it, in general mushrooms growing in the ground are more dangerous than mushrooms growing on living trees, and mushrooms on the forest floor are usually more dangerous than mushrooms on lawns. Since the first report of mushroom poisoning in 1871, much of the information about poisonous mushrooms is inaccurate—including the persistent belief that there are some ironclad "rules" that can be used to tell the difference between edible and toxic varieties. In fact, there is no rule that applies equally to all species. For example, it is not true that a silver spoon or coin put in a pan with cooking mushrooms will turn black if the mushrooms are poisonous. *All* mushrooms will discolor silver in boiling water, if they are rotten, but *no* mushroom ever does as long as it is fresh. Toxic mushrooms will not get darker if soaked in water, nor will they get milky if soaked in vinegar.

Symptoms

The most common symptoms of mushroom poisoning include nausea, stomach cramps, vomiting, and watery or bloody diarrhea.

Treatment

There is no specific antidote for mushroom poisoning, but several advances in treatment have lowered the death rate over the last several years. Early replacement of lost body fluids has been a major factor in improving survival rates. The following list outlines what to do if a child accidentally ingests a toxic mushroom:

1. An adult should collect the mushrooms the child was eating; if possible, a few should be dug up so that even the underground parts can be saved for identification. If there are several kinds of mushrooms around the child, all of the different kinds that the child might have eaten should be collected.

2. An adult should check with the child's doctor, the local poison control center, or the hospital emergency room. If directed to go to the emergency room, the adult should bring the child and the mushrooms.

3. Therapy is aimed at decreasing the amount of toxin in the body. If the child is alert and has not vomited, the adult might be told to administer syrup of ipecac: The child is first given several glasses of water or clear juice to drink, followed by ipecac (one teaspoon to an infant, one tablespoon to children one to 12 years of age, and two tablespoons to children over 12 years of age).

4. The child should throw up everything in the stomach very soon after taking the ipecac. If nothing happens within 20 minutes, the same ipecac dose should be given again.

5. The doctor will check the child's vital signs and consult a local mushroom expert to determine whether or not the mushroom is poisonous and whether any other treatment is necessary.

Once the toxins have been removed, either by vomiting or by stomach pumping, the doctor will probably order continuous aspiration of the upper portion of the small intestine through a nasogastric tube with oral charcoal every four hours for 48 hours to prevent the toxin from being absorbed. This method works best if started within six hours of ingestion.

In the United States, early removal of mushroom poison by using dialysis and correcting any electrolyte imbalance has become part of the treatment program. An enzyme called thioctic acid and corticosteroids also appear to be helpful, as well as high doses of penicillin.

mycoplasma infection   Infection with an organism that causes the contagious disease of childhood MYCOPLASMA PNEUMONIA. While classified as a bacterium, mycoplasma does not have a cell wall and cannot be seen on routine smears, or grown on routine culture plates. Because it lacks a cell wall, it is resistant to antibiotics such as PENICILLIN, which works by attacking the cell walls of bacteria.

Mycoplasmas are found everywhere in nature, some living on decaying matter or occupying harmless places within other organisms. Many others are disease-causing bacteria, but only a handful infect humans. These organisms are halfway between bacteria and viruses, with characteristics of both. Much smaller than bacteria, they reproduce slowly, but unlike viruses, they can be killed by a few antibiotics.

Mycoplasma infections cannot be detected by standard bacterial cultures, and are therefore often misdiagnosed and often not treated appropriately or at all. A DNA analysis technique is required to detect the presence of the mycoplasma a in patients' blood. (See also MYCOPLASMA PNEUMONIA.)

mycoplasma pneumonia   A contagious disease that primarily targets children and teens, caused by *Mycoplasma pneumoniae*. Although anyone can get the disease, it occurs most often in older children and teens. The infections occur sporadically throughout the year, but they are most common in late summer and fall; widespread community outbreaks may occur every five to eight years.

Cause

Mycoplasma pneumonia is caused by *M. pneumoniae* and spread through contact with droplets from the nose and throat of infected people when they cough or sneeze. Scientists believe transmission requires close contact with an infected person. The contagious period is probably less than 10 days.

Symptoms

After an incubation period of from one to 25 days, symptoms of dry cough, fever, sore throat, headache, and malaise appear. Ear infections also may occur. Symptoms may last from a few days to a month or more.

Diagnosis

The disease can be diagnosed based on the symptoms; a nonspecific blood test may help in the diagnosis.

Treatment

Antibiotics including erythromycin or tetracycline (over age 8) are effective.

Prevention

There are no vaccines to prevent the spread of mycoplasma infection, and there are no reliable methods for control. (See also MYCOPLASMA INFECTIONS.)

myopia See NEARSIGHTEDNESS.

nail biting A common habit that is not related to any underlying medical problem. While many children bite their nails in their early years, most grow out of the habit, although it can continue as a nervous mannerism into adulthood.

National Association for the Education of Young Children (NAEYC) The nation's largest and most influential organization of early childhood educators dedicated to improving the quality of programs for children from birth through third grade.

Founded in 1926, the National Association for the Education of Young Children celebrated its 75th anniversary with more than 100,000 members and a national network of nearly 450 local, state, and regional affiliates. These affiliates aim to improve professional practice and working conditions in early childhood education and to build public support for high quality early childhood programs. Membership is open to all who share a desire to serve and act on behalf of the needs and rights of young children. (For contact information, see Appendix I.)

National Association for the Visually Handicapped The only nonprofit health agency in the world solely dedicated to providing assistance to those with partial vision loss (the "hard of seeing"). The association works with millions of people worldwide coping with difficulties of vision impairment and providing anything from large-print books to the latest information on a particular condition.

The association does not receive federal subsidies or United Way funds but rather relies upon the contributions of members and friends. (For contact information, see Appendix I.)

National Federation of the Blind (NFB) The nation's largest membership organization of blind persons, founded in 1940. With 50,000 members, the National Federation of the Blind (NFB) has affiliates in all 50 states plus Washington, D.C., and Puerto Rico, and more than 700 local chapters. The National Federation of the Blind provides information and referral services, scholarships, literature and publications about blindness, aids and appliances and other adaptive equipment for the blind, advocacy services, development and evaluation of technology, and support for blind persons and their families.

Special services of the federation include a Materials Center containing literature about blindness and different aids and appliances used by the blind, and the International Braille and Technology Center for the Blind—the world's largest and most complete evaluation and demonstration center for all speech and Braille technology used by the blind from around the world. NFB-NEWSLINE for the Blind, the world's first free talking newspaper service, offers the blind the complete text of leading national and local newspapers with the use of only a touch-tone telephone. Jobline offers national employment listings and job openings through a telephone menu system available to anyone free of charge.

National Center for Learning Disabilities (NCLD) A nonprofit organization that seeks to raise public awareness and understanding of learning disabilities, provide information and referrals, and arrange educational programs and legislative advocacy. The National Center for Learning Disabilities (NCLD) provides educational tools to heighten understanding of learning disabilities, including the annual publication called *Their World,* quarterly newsletters, articles, specific state-by-state resource listings, and videos about learning disabilities. Founded in 1977, the NCLD's mission is to increase opportunities for all children with learning disabilities to achieve their potential.

National Center for Missing and Exploited Children

(NCMEC)   A private, nonprofit center that provides assistance to parents, children, law enforcement, schools, and the community in recovering missing children and raising public awareness about ways to help prevent child abduction, molestation, and sexual exploitation. It was founded in 1984 by John Walsh, whose six-year-old son Adam was abducted in Florida in 1981.

The National Center for Missing and Exploited Children (NCMEC) has worked on more than 85,500 cases of missing and exploited children, helped recover more than 68,900 children, and raised its recovery rate from 60 percent in the 1980s to more than 93 percent today.

Today the NCMEC staff of 220 analyzes data at its headquarters utilizing state-of-the-art technology, highly trained professionals, and committed staff, interns, and volunteers. John Walsh continued his work to fight for victimized children and to catch criminals through Fox's television program *America's Most Wanted: America Fights Back,* which began in 1988.

National Center on Birth Defects and Developmental Disabilities

One of the centers at the Centers for Disease Control and Prevention (CDC) that collects, analyzes, and distributes data on BIRTH DEFECTS and developmental disabilities, including information on causes, incidence, and prevalence. The center conducts research on preventing defects and disabilities and provides information on prevention activities.

National Childhood Vaccine Injury Act of 1986

A vaccine safety and compensation system established by Congress in 1986 to create a no-fault compensation alternative to suing vaccine manufacturers and providers for citizens injured or killed by vaccines. The act also created safety provisions to help educate the public about vaccine benefits and risks, and to require doctors to report adverse events after vaccination as well as keep records on vaccines administered and health problems which occur following vaccination. Finally, the act also created incentives for the production of safer vaccines.

For any injuries or deaths before October 1, 1988 (no matter how long ago the injury occurred), a citizen may choose to pursue a lawsuit. For injuries or deaths occurring after that date, a citizen is required to apply for federal compensation before pursuing a lawsuit. The government will offer to pay up to $250,000 for a vaccine-associated death, or will offer to pay for all past and future unreimbursed medical expenses, custodial and nursing care, up to $250,000 for pain and suffering; and loss of earned income. If a citizen rejects the award or is turned down, a lawsuit may be filed. Claims must be filed within 24 months of a death and 36 months of an injury. Restrictions apply to lawsuits, if compensation is denied or rejected by the parent. The system is funded by a surcharge on each dose of vaccine sold. (See also VACCINE ADVERSE EVENTS REPORTING SYSTEM.)

National Clearinghouse on Child Abuse and Neglect

An organization established by the Child Abuse Prevention and Treatment Act of 1974 to provide information, products, and technical assistance to help professionals locate information about CHILD ABUSE and neglect and related child welfare issues. The clearinghouse can help consumers find research, statistics, state laws, and resources on such topics as prevention, child protection, out-of-home care, and permanency planning.

The clearinghouse offers the nation's largest database of child maltreatment and related child welfare materials, summaries and analyses of state laws concerned with child abuse and neglect and child welfare, online access to publications, fact sheets, and searchable databases. It also produces the Children's Bureau Express, an online digest of news and resources at http://www.calib.com/cb-express. Resources, which are available both in print and online, are free or available for a nominal fee.

National Council on Child Abuse and Family Violence (NCCAFV) A national nonprofit group in its second decade of its commitment to intergenerational family violence prevention. The National Council on Child Abuse and Family Violence (NCCAFV) provides public awareness and education materials, program and resource development consultation, and technical assistance and training in the United States and internationally.

National Diabetes Information Clearinghouse (NDIC) An information dissemination service of the National Institute of Diabetes and Digestive and Kidney Diseases (NIDDK) that was established in 1978 to increase knowledge and understanding about diabetes among patients, health-care professionals, and the general public. To carry out this mission, the National Diabetes Information Clearinghouse (NDIC) works closely with NIDDK's Diabetes Research and Training Centers; the National Diabetes Education Program (NDEP); professional, patient, and voluntary associations; government agencies; and state health departments to identify and respond to informational needs about diabetes and its management. (For contact information, see Appendix I.)

National Easter Seal Society A nonprofit organization that has been helping individuals with disabilities and special needs and their families live better lives for more than 80 years. Whether helping someone improve physically or simply gain greater independence for everyday living, Easter Seals offers a variety of services to help people with disabilities address life's challenges and achieve personal goals.

The organization was founded in 1919 by Ohio businessman Edgar Allen, who lost his son in a streetcar accident 12 years before. The lack of adequate medical services available to save his son prompted Allen to sell his business and begin a fund-raising campaign to build a hospital in his hometown of Elyria, Ohio. Through this new hospital, Allen was surprised to learn that children with disabilities were often hidden from public view. Inspired by this discovery, Allen founded what became known as the National Society for Crippled Children, the first organization of its kind in the country.

In the spring of 1934 the organization launched its first Easter seals campaign to raise money for its services. To show their support, donors placed the seals on envelopes and letters. *Cleveland Plain Dealer* cartoonist J. H. Donahey designed the first seal based on a concept of simplicity—because those served by the charity asked simply for the right to live a normal life. The lily—a symbol of spring—was officially incorporated as the Easter Seals' logo in 1952 for its association with resurrection and new life, and it has appeared on each seal since.

The overwhelming public support for the Easter seals campaign triggered a nationwide expansion of the organization and a swell of grassroots efforts on behalf of people with disabilities. By 1967 the Easter seal was so well recognized that the organization formally adopted the name "Easter Seals."

Today the Easter Seals Society helps more than one million children with disabilities and their families annually through a nationwide network of more than 450 service sites providing family-focused services tailored to meet the specific needs of the particular community it serves. Primary Easter Seals services include medical rehabilitation, early intervention, physical therapy, occupational therapy, speech and hearing therapy, job training and employment, child care, and adult day services.

National Fragile X Foundation A nonprofit foundation established in 1984 to unite the FRAGILE X SYNDROME community, provide educational and emotional support, promote public and professional awareness, and support research in improved treatments and a cure. (For contact information, see Appendix I.)

National Head Start Association (NHSA) A private nonprofit membership organization representing the children, staff, and Head Start programs in America. The National Head Start Association (NHSA) provides a national forum for the enhancement of Head Start services for poor children up to age five and their families. It is the only national organization dedicated exclusively to the concerns of the Head Start community.

Over the past 25 years NHSA's mission has changed from simply defending Head Start in Congress to actively expanding and improving the program. From planning massive annual training conferences to publishing a vast array of publications, the National Head Start Association continually strives to improve the quality of Head Start's comprehensive services for America's children and families.

National Hydrocephalus Foundation   A nonprofit organization founded in 1980 to familiarize the public with HYDROCEPHALUS, a buildup of cerebrospinal fluid inside the skull. The foundation also seeks to remove stigma from those with hydrocephalus, collect and disseminate information, counsel parents on specific problems encountered as a result of hydrocephalus in their children, work to obtain government funding for research, secure health insurance covering this disease, and form local chapters to help accomplish these goals. The foundation is supported by donations and membership fees and responds in particular to the disorder as a condition in itself, as opposed to hydrocephalus as a secondary condition of another disease. (For contact information, see Appendix I.)

National Information Center for Children and Youth with Disabilities   A national information center that provides information on disabilities and disability-related issues. Services are offered to families, educators, administrators, journalists, and students, with a special emphasis on children and youth. The center can provide information about specific disabilities, special education, individualized education programs, parent materials, disability organizations, professional associations, education rights, early intervention services for infants and toddlers, and transition to adult life. (For contact information, see Appendix I.)

National Institute of Allergy and Infectious Disease (NIAID)   The federal research institute that provides the major support for scientists conducting research into better ways to diagnose, treat, and prevent the many infectious, immunologic, and allergic diseases. The National Institute of Allergy and Infectious Disease (NIAID) has four divisions: AIDS; Allergy; Immunology and Transplantation; and Extramural Activities. (For contact information, see Appendix I.)

National Institute of Child Health and Human Development (NICHD)   Federal institute that is part of the National Institutes of Health, the biomedical research arm of the U.S. Department of Health and Human Services. The mission of the National Institute of Child Health and Human Development (NICHD) is to ensure that every person is born healthy and wanted, that women suffer no harmful effects from the reproductive process, and that all children have the chance to fulfill their potential for a healthy and productive life, free of disease or disability.

NICHD was created by Congress in 1962 and supports and conducts research on topics related to the health of children, adults, families, and populations, including:

- reducing infant deaths
- improving the health of women and men
- understanding reproductive health
- learning about growth and development
- examining birth defects and mental retardation
- enhancing involvement across the life span through medical rehabilitation research.

(For contact information, see Appendix I.)

National Marfan Foundation   A nonprofit organization founded in 1981 by people affected by MARFAN SYNDROME and their families. Its purpose is to provide accurate information about the condition to patients, family members, and health-care providers, provide support to members and patients, and support research. The National Marfan Foundation provides programs of information, awareness, education, service, and research through a variety of projects. It offers pamphlets, booklets, and other materials that explain Marfan syndrome, a medical brochure series targeted to health-care professionals, a quarterly newsletter, and an annual report. (For contact information, see Appendix I.)

National Parent Network on Disabilities (NPND)
A nonprofit organization dedicated to empowering parents of children with disabilities. Located in Washington, D.C., the National Parent Network on Disabilities (NPND) provides up-to-date information on the activities of all three branches of government that affect individuals with disabilities and their families. The NPND's primary activities include advocating for and supporting the development and implementation of legislation that will improve the lives and protect the rights of children, youth, and adults with disabilities. Members include individuals and family members, as well as national, state, and local organizations that represent the interests of individuals with disabilities.

The network was formally established in December 1988, but traces its origins to a much earlier time when pioneer parent leaders sought a structured national presence representing the interests and needs of all parents of children with disabilities and special health-care needs.

In 1976 five parent center coalitions were established with federal funding to provide information, training, and support to parents of children with disabilities. The initial parent center coalitions were effective, and by 1983 the federal government had expanded the program. As of 1995 there were 76 Parent Training and Information Centers (PTIs) located in all states and jurisdictions, serving more than 750,000 parents and their families. In 1989 the NPND established its first office in Washington, D.C.

National Reye's Syndrome Foundation Nonprofit citizen group incorporated in 1974, in Bryan, Ohio, to generate an organized movement to eradicate REYE'S SYNDROME. The foundation is committed to helping to educate the public and medical communities about the risk involved with the use of aspirin through awareness programs, brochures, bulletins, television and radio public service announcements, documentary and slide/tape presentations, and a speaker's bureau available to groups and organizations free of charge. The foundation also tries to give the families emotional support and guidance, and to support research into the cause, management, treatment, and prevention of the disease, as well as study the impact the disease

has had on survivors. (For contact information, see Appendix I.)

National Safe Kids Campaign The first and only national nonprofit organization dedicated solely to the prevention of unintentional childhood injury, the number one killer of children ages 14 and under. More than 300 state and local Safe Kids coalitions in all 50 states, the District of Columbia, and Puerto Rico comprise the Campaign.

The National Safe Kids Campaign communicates prevention messages directly to children and their families through national programs involving media events, device distribution, and hands-on educational activities to get communities more involved in the children's safety. The programs include National Safe Kids Week, Safe Kids Buckle Up, Safe Kids Walk This Way, and Safe Kids At Home.

National Safety Council The nation's leading advocate for safety and health, founded in 1913 and chartered by the U.S. Congress in 1953. The National Safety Council has been working for generations to protect lives and promote health with innovative programs. The Council is a nonprofit, nongovernmental, international public service organization dedicated to improving the safety, health, and environmental well-being of all people.

The National Safety Council started in the workplace—in factories, warehouses, construction sites—making businesses aware of ways to prevent unintentional injuries on the job. Subsequently, its efforts were expanded to include highway, community, and recreation safety; and its mission now encompasses all major causes of preventable injuries and deaths, including occupational and environmental health and general wellness. Along with its national responsibilities, the Council carries out its mission on the community level through a network of chapters.

National Scoliosis Foundation A patient-led nonprofit organization dedicated since 1976 to helping children, parents, adults, and health-care providers to understand the complexities of spinal deformities such as SCOLIOSIS. The foundation is involved in all aspects of scoliosis support, including screening programs, treatment methods, pain management, and patient care. The group aims to promote public awareness, provide reliable information, foster ongoing research, and educate and nurture those affected by scoliosis. It also provides comprehensive education and support for patients and health-care professionals through videos, books, brochures, local chapters, conferences, and postural screening training sessions.

National Tay-Sachs and Allied Diseases Association, Inc. (NTSAD) National association dedicated to the treatment and prevention of Tay-Sachs, Canavan, and related diseases, and to providing information and support services to individuals and families affected by these diseases. The association focuses on public and professional education, research, genetic screening, family services, and advocacy.

The association was founded in 1956 by a small group of concerned parents with children affected by TAY-SACHS DISEASE or a related genetic disorder. Dedicated to the defeat of Tay-Sachs and several allied diseases, the National Tay-Sachs and Allied Diseases Association (NTSAD) was an early pioneer in the development of community education about Tay-Sachs disease, carrier screening programs, and laboratory quality control programs. Today more than one million people have been tested for the Tay-Sachs gene, thousands of Tay-Sachs carriers identified, and hundreds of healthy children born to high-risk couples.

Over the past four decades the organization has grown in size, scope, and stature. NTSAD services now encompass 48 genetic diagnoses and, as science yields discoveries in the arena of the allied diseases, NTSAD is committed to a leadership role in the application of this knowledge to the betterment of children, adults, and families. (For contact information, see Appendix I.)

National Vaccine Injury Compensation Program Program established by the U.S. Congress as part of the NATIONAL CHILDHOOD VACCINE INJURY ACT of 1986 (PL 99-660). The program is designed to ensure an adequate supply of vaccines, stabilize vaccine costs, and maintain an efficient way to help children injured by childhood vaccines.

The program, which went into effect October 1, 1988, is a no-fault alternative to the traditional tort system for resolving vaccine injury claims. Since its inception, the Vaccine Injury Compensation Program (VICP) has helped stabilize the U.S. vaccine market by providing liability protection to both vaccine companies and health-care providers, by encouraging research and development of new and safer vaccines, and by allowing a quicker and less adversarial alternative to lawsuits.

The VICP covers all vaccines recommended by the Centers for Disease Control and Prevention for routine administration to children:

- diphtheria, tetanus, pertussis (DTP, DTaP, DT, TT, or Td)
- measles, mumps, rubella (MMR or any components)
- polio (OPV or IPV)
- hepatitis B
- haemophilus influenza type B (HIB)
- varicella
- rotavirus (no longer given)
- pneumococcal conjugate

In the early 1980s reports of harmful side effects after the DTP (diphtheria, tetanus, pertussis) vaccine posed major liability concerns for vaccine companies and health-care providers and caused many parents to question the safety of the DTP vaccine. Parents began filing lawsuits against vaccine companies and health-care providers. Vaccination rates among children began to fall, and many companies that produce vaccines decided to stop, creating significant vaccine shortages and a real threat to the nation's health.

Eventually a coalition of physicians, public health organizations, leaders of industry, government representatives, and private citizens developed the idea of a no-fault alternative to lawsuits for resolving vaccine injury claims—the National Vaccine Injury Compensation Program (VICP).

The program is administered jointly by the U.S. Department of Health and Human Services, the U.S. Court of Federal Claims, and the U.S. Department of Justice. The VICP is located in the Division

VACCINE INJURY CHART

Vaccine	Injury	Onset
Tetanus (DTaP, DTP, DT, Td, TT)	Anaphylaxis or anaphylactic shock	0–4 hours
	Brachial neuritis	2–28 days
Pertussis antigen-containing (DTaP, DTP, P, DTP-HIB)	Anaphylaxis/anaphylactic shock	0–4 hours
	Encephalopathy (or encephalitis)	0–72 hours
MMR or in any combination (MMR, MR, M, R)	Anaphylaxis or anaphylactic shock	0–4 hours
	Encephalopathy	5–15 days
Rubella (MMR, MR, R)	Chronic arthritis	7–42 days
Measles (MMR, MR, M)	Thrombocytopenic purpura	7–30 days
	Vaccine-strain measles viral infection in an immunodeficient receipt	0–6 months
OPV	Paralytic polio (recipient and community contact cases)	0–30 days/0–6 months
	Vaccine-strain polio viral infection	0–30 days/0–6 months
IPV	Anaphylaxis or anaphylactic shock	0–4 hours
Hepatitis B	Anaphylaxis or anaphylactic shock	0–4 hours
HIB (conjugate)	No condition specified	Not applicable**
Varicella	No condition specified	Not applicable**
Rotavirus	No condition specified	Not applicable**
Live, oral, rhesus-based rotavirus vaccine	Intussusception	0–30 days
Pneumococcal conjugate vaccines	No condition specified	Not applicable**
New vaccines	No condition specified	Not applicable**

**No condition has been identified requiring inclusion on the Vaccine Injury Table; therefore, compensation for alleged injuries must be pursued on a causation in fact basis.

of Vaccine Injury Compensation, Health Resources and Services Administration. The nine-member Advisory Commission on Childhood Vaccines (ACCV) administers the VICP.

Qualifying for Compensation

The coalition devised a "vaccine table of injuries" chart (see Vaccine Injury Chart) that lists specific injuries or conditions caused by vaccines, and the time frames in which they must occur after vaccine administration, in order to qualify for compensation. However, if an adverse event is not listed on the table, an individual may still file a claim but must prove that the vaccine caused the injury. Compensation may not be awarded if the court determines that the injury or death was not caused by the vaccine. There are three means of qualifying for compensation:

1. A petitioner must show that an injury listed on the Vaccine Injury Chart occurred.

2. Or, a petitioner must prove that the vaccine significantly aggravated a preexisting condition.

3. Or, a petitioner must prove that the vaccine caused the condition.

nearsightedness The popular name for myopia, which refers to the inability to see distant objects clearly. Nearsightedness does not usually occur in infancy but begins to appear in some children as early as age two. The number of children with the problem rises steadily, peaking during the teen years.

It is caused by a mistake in the way the eye bends the light rays that the brain translates into visual images. Normally, light rays focus precisely on the retina at the back of the eyeball. In children who are nearsighted, the eyeball is too long from front to back so that the rays converge in front of the retina. This causes blurring of objects more than a few feet away from the affected child, and the farther away the objects are, the more indistinct they are.

Symptoms

Often young nearsighted children do not realize that they have a visual problem. Symptoms include squinting, holding the head at an unusual angle, eye rubbing, sitting too close to the TV, and clumsiness. Many parents do not notice the problem until the child starts school, when it quickly becomes apparent that there are problems in seeing the blackboard. Many parents first discover a problem during a school vision screening.

Treatment

Correction for nearsightedness includes wearing glasses or contact lenses. Because a child's eyes grow and change quickly during the first seven years of life, youngsters this age may need vision checks every six months. Because contact lens require more difficult care, they are rarely prescribed for young children.

necrotizing enterocolitis (NEC) This gastrointestinal disease primarily affects premature infants, infecting, inflaming, and eventually destroying part of the infant's bowel. Although it affects only one infant in 2,000 to 4,000 births, (up to 5 percent of neonatal intensive care unit admissions), it is the most common and serious gastrointestinal disorder among hospitalized preterm infants.

Necrotizing enterocolitis (NEC) typically begins within the first two weeks of life, because premature infants have immature bowels that are sensitive to changes in blood flow and prone to infection. They may have difficulty with blood and oxygen circulation and digestion, which increases their chances of developing NEC. However, the exact cause of NEC is unknown. Experts suspect that the intestinal tissues of premature infants are weakened by too little oxygen or blood flow, and when milk feedings are begun, the added stress of moving food through the intestine allows bacteria to damage the intestinal wall. The damage may affect only a short segment of the intestine, or it may progress quickly to involve a much larger portion.

The infant will begin to look sick if bacteria continue to spread through the wall of the intestines and into the blood, and may develop mineral imbalances. In severe cases the intestine may perforate, allowing bacteria to leak into the abdomen and causing life-threatening PERITONITIS. Because the infant is physically immature, even with quick treatment there may be serious complications.

Some experts believe that NEC can be triggered by the type of infant formula and its rate of delivery, or the immaturity of the mucous membranes. (Babies who are fed breast milk can also develop NEC, but their risk is lower.) Another theory is that babies who have had difficult deliveries with low oxygen levels can develop NEC. When there is not enough oxygen, the body sends the available oxygen and blood to vital organs instead of the gastrointestinal tract, and NEC can result. Babies with an increased number of red blood cells also seem to be at higher risk, because too many red blood cells thicken the blood and hinder the transport of oxygen to the intestines.

NEC sometimes seems to occur in epidemics, affecting several infants in the same nursery, which suggests that in some cases the infection could be spread from one baby to another, despite the fact that all nurseries have very strict precautions to prevent the spread of infection.

Symptoms

The symptoms of NEC may vary from one baby to the next, and may mimic other digestive problems, but they include:

- poor tolerance to feedings
- food stays in stomach longer than expected
- decreased bowel sounds
- bloating and abdominal tenderness
- greenish vomit
- red abdominal skin
- increase or drop in number of stools
- bloody stools

Other symptoms include periodic stoppage of breathing, slowed heart rate, diarrhea, lethargy, and fluctuating body temperature. Advanced cases may show fluid in the abdominal cavity, infection of the membrane lining the abdomen, or shock.

Diagnosis

NEC is usually confirmed by the presence of an abnormal gas pattern seen on an X ray. A surgeon may need to withdraw fluid from the abdomen to determine whether the intestines have perforated.

Treatment

Most babies with NEC do not need surgery. Treatment includes stopping feedings, sending a tube through the nasal passages to the stomach to remove air and fluid from the stomach and intestine, intravenous fluids, antibiotics, and frequent examinations of the abdomen. If the swollen abdomen interferes with breathing, extra oxygen or a ventilator is used to help the baby breathe.

If the treatment is successful, the baby may be able to be fed normally within 72 hours, although in most cases feedings are withheld and antibiotics are continued for seven to 10 days. Severe cases may require the removal of part of the intestine.

Most infants recover completely, but sometimes the bowel may be so scarred and narrowed that it causes future intestinal obstruction or interferes with the absorption of nutrients. This is more common in children who required surgery for NEC and had part of their intestine removed.

neonatal acne   See ACNE, INFANT.

nephritis   Inflammation of the kidneys that usually occurs as a result of infection elsewhere in the body. Pyelonephritis is a type of kidney inflammation caused by direct bacterial infection of the kidney from the lower urinary tract. Glomerulonephritis is another type that may be caused by infection elsewhere in the body, or as the result of certain inherited disorders or immune system diseases. All types of nephritis can cause the kidneys to fail so that they can no longer filter blood and regulate the body's fluid balance.

During kidney failure, the kidneys cannot absorb the correct amount of protein and other essential nutrients and instead release them into the urine.

Symptoms

Bloody or cloudy urine is the primary symptom of nephritis, although the blood is not always visible without a microscope. Other symptoms include nausea, fever, appetite loss, weakness, and side pain. Complications may include high blood pressure and fluid buildup that requires hospitalization.

Diagnosis

Blood tests can reveal the presence of antibodies to certain bacteria (especially streptococcal bacteria). Occasionally a doctor may need to remove a kidney tissue sample for examination in the lab.

Treatment

An active infection will require antibiotics; otherwise, treatment includes drugs to keep the body functioning until the inflammation fades away.

neural tube defects (NTD)   A group of birth defects that occur in the first month of pregnancy, when the structure that develops into the brain and spinal cord is forming. Normally, this structure folds into a tube by the 29th day after conception, but if the tube does not close completely, the baby has a neural tube defect. Many babies with these defects are stillborn or die soon after birth.

The two most common forms of neural tube defects (NTDs) are SPINA BIFIDA and ANENCEPHALY. Spina bifida occurs when the spinal column does not close completely around the spinal cord. The seriousness of this condition can range from mild to severe and can be associated with loss of bladder and bowel function, paralysis, and sometimes death. Anencephaly, which occurs in three out of 10,000 births, involves the lack of development of parts of the brain or a complete loss of brain tissue.

Neural tube defects affect about 2,500 babies a year in the United States—one out of every 2,000 live births. Studies have shown that many of these defects may be prevented if the mother gets enough folic acid before and during pregnancy, especially during the first trimester. Specifically, women who get 400 micrograms (0.4 milligrams) of folic acid (also known as folate, a B vitamin) each day before conception and during early pregnancy reduce the risk that their baby will be born with a serious neural tube defect by up to 70 percent.

Women must make sure that they are receiving enough folic acid before they become pregnant, because the neural tube closes during the period about a week after the first missed menstrual period. This is why mothers cannot wait to start taking folic acid when they first realize they are pregnant. For this reason, it is recommended that women of reproductive age take folic acid throughout their reproductive years.

Folic acid is found naturally in green, leafy vegetables and in orange juice. In 1998 the U.S. Food and Drug Administration required the addition of folic acid to enriched grain products (such as breakfast cereals, breads, pastas, and rice), designed to provide an additional 100 micrograms of folic acid to a woman's daily diet. Still, to reach the recommended level of 400 micrograms daily, a vitamin supplement is usually necessary.

neurocutaneous syndromes A group of genetic neurological skin disorders affecting the brain, spine, and peripheral nerves that can cause tumors to grow inside the brain, spinal cord, organs, skin, and skeletal bones. The most common syndromes involving children include NEUROFIBROMATOSIS, STURGE-WEBER SYNDROME, TUBEROUS SCLEROSIS, ataxia-telangiectasia, and VON HIPPEL-LINDAU DISEASE.

The first symptoms most commonly noted in children are skin lesions, including birthmarks, tumors, and other growths. All of the these diseases are believed to begin as a result of abnormal development of embryonic cells (primitive cells that are present in the earliest stages of an embryo's development). Although there is no cure for these conditions, treatments are available that help to manage symptoms and complications.

Symptoms vary widely among these conditions and from child to child. Because neurocutaneous syndromes affect children in different ways, the full extent of these diseases may only appear as the child gets older. There are no cure for these conditions, which means that educational, social, and physical problems must be managed throughout a child's life.

Support groups can be extremely helpful in providing a supportive social environment and information. Psychotherapy can boost an affected child's self-esteem and coping skills and can help family members deal with the stress involved in caring for a child with a chronic illness or disability. Physical, occupational, or speech therapy can help the child improve some of the developmental delays caused by a specific illness.

neurofibromatosis (NF) One of the most common NEUROCUTANEOUS SYNDROMES that primarily affects the growth and development of nerve cells, causing tumors or neurofibromas that produce skin changes, bone deformities, eye problems, and other complications, especially in the brain. In 1882 neurofibromatosis (NF) was first described in medical literature by Dr. Friedrich von Recklinghausen, and the disease was known as Von Recklinghausen's disease for many years. NF affects more than 100,000 Americans, making this condition more common than CYSTIC FIBROSIS, hereditary MUSCULAR DYSTROPHY, Huntington's disease, and TAY-SACHS DISEASE combined.

NF is not the "Elephant Man's disease," although it was at one time believed to be. Scientists now believe that John Merrick, the so-called Elephant Man, had Proteus syndrome, which is an entirely different disorder.

Cause

Although neurofibromatosis is usually inherited, between 30 percent and 50 percent of new cases occur from spontaneous mutations within a child's genes. However, once the gene is altered, it can then be passed on to succeeding generations. A parent with neurofibromatosis has a 50 percent chance of having a child with the disease, and the type of NF inherited by the child is always the same as that of the affected parent. NF is found throughout the world and affects both sexes equally; it has no particular racial, geographic, or ethnic distribution. Therefore, NF can appear in any family.

Types

The disorder was originally divided into two different types—neurofibromatosis type 1 and type 2 (NF1 and NF2)—but in fact these two types are actually two totally separate disorders caused by two different genes.

Neurofibromatosis type 1 occurs far more frequently (about 90 percent of all cases) and is a very common genetic disorder, occurring in about one in 4,000 babies born in the United States. When diagnosing NF1 (also called von Recklinghausen disease), doctors will take a thorough medical history because children with NF1 often have a parent with the disease.

Neurofibromatosis type 2 is less common, occurring in about one in 140,000 births. Also known as bilateral acoustic NF, it is characterized by multiple tumors on the cranial and spinal nerves, and by other lesions of the brain and spinal cord. Tumors affecting both of the auditory nerves are the hallmark.

Symptoms

The symptoms of NF1 and NF2 are quite different from each other, and are described below.

NF1   The classic sign of NF1 is a skin pigment problem (café-au-lait spots) of light brown, coffee-colored patches that may look like freckles at first but often increase in size and number during the first few years of life. A child diagnosed with NF1 will usually have at least six café-au-lait spots that are larger than freckles.

Another common symptom of NF1 is Lisch nodules (tiny, benign tumors on the iris of the eye that do not cause problems but that can help confirm the diagnosis). Tumors along the optic nerves can rarely occur, and they will affect vision. Benign tumors called neurofibromas are found on or under the skin or along the nerves of the body and usually appear at puberty. Bone deformities may also occur, as can curvature of the spine (SCOLIOSIS).

Between 30 percent and 40 percent of children with NF1 also have a high incidence of seizures, learning disabilities, attention deficit disorder, and speech problems.

NF2   NF2 causes tumors on the hearing nerve leading to hearing loss, ringing of the ears, and problems with balance that usually becomes apparent in the teen years or early 20s.

Although tumors on the eighth cranial nerve are most common, children with NF2 can develop tumors on other nerves, called "schwannomas" because they begin in Schwann cells. Schwann cells support, protect, and insulate nerve cells. The symptoms of a schwannoma will depend on its location; those that begin on cranial nerves (such as eighth cranial nerve tumors) affect the head and neck unless they grow large enough to push on the brain stem and affect the body also. Those that grow on the nerves as they exit the spinal cord may cause numbness of a part of the body; some tumors may grow large enough to press on the spinal cord and cause weakness and numbness in the legs. Those that grow in the bundles of nerves gathered in the armpits and groin area may cause weakness in one arm or leg. Schwannomas may even grow in tiny nerves in the skin; they rarely cause neurological symptoms, but they may rub on clothing or be cosmetically disfiguring.

Other symptoms of NF2 may include facial weakness, headache, vision changes, and a lump or swelling under the skin caused by the development of a neurofibroma. In a family member at risk for NF2, a positive diagnosis can be made if mild signs of NF are found elsewhere, such as one or two café-au-lait spots or a small lump under the scalp or skin.

Diagnosis

A genetic test is available for NF2. Otherwise, a doctor can diagnose the condition from available symptoms.

Treatment

Treatment of a child with NF1 involves managing symptoms. Children with complications of the eye, nervous system, spine, or bones will be referred to an appropriate specialist for treatment. Surgical removal of neurofibromas is required if they are causing chronic pain, become infected, are pressing or growing into vital body organs, or for cosmetic reasons.

Children with NF1 are usually checked for height, weight, head circumference, blood pressure, vision and hearing, evidence of normal sexual development, signs of LEARNING DISABILITY and HYPERACTIVITY, and evidence of SCOLIOSIS, in addition to examination of the skin for café-au-lait spots and neurofibromas. The causes of any unusual growth pattern are generally investigated, and early or late onset of puberty also suggests further study. Further diagnostic evaluations, including blood tests and X rays, are usually needed only to investigate suspected problems.

Healthy children with NF1 are usually examined every six or 12 months.

The only treatments available for the tumors of NF2 are surgery and radiation therapy. Most people with NF2 require at least one operation during their lifetime. Since the tumors of NF2 lie on nerves near the brain and spinal cord, their surgical removal can be risky and may further injure nerves, causing neurological problems. For these reasons, the risk of surgical damage should always be carefully weighed against the potential benefits of the proposed procedure. When surgery is no longer an option for a particular person because of medical problems or the size or location of a tumor, radiation therapy may be considered. As with surgery, radiation therapy has both risks and benefits, which must be carefully considered.

Neurofibromatosis can be stressful for many affected children, who may experience social isolation and loneliness or worry about possible future complications. Anxiety about the need for medical treatments, a sense of losing control, and the feeling of being different from others are often experienced.

newborn screening tests   Every American newborn is tested by law for certain harmful or potentially fatal disorders that are not otherwise apparent at birth. Many of these are metabolic disorders (often called INBORN ERRORS OF METABOLISM) that interfere with the way the body uses nutrients to maintain tissues and produce energy. Other disorders that may be detected through screening include problems with hormones, vitamin levels, or the blood.

Because metabolic and other inherited disorders may hinder an infant's normal physical and mental development, early diagnosis can be crucial. With a simple blood test, doctors often can tell whether newborns have certain conditions that could eventually cause problems. Even though these conditions are considered rare, early diagnosis and proper treatment can make the difference between lifelong impairment and healthy development.

Different states have different newborn screening laws, but most states require basic screening programs. The list below is given in order from the most common (all states screen for the first two) to least common (ranging from three-fourths or one-half of states to just a few).

Phenylketonuria (PKU)   When this disorder is detected early, mental retardation can be prevented simply by feeding a special formula low in phenylalanine. This special diet will need to be followed throughout childhood and adolescence and perhaps into adult life.

Congenital hypothyroidism   This is the disorder most commonly identified by routine screening. Affected babies do not have enough thyroid hormone, which can lead to retarded growth and brain development. The thyroid, a gland at the front of the neck, releases chemical substances that control metabolism and growth. If the disorder is detected early, a baby can be treated with oral doses of thyroid hormone to permit normal development.

Galactosemia   Babies with this condition lack the enzyme that converts galactose (one of two sugars found in lactose) into glucose, a sugar the body is able to use. As a result, milk (including breast milk) and other dairy products must be eliminated from the diet, or galactose can accumulate and damage the body's cells and organs. This could lead to blindness, severe mental retardation, growth deficiency, and even death.

Sickle-cell disease   This inherited blood disease features red blood cells that stretch into abnormal "sickle" shapes, causing episodes of pain, damage to vital organs such as the lungs and kidneys, and even death. Young children with sickle-cell disease are especially prone to certain dangerous bacterial infections, such as PNEUMONIA and MENINGITIS. Studies suggest that newborn screening can alert doctors to begin antibiotic treatment before infections occur and to monitor symptoms of possible worsening more closely. The screening test can also detect other disorders affecting hemoglobin (the oxygen-carrying substance in the blood). It is especially common in African Americans (about one in every 500 African-American births) and one in every 1,000 to 1,400 Hispanic-American births; it also occurs with some frequency among people of Hispanic, Mediterranean, Middle Eastern, and South Asian descent.

Biotinidase deficiency   Babies with this condition do not have enough biotinidase, an enzyme that recycles biotin (a B vitamin). The deficiency may cause seizures, poor muscle control, immune system impairment, hearing loss, MENTAL RETARDATION, coma, and even death. If the deficiency is detected in time, however, problems can be prevented by giving the baby extra biotin.

Congenital adrenal hyperplasia This group of disorders involves a deficiency of certain hormones produced by the adrenal gland that can affect genital development and may cause a fatal loss of salt from the kidneys. Lifelong supplementation of the missing hormones controls the condition.

Maple syrup urine disease Babies with this inborn error of metabolism lack an enzyme needed to process three amino acids essential for the body's normal growth. When these amino acids are not processed properly, they can build up in the body, causing urine to smell like maple syrup or sweet, burnt sugar. These babies usually have little appetite and are extremely irritable. If not detected and treated early, this condition can lead to mental retardation, physical disability, and death. A carefully controlled diet that eliminates certain high-protein foods containing those amino acids can prevent complications.

Homocystinuria This metabolic disorder is caused by a deficiency of one of several enzymes needed by the brain for normal development. If untreated, it can lead to dislocated lenses of the eyes, mental retardation, skeletal abnormalities, and abnormal blood clotting. However, a special diet combined with dietary supplements may help prevent most of these problems.

Tyrosinemia Babies with this disorder have trouble processing the amino acid tyrosine, which builds up in the body, causing mild retardation, language problems, liver problems, and death from liver failure. A special diet, or even a liver transplant, may be needed to treat the condition.

Cystic fibrosis An inherited disorder that causes cells to release a thick mucus that can lead to chronic respiratory disease, problems with digestion, and poor growth. There is no known cure; treatment is focused on preventing the associated serious lung infections and providing adequate nutrition. Detecting the disease early may help doctors reduce the lung and nutritional problems associated with cystic fibrosis, but the real impact of newborn screening is yet to be determined.

Toxoplasmosis This parasitic infection is transmitted through a mother's placenta to an unborn child, where it can invade the brain, eye, and muscles, causing blindness and mental retardation.

Who Should Be Screened

If parents have a positive family history of an inherited disorder, have previously given birth to an affected child, or have reason to believe that a child may be at risk for a certain condition, additional testing may be needed. If a hospital cannot or will not provide expanded screening and the child's doctors believe additional testing would be a good idea, an independent laboratory can provide supplemental testing for more than 30 metabolic disorders through a mail-order service available anywhere in the United States. The labs send out kits that are used to collect additional blood at the time of a baby's regular screening, which is then mailed back for analysis. The cost ranges from $25 to $50.

nightmares Frightening dreams that usually force at least a partial awakening. Nightmares are experienced by almost all children at one time or another; one out of every four children has nightmares more than once a week. Most children have nightmares between the ages of three or four and seven or eight, which seem to be a part of normal development and do not generally signal a mental problem.

Most nightmares occur late during the sleep cycle (usually between 4 A.M. and 6 A.M.). Nightmare themes may vary widely from child to child, and from time to time for the same child, but the most common theme is being chased. Children are commonly chased by an animal or some fantasy figure. The nightmares of early childhood probably reflect the struggle to learn to deal with normal childhood fears and problems. Many children also experience nightmares after they have suffered a traumatic event, such as surgery, the loss of a loved one, or a severe accident. The content of these nightmares is typically directly related to the traumatic event, and the nightmares often occur over and over. Finally, some children experience frequent nightmares that seem unrelated to their waking lives; these individuals tend to be more creative, sensitive, trusting, and emotional than average.

After a nightmare, the child may wake up and seek comfort from parents; usually, the child can relate what happened in the dream and why it was scary. Children may have trouble going back to sleep after a nightmare and may have the same dream again on other nights.

Nightmares decrease in frequency as children get older, and often stop completely in adolescence, although some—especially those who are imaginative and creative—may continue to have nightmares into adulthood.

Treatment

Experts usually suggest that parents encourage young children to discuss their nightmares with their parents or other adults, but that children generally do not need treatment. However, if a child is suffering from recurrent or very disturbing nightmares, the help of a therapist may be needed to have the child draw the nightmare, talk with the frightening characters, or imagine how the nightmare could change to help the child feel safer and less frightened.

Nightmares that replay a traumatic event actually reflect a normal mental healing process and will occur less often and be less frightening if the child is recovering. Nightmares in children can occur up to six months after a stressful physical or emotional event. However, if nightmares continue and interfere with a child's sleep, they can affect the child's ability to function during the day. For this reason, parents may want to consult a doctor to see whether any treatment is appropriate to help the child. (See also NIGHT TERRORS.)

night terrors A relatively common sleep problem that occurs primarily in young children between the ages of three and five years. Two percent to 3 percent of all children will experience episodes of night terrors, but by the time they reach school age, most have outgrown these nighttime events. Although it may be frightening to watch, night terrors are not unusual nor dangerous to a child. As the brain matures and a child's sleep pattern matures, the terrors go away.

Night Terrors vs. Nightmares

A night terror is different from a NIGHTMARE, which occurs during the dream phase of sleep (REM sleep). A nightmare frightens a child, who usually wakes up with a vivid memory of a long scary dream. Night terrors, on the other hand, occur during a phase of deep non-REM sleep, usually an hour or two after the child goes to bed. During a night terror, which may last anywhere from a few minutes up to an hour, the child is still asleep, although her eyes may be open. When she does wake up, she will have absolutely no recollection of the episode other than a sense of fear.

Cause

Several factors may contribute to a child's night terrors. They often seem to run in families and may be triggered by fatigue and psychological stress.

Treatment

It is important that a child prone to night terrors get plenty of rest and minimize stress whenever possible. Because children usually have night terrors at the same time each night (usually within the first few hours after falling asleep) parents can try waking a child about 30 minutes before the night terror usually happens. After about five minutes, the child can be allowed to fall back to sleep.

Because a child may get out of bed and run around, parents should gently restrain a child experiencing night terrors. Once a night terror has started, the child should not be shouted at or shaken awake, as these methods will just worsen the terror.

nonsteroidal anti-inflammatory drugs (NSAIDs) A type of painkiller and fever reducer that reduces inflammation in the body. Examples of nonsteroidal anti-inflammatory drugs (NSAIDs) include ibuprofen (such as Motrin or Advil) and naproxen (Aleve). Ibuprofen is available without prescription to treat fever in children over a year old. Nonaspirin NSAIDs are given to children to lower fever and treat pain instead of aspirin, which has been associated with the development of REYE'S SYNDROME.

nonverbal learning disabilities (NLD) A form of LEARNING DISABILITY that primarily affects social functioning in areas such as interpersonal skills, social perception, and interaction. Also called "right-hemisphere learning disorders," this problem often goes unrecognized for a large part of a child's schooling. Since abnormalities of the right hemisphere interfere with understanding and adaptive learning, experts believe that nonverbal learning disabilities are more debilitating than verbal disabilities.

Experts suspect that nonverbal learning disabilities are caused by a problem in the right hemisphere of the brain, either from brain injury or damage before birth. The damage primarily affects visual-spatial perception, processing, and reasoning. Children with nonverbal learning disabilities (NLD) often are very good verbally and may develop reading and speaking skills earlier than their peers; consequently, their nonverbal learning difficulties may be overlooked. Both parents and teachers will often suspect that something is wrong early on, but they cannot quite figure out what it is.

Nonverbal learning disorders remain predominantly misunderstood and largely unrecognized. Although NLD syndrome was discovered in the early 1970s, even today education professionals are largely unfamiliar with nonverbal learning disorders. Typically, parents are assured that everything is fine and that their child is "just a perfectionist," or is immature, bored, or a bit clumsy. Rarely are a parent's or teacher's concerns accepted until the child reaches a point in school where he is no longer able to function. These children are often labeled "behavior problems" or "emotionally disturbed" because of their frequent inappropriate and unexpected conduct, despite the fact that NLD has a neurological rather than an emotional origin.

It is especially important to identify children with nonverbal learning disorders because overestimates of the child's abilities and unrealistic demands made by parents and teachers can lead to ongoing emotional problems. Unfortunately, there are few resources available for the child with NLD syndrome through schools or private agencies, and it is hard to find a professional who understands nonverbal learning disabilities.

Nonverbal learning disorders are much less common than language-based learning disorders (affecting only between .1 percent and 1 percent of the general population). Unlike language-based learning disabilities, the NLD syndrome affects girls as often as boys. Although there are not many people with NLD, experts suspect that as school assessment procedures improve, a higher proportion of children will be identified with NLD.

Symptoms

Children with NLD may have trouble perceiving and understanding the subtle visual cues important to nonverbal communication that form the basis of social interaction and interpersonal relations. They may misread overt signals of impatience, annoyance, or the desire to end an interaction and consequently may respond in ways that are perceived by others as inappropriate. A child with NLD syndrome may have trouble adapting to new situations or accurately reading nonverbal signals and cues. Although these students make progress in school, they have trouble "producing" in situations where speed and adaptability are required.

There are three categories of dysfunction:

- lack of coordination, severe balance problems, or difficulties with fine motor skills
- poor visual recall, faulty spatial perceptions, or problems with spatial relations
- lack of ability to comprehend nonverbal communication, trouble adjusting to new situations, or significant problems with social judgment and social interaction

Children with nonverbal learning disorders commonly appear awkward and uncoordinated in both fine and gross motor skills. They may have had extreme difficulty learning to ride a bike or to kick a soccer ball. Fine motor skills, such as cutting with scissors or tying shoelaces, seem to be impossible for them. Young children with NLD are less likely to explore their environment because they cannot rely on their own perceptions. These children do not learn much from experience or repetition and cannot generalize information.

In the early years, children may appear confused much of the time despite a high intelligence and high scores on receptive and expressive language measures. Closer observation will reveal a social ineptness due to misinterpretations of body language and tone of voice. These children do not perceive subtle cues in their environment, such as the idea of personal space, the facial expressions of others, or nonverbal displays of pleasure or displeasure. These are all social skills that are normally grasped intuitively through observation, not directly taught.

Instead, these children cope by relying on language as their principal means of social relating, information gathering, and relief from anxiety and often develop an exceptional memory for rote material. Since the nonverbal processing areas of the brain are not giving automatic feedback, they rely solely on memory of past experiences, each of which they labeled verbally to guide them in future situations. This, of course, is less effective and less reliable than being able to sense and interpret another person's social cues. Normal conversational "give and take" seem impossible for these children.

It is hard for these children to change from one activity to another or to move from one place to another. A child with NLD needs to concentrate merely to get through a room. Owing to the inability to handle such information processing demands, these children will instinctively avoid any kind of novelty.

Problems with NLD grow more apparent and more profound during the latter stages of childhood development and into adolescence, as pressures on social interaction increase and the requirements for appropriate social performance become more subtle and complex.

Cause

Non-language-based learning disorders are believed to be inherited, but a specific genetic problem has not yet been discovered. Nonverbal learning disabilities involve the performance processes that originate in the right cerebral hemisphere of the brain, which specializes in nonverbal processing. Brain scans of children with NLD often reveal mild abnormalities of the right cerebral hemisphere. Current evidence suggests that a contributing cause of the NLD syndrome involves early damage of the right cerebral hemisphere or white matter disease that forces the left hemisphere system to function on its own. A number of children suffering from NLD have at some time early in their development:

- sustained a moderate to severe head injury
- received repeated radiation treatments on or near their heads over a prolonged period of time

- had congenital absence of the corpus callosum
- been treated for hydrocephalus
- had brain tissue removed from the right hemisphere

Prognosis

How well these children progress seems to depend on early identification and accommodation. Typically, children with this condition are regularly punished for circumstances they cannot help without ever really understanding why, and they are often left with little hope that the situation will ever improve. As a result, these children tend to have serious forms of depression, withdrawal, anxiety, and in some cases, suicide.

Diagnosis

Whereas language-based disabilities are usually obvious to parents and educators, nonverbal learning disorders routinely go unrecognized. Many of the early symptoms of nonverbal learning disabilities (the language-based accomplishments) make parents and teachers proud. This child may speak like an adult at two or three years of age, and during early childhood, he is usually considered "gifted" by his parents and teachers. Sometimes the NLD child has a history of rote reading at a very young age. This child is generally an eager, enthusiastic learner who quickly memorizes rote material.

Extraordinary early speech and vocabulary development are not often suspected to be a coping strategy used by a child with problems in the right-hemisphere brain system and limited access to nonverbal processing abilities. The NLD child is also likely to acquire an unusual aptitude for spelling, but few adults will consider this to be a reflection of the overdependence on auditory perceptions.

Likewise, remarkable rote memory skills, attention to detail, and a natural facility for decoding, encoding, and early reading development are not generally cause for alarm. Yet these are some of the important early indicators that a child is having trouble relating to and functioning in the nonverbal world.

Dysfunctions associated with NLD are less apparent at the age of seven to eight years than at 10 to 14 years, and they become progressively more apparent and more debilitating with each year. During late elementary school, the child will begin to not complete or turn in written assignments. The child produces limited written output and the process is always slow and laborious. By the time the problem is revealed, the child may have already shut down in response to impossible academic pressures and performance demands.

Treatment

Parents and the school should not underestimate the gravity of this disability. The main problem in the painstaking approach to teaching the child is the caregiver's faulty impression that the child is much more adept than he is. Everyone tends to overestimate the intelligence of NLD adolescents. The child should be shielded from teasing, persecution, and other sources of anxiety.

Independence should be introduced gradually, in controlled, nonthreatening situations. The more completely the strengths and weaknesses of the child are understood, the better prepared the care providers will be to promote the child's independence. These children should never be left to their own devices in new activities or situations that lack sufficient structure. Goals and expectations must be attainable.

Occupational therapy is a good idea for the younger child. Use of a computer word processor can help, since the spatial and fine motor skills needed for typing are not as complicated as those involved in handwriting. Tasks requiring folding, cutting with scissors, or arranging material (maps, graphs, mobiles) will require considerable help. Timed assignments will need to be modified or eliminated.

Adults need to check often that the child understands, and that information is presented clearly. All expectations need to be direct and explicit, and the student's schedule needs to be as predictable as possible. He should be prepared in advance for changes in routine, such as: assemblies, field trips, minimum days, vacation days, finals, and so on.

This type of child needs to be assigned to one case manager at school who will oversee progress and can make sure all of the school staff are making the necessary accommodations and modifications. Inservice training and orientation for all school staff that promotes tolerance and acceptance is a vital part of the overall plan for success, as everyone must be familiar with and supportive of the child's academic and social needs.

This child needs to be in a learning environment that provides daily, nonthreatening contact with nondisabled peers—not a "special" or alternative program in order to boost social development. This child will benefit from cooperative learning situations when grouped with good role models.

Transitions will always be difficult for this child, so he will need time during the school day to collect his thoughts before "switching gears."

Teachers will need to present strategies for conversation skills, how and when to change the subject, tone and expression of voice, and nonverbal body language (facial expressions, correct social distance). Isolation, deprivation, and punishment are not effective methods to change the behavior of a child who is already trying his best to conform, but who misinterprets nonverbal cues.

Norwalk agent virus infection Infection by a family of several small viruses that can cause viral gastroenteritis with diarrhea. Although viral gastroenteritis may be caused by a number of viruses, the Norwalk family is responsible for about a third of all cases in children (except for infants). Norwalk virus is also the most common cause of viral contamination in shellfish. Although anyone can get Norwalk virus, those at highest risk are children under age four. Norwalk virus was first identified as the cause of an outbreak of gastroenteritis among children at a school in Norwalk, Ohio, and among their teachers and their families.

Norwalk and Norwalk-like viruses are being recognized more frequently as important causes of food-borne disease in the United States. However, since no routine diagnostic test is available, the true prevalence is not known. Outbreaks commonly occur in schools, camps, hospitals, and, in particular during 2002 and 2003, on cruise ships. Many oyster-related outbreaks of intestinal illness linked to Norwalk-like viruses have been reported in Louisiana, Florida, Maryland, and other states where oyster harvesting is common. In 1993, 73 people in Louisiana and about 130 others in the United States who ate oysters from Louisiana became ill. A malfunctioning sewage system was the cause of an outbreak in 1996, and an outbreak in 1997 was linked to sewage from oyster-harvesting boats.

In 2003 the U.S. Centers for Disease Control and Prevention (CDC) has assisted with four outbreaks of Norwalk virus-related gastrointestinal illness aboard cruise ships. The *Sun Princess* (Princess Cruise Lines) sailed from Los Angeles to Hawaii on January 25, 2003, for a 15-day cruise, but three days later, 267 of 2,029 passengers and 29 of 877 crew became sick with gastrointestinal illness. Princess Cruises terminated the cruise on February 4 as a precautionary measure and returned passengers home by airline.

On a *Sundream* (Sun Cruises, U.K.) cruise between January 20 and February 3, 2003, gastrointestinal illness was reported in 95 of 1,085 passengers and 12 of 403 crew. The ship made one stop in St. Thomas, U.S., en route to Venezuela. The *Olympia Voyager* (Royal Olympic Cruises, Greece) left port from Port Everglades, Florida, and ended in Houston, and between January 15 and February 3, 2003, gastrointestinal illness was reported among 35 of 756 passengers and 5 of 356 crew. Cleaning and disinfection were initiated during the first week of the cruise and no new cases were identified on the second week.

At virtually the same time, the *Carnival Spirit* reported 102 of 2,143 passengers and 10 of 902 crew ill on a cruise between January 27 and February 4, 2003. Stool specimens were submitted to the CDC for analysis.

Extensive cleaning and disinfection were carried out on all cruise ships immediately following reports of illness, and the CDC continued to monitor the situation.

Cause

Outbreaks of Norwalk gastroenteritis often occur in settings where there is close contact between many children. The virus is found in stool and on hands and surfaces that have had contact with stool and can be transmitted by eating contaminated food or drinking tainted water. In addition, the virus can be transmitted from person to person.

Water is the most common source of outbreaks and may include water from city supplies, wells, recreational lakes, swimming pools, and water stores in cruise ships. Shellfish and salad ingredients are foods most often implicated in Norwalk outbreaks. The virus is destroyed by cooking but not by freezing

Everyone who ingests the virus and who has not recently had an infection with the same strain is susceptible to infection and can develop symptoms. Infection is most common in older children (and adults).

Symptoms

Within two to three days of infection, symptoms of vomiting, abdominal cramps, mild diarrhea, fatigue, and muscle aches appear. Most people experience only a mild illness and recover within 48 hours. About three months after infection, children will develop a short-term immunity. After this period of time, however, it is possible to be reinfected. Severe illness or hospitalization is very rare.

Diagnosis

Research labs can look for virus in stool specimens; a blood test can uncover antibodies to the virus. Specific diagnosis of the disease can only be made by a few labs.

Treatment

Because the diarrhea is caused by a virus, there is no cure. When a person becomes infected, the body develops antibodies that destroy the virus. Rest, clear fluids, and acetaminophen for headaches and body aches will help. Patients who do not experience vomiting can continue to eat solids.

Prevention

There are no specific preventive measures, since scientists do not know enough about how the virus is transmitted. However, it is wise to follow guidelines for avoiding food-borne illness and follow precautions for food and beverage safety when traveling to tropical countries. Hands should be washed before preparing or serving foods, and someone else should prepare food if the cook has cramps, nausea, vomiting, diarrhea, or open sores on the hands. Children and their caregivers should wash thoroughly before eating and after toileting.

nosebleed Blood can flow from the nose for many reasons, most of which are not serious, but almost all children will have at least one nosebleed in their childhood. Preschoolers may have several benign nosebleeds a week, but they become much less common after puberty. In any case, the amount of blood lost from most nosebleeds is quite minor.

The nose bleeds so readily because blood vessels in the nose are fragile and close to the surface and are very susceptible to minor trauma, cracking, and drying. Nosebleeds are also more common among those with nasal allergies or colds. A child who pokes a finger or a foreign object in the nose may likely trigger a bout of bleeding. A cold or nasal allergy also produces swelling and irritation in the nasal passages, making the nose more likely to bleed. Sneezing hard or blowing the nose, dry air, or irritating fumes all can cause a nosebleed. In young children, irritation from gastroesophageal reflux can trigger a bleed. Nosebleeds are more common in winter or in dry climates, when the dry air dries out the nasal passages.

Treatment

With proper treatment, a nosebleed usually lasts less than 10 minutes. The child should be kept quiet with head tilted forward as direct pressure is applied to the nose. In a child the caregiver should gently pinch the soft part of the child's nose against the center, using a thumb and forefinger, and held in place for five to 10 minutes. If the bleeding has not yet stopped entirely, the procedure may be repeated once. In most cases the bleeding will have stopped, but if it does not, a physician should be contacted immediately. In an emergency a doctor can apply nose drops designed to constrict the blood vessels, or a special dressing to stop the bleeding.

Prevention

Because a moist nasal passage is less inclined to bleed, saline nose drops or a humidifier for the home can help prevent nosebleeds. Avoiding nose-picking, sneezing, and nasal congestion also can prevent some nosebleeds. If one blood vessel continually triggers nosebleeds, a doctor may try to cauterize it to prevent further bleeding.

notifiable disease   See REPORTABLE DISEASE.

nurse practitioner (NP)   A registered nurse (RN) with additional education and training in a specialty area such as family practice or pediatrics. Also called "advanced practice nurses" (APNs), nurse practitioners have a master's degree in nursing (MS or MSN) in the specialty area of their interest. For example, a pediatric NP has advanced education, skills, and training in caring for infants, children, and teens. If accredited through the national board exam, the APN will have an additional credential such as Certified Pediatric Nurse Practitioner (CPNP) or Certified Family Nurse Practitioner (CFNP). NPs follow the rules and regulations of the Nurse Practice Act of the state where they work; many are also nationally certified in their area of specialty.

These nursing professionals work closely with doctors to provide high quality care. Many others are involved in education, research, and legislative activities to improve the quality of health care in the United States. Pediatric and family practice NPs can provide regular pediatric health care, including:

- take a child's health history and perform a physical exam
- plan a child's care with parents and the child's health-care team
- perform some tests and procedures
- answer questions about your child's health problems
- treat common childhood illnesses
- change the care plan with your child's doctor as needed
- teach your family about the effects of illness on your child's growth and development
- teach your child about self-care and healthy lifestyle choices
- write prescriptions and order medical tests
- teach other health-care members and local groups about child health care
- provide referrals to community groups.

nut allergy   More than three million Americans are currently allergic to nuts and peanuts, including one out of every 200 children, and the numbers are increasing at an alarming rate. (Peanut allergies and nut allergies are actually different allergies. Peanuts do not grow on trees and are not true nuts. It is possible to be allergic to tree nuts and not peanuts, or to peanuts and not tree nuts, or to both.) Peanut and tree nut allergies are the leading cause of severe or fatal food-allergic reactions; they are also a cheap source of dietary protein predominantly eaten in peanut butter and snack nuts. Unfortunately, more and more nut products are finding their way into food products either directly or by indirect contamination of food products during the manufacturing process.

Nuts and peanuts may masquerade on a food label as "hydrolyzed vegetable protein" or "groundnuts," and it is important to realize that for the sensitive person, this lifelong allergy can be fatal in even trace amounts.

Life-threatening nut and peanut allergies can kill in two ways. As the food is swallowed, it produces immediate swelling that spreads to the vocal cords. When the vocal cords swell shut, the child is unable to breathe and can die with terrifying rapidity. The second reaction is anaphylactic shock: The child swallows and digests the food and up to two hours later can go into shock and die.

Most of the time, children with known nut allergies have an allergic reaction when nuts masquerade as a hidden ingredient, perhaps in a cake, cupcake, or even something as innocuous as chili. Many food servers do not realize that being asked if something has nuts in it also refers to nuts in ALL forms, including peanut butter or walnut oil.

Risk Factors

Certain children are more likely to develop a nut or peanut allergy, including those with asthma or a family history of asthma, eczema, or hay fever, or those with infantile digestive problems and possible genetic links to nut sensitivities.

Prevention

Parents can try to prevent nut and peanut allergies from developing in their children, such as maintaining a smoke-free environment at home (beginning before birth), breast-feeding (while avoiding nuts and peanuts during nursing), and delaying the introduction of nuts and peanuts in those children at risk for allergies.

obesity Childhood obesity in the United States is becoming a serious national problem as the number of overweight and obese children continues to rise. This is particularly important because obesity is linked to the development of diabetes, heart disease, and cancers caused by or linked to unhealthy diet and lack of physical activity.

Since 1980 the percentage of overweight children in the United States has nearly doubled, and nearly tripled among adolescents. By 1999, 10 percent of two to five year olds and more than 25 percent of white children aged six to 19 are overweight; more than 33 percent of black and Hispanic children are overweight. If trends in obesity continue, one in three American children born in 2000 will go on to develop diabetes in their lifetimes. In fact, increasing numbers of diabetes cases diagnosed in childhood are type 2 diabetes—once thought to be exclusively an adult disease associated with obesity. Overweight and obese children are also at risk for other serious health conditions, such as high blood pressure and high cholesterol (once considered exclusively adult issues). They also are prone to low self-esteem from being teased, bullied, or rejected by their peers.

To address the issue of obesity among school-age children, many public schools have been making an effort to change the way kids eat. Some of the major urban school districts such as those in Los Angeles, New York, and Philadelphia are banning the sale of soda in their schools. Starting in September 2003, New York City's school system—the country's largest—stopped selling hard candy and doughnuts from in-school vending machines. In addition, fat and salt were trimmed from 800,000 lunches served daily in the schools.

The food and beverage industry is also considering significant changes. Kraft Foods announced that it will alter how it produces, packages, and promotes its products, using recommendations from a panel of international experts in behavior, intervention programs, lifestyle education, nutrition, obesity, physical activity, and public health. Among Kraft's plans are to cut portion sizes in single-serve packages, stop all of its in-school marketing, provide some healthier choices, and offer nutrition labeling in all markets worldwide.

The Food and Drug Administration (FDA) announced that all food labels must list the exact amount of unhealthy trans fat (also called trans-fatty acids). Although companies have until 2006 to make the change, the expanded information will eventually help consumers make more healthy decisions about the foods they opt to eat. Some fast-food restaurant chains have changed the oil used to cook French fries, cutting the trans-fatty acids by half.

To help keep children at a healthy weight, parents should:

- avoid serving too much fruit juice or fruit juice drinks, which have lots of simple sugar
- not use food as a bribe, reward, or incentive for children
- not insist that children clean their plates. Instead, parents should reinforce the idea that they should only eat when they are hungry.
- not completely eliminate all sweets and favorite snacks from an overweight child's diet, which could make a child overeat these forbidden foods outside the home
- schedule family meals together
- serve a variety of healthy foods in moderation

Exercise

Because so many overweight children lead sedentary lifestyles, it can be important to make sure they have enough exercise. Families that make time for TV, computer, video games, and meetings can make time for exercise. Adults who model exercise will also tend to have children who participate in exercise as well.

obsessive-compulsive disorder (OCD) An anxiety disorder in which the brain gets "stuck" on a particular thought or urge and cannot let go, leading to obsessive thinking or beliefs. All children worry, but a child who cannot stop thinking about these worries—and who may begin to perform certain rituals over and over again—may be diagnosed with obsessive-compulsive disorder (OCD).

About one million children and teens in the United States experience OCD—or one in every 200 American children. It is more common than many other childhood disorders or illnesses, but the child often hides the behavior because it causes pain and embarrassment.

For years thousands of children were undiagnosed because OCD had been considered an "adult" problem. Instead of getting treatment, children with OCD were called dumb, lazy, or easily distracted and were often misdiagnosed as learning-disabled or autistic. Even today many children's symptoms are overlooked. The danger of leaving the disorder untreated (besides school failure and lack of friends) is that children with OCD grow up to ease their pain by abusing drugs and alcohol.

Cause

OCD is not a neurosis as it was long thought to be, nor is it caused by overcontrolling parents. The disorder is related to a chemical problem in the brain that occurs when part of the brain that filters information does not function properly, causing certain thoughts to return over and over. It can run in families, although it seems that genes are only partly responsible for the condition. (If one identical twin has OCD, there is only a 13 percent chance that the other twin also has the condition.) No one knows for sure what triggers OCD, but some experts believe that OCD may be linked to infections with streptococcal bacteria.

Some experts suspect that there may be different types of OCD, and that some types are inherited while other types are not. Preliminary research suggests that OCD that begins in childhood may be different from OCD beginning in adulthood. Individuals with childhood-onset OCD appear much more likely to have blood relatives affected with the disorder than do those whose OCD first appears in adulthood. If one parent has OCD, the likelihood the child will be affected is about 2 to 8 percent; if the parent also has blood relatives with the disorder, the risk for the child increases somewhat. If the parent's OCD began in adulthood, then any children are at lower risk than if the parent's condition began in childhood.

Symptoms

Not all children with OCD behave the same way. The most common symptom is fear of germs. For schoolchildren, that often means an inability to touch chalk, erasers, and papers; some will not take their backpacks or shoes into the house. However, most children with OCD perform well in school. Sometimes a child's A's are the result of an obsession for perfection. These children seemingly are never satisfied with their work and insist on doing it over and over. A child may stay up all night doing a simple assignment. Other symptoms range from mild to severe, forcing children to endlessly wash hands, kiss doorknobs, walk on the sides of their feet, insist that the window blinds be at a specific height, or repeatedly rebutton clothes or retie shoes. Some are haunted with images of violence and danger. Children with OCD struggle in school, where they are often teased and may suffer emotional and physical dysfunction.

The most common obsessions in children and teenagers with OCD include:

- fear of dirt or germs
- fear of contamination
- fear of illness or harm
- need for symmetry, order, and precision
- religious obsessions
- preoccupation with body wastes
- sexual or aggressive thoughts

- preoccupation with household items
- intrusive sounds or words

The following compulsions have been identified as the most common in children and adolescents with OCD:

- grooming rituals (excessive hand-washing, showering, and teethbrushing)
- repetition (such as going in and out of doors, needing to move through spaces in a special way, checking to make sure that an appliance is off or a door is locked, and checking homework)
- rituals to counteract contact with a "contaminated" person or object
- "touching" rituals
- rituals to prevent harming self or others
- arranging objects and counting rituals
- hoarding and collecting things
- cleaning rituals related to the house or other items

The disorder is often accompanied by TOURETTE'S SYNDROME, a neurological disorder characterized by involuntary movements and vocal tics. Between 35 percent and 50 percent of people with Tourette's syndrome also have OCD, but only a small percentage of children with OCD also have Tourette's syndrome.

Other conditions that often occur in conjunction with OCD include other ANXIETY DISORDERS (such as panic disorder or SOCIAL PHOBIA), depression, disruptive behavior disorders (ATTENTION DEFICIT HYPERACTIVITY DISORDER and OPPOSITIONAL DEFIANT DISORDER), LEARNING DISABILITY, TRICHOTILLOMANIA (compulsive hair pulling), body dysmorphic disorder (imagined ugliness), and habit disorders such as NAIL BITING or skin picking.

Diagnosis

OCD can be detected with positron emission tomography (PET) scans or magnetic resonance imaging (MRI), which can show the chemical functioning or structure of the brain. Research suggests that OCD patients have patterns of brain activity that differ from people without the condition.

Treatment

Most children, but not all, show improvement with behavioral therapy, medication, or both, given in a consistent, logical, and supportive manner. Cognitive-behavioral therapy (CBT) helps children learn to change their thoughts and feelings by changing their behavior. With this treatment, the child is exposed to his fears to decrease his anxiety about it while blocking his response or rituals. For example, a child who is afraid of germs might be exposed to something he considers dirty while not being allowed to wash. In some treatment methods, the child gives OCD a nasty nickname and visualizes it as something he can control. Behavioral treatment with children works best when the whole family is involved.

Although many children respond to therapy alone, others need a combination of therapy and medication. Medication is often combined with CBT to get more complete and lasting results. Research shows that the newest antidepressant, called selective serotonin reuptake inhibitors (SSRIs), are most effective in children with OCD. These include medications such as fluoxetine (Prozac), fluvoxamine (Luvox), paroxetine (Paxil), citalopram (Celexa), and sertraline (Zoloft). Another medication that may be prescribed is clomipramine (Anafranil). Most experts agree that medication should be used to treat children as a second choice to behavior therapy. Medication can reduce the impulse to engage in ritualistic behavior while therapy helps the child and family learn strategies to manage the waxing and waning of OCD symptoms.

Only four OCD medications have U.S. Food and Drug Administration (FDA) approval for use in children and adolescents: clomipramine (Anafranil), fluvoxamine (Luvox), sertraline (Zoloft), and Prozac. Clomipramine has approval for children age 10 and over; fluvoxamine has approval for children aged eight and above. The FDA grants specific approval for use in children after large studies using pediatric patients have been completed. Because these large studies are very expensive and difficult to accomplish, they have not been conducted with all OCD medications. Doctors may still legally prescribe any of the five available medications to children of any age they deem appropriate (called "off label use"). However, most physicians prefer to use medication the FDA has specifically approved for use in children.

Because OCD is a chronic condition that medications do not typically cure, a child may need to take medication indefinitely. Typically, when medication is withdrawn, the OCD symptoms return to their pre-drug level. Many physicians recommend that if the medication is working well, it should continue for at least a year. After a year, the dose can be slowly lowered to see if it is still helpful; this is often done during summer vacation or when an increase in OCD symptoms would be least likely to be disruptive. If OCD symptoms return, the dose is raised again.

Obsessive-Compulsive Foundation (OCF) An international nonprofit organization of more than 10,000 members with OBSESSIVE-COMPULSIVE DISORDER (OCD) and related disorders, their families, friends, professionals, and other concerned individuals. Founded by a group of individuals with OCD in 1986, the mission of the OCF is to educate the public and professional communities about OCD and related disorders; to help people with OCD and related disorders, their family and friends; and to support research into the causes and effective treatments of OCD and related disorders. (For contact information see Appendix I.)

occupational therapist A medical professional trained in occupational therapy who uses "occupation" (purposeful activity) to help children with physical, developmental, or emotional disabilities lead independent, productive, and satisfying lives. An occupational therapist may evaluate children with developmental or neuromuscular problems in order to plan treatment activities, or conduct group or individual treatment to help children in a mental health center learn to cope with daily activities. They also may recommend changes in layout and design of the home or school to allow children with injuries or disabilities greater access and mobility.

Occupational therapists work in a variety of different settings, including hospitals, rehabilitation centers, schools, private practice, and government agencies.

oppositional defiant disorder (ODD) A behavior disorder characterized by uncooperative, defiant, negative, irritable, and annoying behavior toward parents, teachers, and other authority figures in children and teens. Oppositional defiant disorder (ODD) is reported to affect between 2 and 16 percent of children and adolescents in the general population, usually appearing by age eight. ODD is more common in boys than in girls and may be more common among those children whose parents are having marital problems. Oppositional defiant disorder often coexists with other mental health disorders such as mood disorders, anxiety disorders, conduct disorder, and ATTENTION DEFICIT HYPERACTIVITY DISORDER.

Symptoms
Most symptoms seen in teens with oppositional defiant disorder also occur occasionally in healthy adolescents, but those with ODD experience more frequent symptoms that interfere with learning, school adjustment, and relationships. Children with ODD argue excessively, refuse to comply with appropriate requests, and always question rules and refuse to follow them. Their behavior is intended to annoy or upset others, and the child often blames others and is easily annoyed by them. Often, the ODD child has an angry attitude, speaking harshly, or unkindly and deliberately behaving in ways that seek revenge.

Treatment
Treatment may include individual therapy, family therapy, peer group therapy, or medication.

Individual psychotherapy Therapists often use cognitive-behavioral approaches with an ODD child to improve problem solving skills, communication skills, impulse control, and anger management skills.

Family therapy Family therapy is often focused on making changes within the family system, such as improving communication skills and family interactions. Parenting children with ODD can be very difficult and trying for parents. Parents need support and understanding as well as techniques that aid in developing more effective parenting approaches.

Peer group therapy This method of treatment focuses on helping the affected child develop social skills and interpersonal skills.

Medication While not considered effective in treating ODD, medication may be used if other symptoms or disorders are present and responsive to medication.

orthopedic surgeon A physician who specializes in orthopedic surgery and who understands the musculoskeletal system. Orthopedists may diagnose a condition, identify and treat an injury, and provide rehabilitation. The orthopedist may have completed up to 14 years of formal education. After becoming licensed to practice medicine, the orthopedic surgeon may become board certified by passing both oral and written examinations given by the American Board of Orthopaedic Surgery.

Many orthopedic surgeons choose to practice general orthopedics, while others specialize in certain areas of the body (such as foot or hand), or in a specialized area of orthopedic care (such as sports medicine or trauma medicine). Some orthopedists may specialize in several areas and may collaborate with other specialists, such as neurosurgeons or rheumatologists.

osteomyelitis A serious bone infection that occurs primarily in children between ages five and nine, although it can appear in infants and teenagers as well. The infection that causes osteomyelitis often begins in another part of the body and spreads to the bone via the bloodstream. In children, osteomyelitis typically appears in the long bones. If untreated, the infection can damage the bones and joints, interfering with growth and causing permanent disability. If a joint is infected, the condition is called "pyogenic arthritis." If the bone tissue dies as a result of the lost blood supply, it may lead to a chronic infection that can persist intermittently for years. Osteomyelitis typically affects two out of every 10,000 people.

Risk Factors
Osteomyelitis is more common in children who have been recently injured, who have diabetes, who have had their spleen removed, who are undergoing hemodialysis, or who abuse drugs.

Symptoms
Symptoms of bone infection include pain, swelling, and tenderness in an arm or leg (babies refuse to move the affected arm or leg). This may be followed by fever, nausea and vomiting, or swollen lymph glands. If a joint is affected, the child may have a swollen knee, elbow, wrist, or ankle.

Diagnosis
The doctor will examine the child and take a blood test to check for a high white blood count (indicating an infection). A needle aspiration of the area around the infected bone can help identify possible bacteria (the child may be anesthetized for this test). A bone scan can reveal infected bone and is often more useful than a standard X ray, which may not show bone changes until at least a week after the infection has begun.

Treatment
High doses of antibiotics are given for up to six weeks until symptoms improve and an X ray shows the bone is healing. If antibiotics fail to treat the infection, the abscess may need to be surgically drained.

otitis externa See EAR INFECTION.

otitis media See EAR INFECTION.

papilloma virus, human (HPV) A very common and extremely contagious virus that can cause abnormal tissue growth on the feet, hands, vocal cords, mouth, and genital organs. More than 60 types of human papilloma virus (HPV) have been identified; each type infects certain parts of the body. Some cause WARTS, including PLANTAR WARTS on the feet, common hand warts, juvenile warts, and genital warts (see WARTS, GENITAL). They also cause other invisible genital HPV infections. A wide variety of benign and cancerous growths also may be associated with HPVs, which has been demonstrated to cause vulvar or cervical cancer in some women.

Up to one out of 10 Americans have genital HPV infections, and between 500,000 and a million new cases of genital warts occur every year. Some studies show that about one-third of all sexually active teenagers have genital HPV infections. Because they do not have symptoms or do not recognize them, millions of others do not know that they carry HPV. The majority of those now seeking treatment for genital warts are teens and young women between the ages of 15 and 29.

Symptoms

HPV infections cause a variety of problems, but there may be no symptoms of infection at all. Genital warts caused by HPV may be found on the vulva, in the vagina, and on the cervix, penis, anus, and urethra of infected women and men, but they are found very rarely in the mouth or throat. They often are flesh-colored and soft and may look like miniature cauliflowers. Usually they grow in more than one location and may cluster in large masses. Genital warts usually are painless but may itch. If allowed to grow, they can block the openings of the vagina, urethra, or anus and become very uncomfortable. Depending on their location, genital warts can cause sores and bleeding.

Genital warts often grow more rapidly during pregnancy. An increase in the size and number of genital warts occurs when a person's immune system is weakened by diabetes, an organ transplant, Hodgkin's disease, HIV/AIDS, or other conditions. There are other genital HPV infections that cannot be seen with the naked eye. Some are more dangerous than genital warts because they are associated with cancers of the cervix, vulva, vagina, or penis.

Cause

Genital HPVs can spread whether or not warts are present, usually by vaginal or anal intercourse. Because genital HPV infections are often unseen, they can be spread by sex partners who do not know they are infected. It may also be possible by contact with the virus through such potential vehicles as toilet facilities, steam room benches, shared swimsuits, or underwear.

People most at risk for genital HPV infections are people who:

- have weakened immune systems
- are sexually involved with a number of different partners
- have sex partners who are sexually involved with a number of different partners
- have infected partners

Diagnosis

Medical examination is the first step in determining if there is a genital HPV infection. Many times a woman does not notice warty lesions, but her physician may see something unusual while performing a routine gynecologic examination or Pap smear. Pap smear results can be used to screen for tissue changes in the cervix and help corroborate findings of other tests such as colposcopy, which allows a doctor to see the cervix with a special microscope and to sample any suspicious tissue.

Treatment

HPV is a persistent and hard-to-cure organism, so treatment must usually be repeated. Moreover, an infected woman should be monitored throughout her life for recurrence or development of precancerous changes, whether or not warts are apparent. Because the virus remains in the lesions it creates, treatment for HPV consists of controlling infection by removing visible warts or precancerous lesions.

They can be removed by surgery, by freezing, or by locally applied chemicals. The method depends on the extent of infection, accessibility of lesions, and malignancy potential.

Surgery is sometimes used to cut away warts if treatment without anesthesia would cause discomfort, or warts are so extensive that simultaneous reconstructive surgery is required. Surgery may permit a more thorough removal of infected sites, although its cost must be weighed against potential benefits and risks. Surgery may either mean an excisional biopsy done as an outpatient procedure or a more involved procedure performed under anesthesia.

In superficial cryotherapy, liquid nitrogen is applied by cotton swab to minor external warts. Extensive lesions can be frozen faster and to a greater depth with a cold cautery device which pinpoints warts. Cold cautery cryotherapy is usually performed within a week after menstruation, and it cannot be used in pregnant women. After cryotherapy women may experience cramping, abdominal pain, infection, or rarely, cervical scarring. Painkillers given before cryotherapy will ease pain, and ice packs applied externally after the procedure will reduce any swelling or inflammation. Considerable watery vaginal discharge for 10 to 20 days after cryotherapy is normal, but fever, pain unrelieved by analgesics, or unusually prolonged discharge should be reported to the doctor.

Laser treatment involves a high-intensity beam of light that vaporizes lesions, particularly those that are external or in less accessible locations. In the hands of a well-trained physician, laser therapy is highly effective in removing multiple lesions. The procedure is usually more expensive than other types of treatment and carries risks of removing too much tissue, and delayed healing, scarring, or pain.

Acids such as trichloroacetic acid (TCA) or bichloroacetic acid (BCA) may be painted on visible warts using a small cotton swab or wooden applicator. To be effective, TCA or BCA must be applied in proper concentrations, but these sometimes cause a burning sensation after treatment. Local and systemic painkillers will help relieve pain. Scarring and chronic pain are potential aftereffects.

5-Fluorouracil (5-FU) cream applied to the vulva on a regular regimen can help control external lesions. However, it should not be used by pregnant women and may cause serious skin irritation.

Interferon, a newer drug approved for injection into a muscle or select lesions, can be used, but it is expensive, has significant systemic side effects, and cannot be used during pregnancy. Podophyllin was once a popular treatment, but it is used less often now because it cannot be used during pregnancy or for most internal lesion sites and because it may cause cancer or toxic reactions.

After any HPV treatment, the treated area should be kept clean and dry with cornstarch dusting, cotton underwear, and loose clothing. Sexual intercourse should be avoided until healing has occurred externally and internally, usually within two to four weeks. Follow-up colposcopy and Pap smears are usually scheduled at three-month intervals after treatment of HPV, and yearly thereafter. These tests monitor that the cervix remains free of precancerous or cancerous tissue. A woman with HPV should notify any sexual partners of her infection, use latex condoms with every partner (unless in a mutually monogamous relationship), and urge that the partner be treated for HPV if his physician has identified HPV lesions.

Prevention

Condoms are recommended for all sexual contacts other than a monogamous relationship. Condoms prevent transmission of infection to a partner and lower the risk of becoming infected with a different form of HPV or other sexually transmitted diseases.

Applying spermicides with nonoxynol-9 to affected or treated areas may be helpful in reducing transmission of the virus. Everyone with genital lesions, and all partners of persons with genital lesions, should alert new sexual partners about HPV infection risk and take precautions to limit spread of HPV.

parabens, sensitivity to   The parabens (methyl-, propyl-, and butyl-) are the most common preservatives used in foods, drugs, and cosmetics, but they can cause a severe redness, swelling, itching, and pain. They can also cause anaphylactic shock in susceptible individuals.

Parabens can be found in mayonnaise, salad dressings, spiced sauces, mustard, processed vegetables, frozen dairy products, some baked goods, jellies and jams, soft drinks, fruit juices, syrups, and candies. In medications, they are used in many dermatologic creams; eye, ear, and nose drops; rectal and vaginal medications; bandages; and local anesthetics. Cosmetics containing parabens include foundations, powders, cover-up sticks, bronzers, makeup removers, blushes, highlighters, lipsticks, quick-dry nail products, mascaras, eye shadows, and eyeliners. However, considering how widespread the use of parabens is, sensitivity to this preservative is low. (See also ALLERGIES.)

parainfluenza   A common virus that causes respiratory infections in infants and young children. Types I and II may cause CROUP; type III also may cause BRONCHIOLITIS and bronchopneumonia. Types I, III, and IV are associated with sore throats and the common COLD.

The parainfluenza virus is part of the group of germs that includes the RESPIRATORY SYNCYTIAL VIRUS and the agents causing MEASLES and MUMPS.

Between 90 percent and 100 percent of children over age five have antibodies to type III, and about 75 percent have antibodies to type I and type II. The different types occur at different times of the year and have different symptoms. Type I causes biennial outbreaks of croup in the fall during odd-numbered years. Type II causes annual or biennial fall outbreaks, while type III occurs mostly during the spring and early summer months each year, although the virus can be found throughout the year.

Symptoms
Symptoms vary depending on the type of infection. Cold-like symptoms such as a runny nose and mild cough are common. Life-threatening respiratory symptoms may occur in young infants with bronchiolitis.

Treatment
Most infection in adults and older children are mild and do not require treatment. Treatment may be necessary if breathing difficulties or respiratory distress develop.

Complications
Secondary bacterial infections are the most common complication. Airway obstruction in croup and bronchiolitis can be severe and potentially life threatening.

Prevention
No vaccine is currently available to protect against infection; however, researchers are developing vaccines against type I and type III infection. Passively acquired maternal antibodies may play a role in protection from types I and II in the first few months of life. Frequent hand-washing and use of separate cups, glasses, and utensils should decrease the spread of virus. Excluding children with colds or other respiratory illnesses (without fever) who are well enough to attend child-care or school settings will probably not decrease the spread of the parainfluenzas, because the viruses are often spread in the early stages of illness.

parasomnia   Sleep disorders that include sleepwalking, NIGHT TERRORS, BED-WETTING, and narcolepsy. There are three categories of parasomnia—rhythmic, paroxysmal, and static disorders.

Rhythmic Disorders
Rhythmic disorders, such as head-banging, head-rocking, and body-rocking, involve movements that range from mild to seizure-like thrashing. Other rhythmic disorders include shuttling (rocking back and forth on hands and knees) and folding (raising the torso and knees simultaneously). During the rhythmic movements, the child may moan or hum. These movements seem to occur during the transition between wakefulness and

sleep or from one stage of sleep to another. There is no known cause for this type of disorder, but medical or psychological problems are rarely associated with it. Children who experience rhythmic disorders may have morning headaches, nasal problems, and ear infections.

Another rhythmic disorder is restless legs syndrome (RLS), a sensory and motor abnormality that seems to have a genetic basis. In RLS the child's legs move repeatedly. Many people who have RLS also have periodic leg movement syndrome (PLMS)—this occurs during sleep when the legs move involuntarily.

Treatment for RLS can include music therapy, psychotherapy, hypnotism, motion-sickness medications, tranquilizers, or stimulants.

Paroxysmal Disorders

Paroxysmal disorders are those that come on or recur suddenly. They include night terrors, NIGHT-MARES, sleepwalking, and bed-wetting.

Night terrors (pavor nocturnus) are characterized by a sudden arousal from sleep with a piercing scream or cry. During the episode, heart and breathing rates may increase and the child's eyes may be open, but he probably will not remember what happened, other than waking up and feeling scared. Night terrors occur in the first third of the sleep cycle, when the child is in deep sleep. Instead of waking or moving into another stage of sleep, the child gets "stuck" between stages. This can occur in as many as 15 percent of young children and can be caused by being overly tired or having an interrupted sleep cycle. By themselves, night terrors are not dangerous, but a child in the midst of a night terror could jump out of bed and hurt himself.

Experts are not sure what causes night terrors. After evaluation to rule out any possible physical causes, such as certain neurological conditions, medication may be used as treatment.

Nightmares differ from night terrors in that they are usually psychologically based, are more often remembered, and are not usually dangerous. Nightmares also occur only during REM (rapid eye movement) sleep, when the sleeping child's eyes move quickly, and heart rate and breathing may be erratic.

Sleepwalking is not dangerous when it occurs only rarely, but it can be hazardous if the child often gets out of bed or walks long distances in his sleep. Because the child is not awake during an episode, dangerous objects should be removed from his bedroom, and windows should be locked. Following a medical evaluation, medication or a consistent sleep-wake cycle may help cut down or eliminate sleepwalking.

Bed-wetting (enuresis) is a common problem that is classified as a parasomnia because it occurs at night and can affect sleep. Bed-wetting also can negatively affect a child's self-esteem. It typically occurs in children between ages three and eight and eventually stops on its own, although in a few cases it can sometimes continue into adolescence (1 percent of 18 year olds bed-wet). A child who regularly wets the bed should see a doctor to rule out any physical cause.

Static Disorders

Static sleep disorders are not disruptive and will not normally hurt a child; they include sleeping with open eyes (common in infants and young children) or in odd positions (such as upside down). Even though static disorders are not harmful, children who sleep in odd positions or with their eyes open should be examined by a doctor. Parents who worry about a child's sleeping patterns should talk to the child's doctor, who may suggest a referral to a sleep specialist. In the meantime, parents can establish good sleep habits, such as following fixed sleep and wake-up times, maintaining a consistent play and meal schedule, avoiding stimulants such as caffeine. The bedroom should be quiet and conducive to sleeping, and the child should use his bed only for sleeping—not for homework, playing, or watching TV.

paratyphoid fever Another name for SALMO-NELLA POISONING.

passive smoking See SECONDHAND SMOKE.

peanut allergy See NUT ALLERGY.

Pediatric AIDS Foundation The leading world-wide nonprofit organization dedicated to identifying, funding, and conducting pediatric HIV/AIDS research. The foundation's mission is to identify, fund, and conduct critical pediatric research that will lead to better treatments and prevention of HIV infection in infants and children, to reduce and prevent HIV transmission from mother to child, and to accelerate the discovery of new treatments for other serious and life-threatening pediatric diseases.

The Pediatric AIDS Foundation was cofounded in 1988 by Elizabeth Glaser, Susan DeLaurentis, and Susie Zeegen. As mothers, the three friends decided to take action after Elizabeth and her husband Paul discovered that she, their daughter Ariel and son Jake were all HIV-infected. Elizabeth Glaser died in 1994. (For contact information, see Appendix I.)

pediatric dentists   Dentists who limit their practice to treating only children, and who have received two to three years of special training in pediatric dentistry after dental school. In just the way that pediatricians specialize in children's health, pediatric dentists specialize in caring for children's teeth. A pediatric dentist can provide both primary and specialty dental care for infants and children through adolescence. Pediatric dentists are trained to look at the whole child and to help educate parents at the same time. They are an especially good choice for children with emotional, physical, or mental problems, because these specialists are trained and qualified to treat special young patients.

pediatrician   A physician who provides preventive health maintenance for healthy children and medical care for those who are seriously or chronically ill. Physicians trained in pediatrics are experts in emotional and behavioral/developmental assessment and can be powerful advocates for troubled children and adolescents. They diagnose and treat infections, injuries, genetic defects, malignancies, and many types of organic disease. They also try to reduce infant and child mortality, control infectious disease, foster healthy lifestyles, and ease the day-to-day difficulties of children and adolescents with chronic conditions.

More and more, pediatricians are also involved with the prevention, early detection, and management of behavioral, developmental, and functional social problems. With structured evaluation and early intervention, the primary care pediatrician can identify and address the developmental and behavioral issues related to poverty, violence, personal and familial substance abuse, and single-parent households.

After graduating from medical school, primary care pediatricians complete three years of pediatric residency, where they work with newborns, children, adolescents, and young adults in both community and hospital-based settings. The three-year residency includes mandated rotations in general pediatrics, normal newborn care, and a period of time in subspecialty areas, such as allergy/immunology, cardiology, critical care neonatal and child/adolescent, endocrinology/metabolism, gastroenterology, hematology/oncology, nephrology, neurology, and pulmonology. Further options for subspecialty education include adolescent medicine, ambulatory pediatrics, behavioral pediatrics, developmental disabilities, emergency medicine, genetics, infectious disease, and rheumatology.

After a pediatric residency, a pediatrician can be board certified after completing a comprehensive written examination. Recertification is required every seven years.

One in three pediatricians also completes a three-year fellowship to prepare for subspecialty practice in either adolescent medicine, cardiology, critical care medicine, emergency medicine, endocrinology, gastroenterology, hematology/oncology, infectious diseases, neonatal/perinatal medicine, nephrology, pulmonology, or rheumatology. Certificates of added qualification are available in sports medicine, medical toxicology, and clinical laboratory immunology.

pediculosis   See LICE.

pelvic inflammatory disease (PID)   Infection of the female reproductive organs (ovaries, uterus, or fallopian tubes), one of the most common causes of pelvic pain and infertility in women. In the United States, the highest rates of pelvic inflammatory disease (PID) occur among teenage girls. One case of PID does not confer immunity; it is possible to have many reinfections.

Cause

While it may not have an obvious cause, PID often occurs from an untreated sexually transmitted disease such as GONORRHEA or CHLAMYDIA. It also may occur after childbirth, abortion, or miscarriage. Young, sexually active girls and those who use the intrauterine birth control device are at higher risk.

The bacteria travel from the cervix to the fallopian tubes and ovaries, leading to permanent scarring of the tubes. The more times a girl contracts PID, the higher the chance she will become sterile because of scarring. Younger girls are more at risk for the disease because their reproductive organs are not good at fighting off infection.

Symptoms

Most girls have no symptoms in the early stages. As the disease progresses, symptoms may include burning during urination, pelvic pain, heavy menstrual flow with severe cramps, bleeding between periods, pain during sex, unusual vaginal discharge, fever, low backache, nausea, and vomiting. The cervix is tender if palpated. The very youngest girls tend to have the most severe symptoms.

Diagnosis

Diagnosing PID is not always a simple procedure because the site of the infection cannot be examined easily and PID symptoms often imitate other conditions such as appendicitis. A sample from the cervix can be cultured, and blood counts will help reveal the infection. If the diagnosis is still unclear, a physician can examine the fallopian tubes with a laparoscope in the hospital to assess their condition.

Treatment

Many girls are admitted to the hospital for intravenous antibiotic treatment. Mildly ill patients can be treated at home with oral antibiotics. In most cases, antibiotics are prescribed for at least 10 to 14 days to make sure the infection is completely cured; those treated at home must be monitored closely and reevaluated within 72 hours. A pelvic abscess or excessive scar tissue may require surgery.

Prevention

PID can be prevented by avoiding exposure to sexually transmitted diseases (STDs). All sexually active teens should be screened regularly for STDs.

PID is not contagious, but the bacteria that can lead to PID are highly contagious; all sexual partners of someone diagnosed with chlamydia or gonorrhea should be notified and treated with antibiotics, even if they have no signs or symptoms.

Although birth control pills do not protect against STDs, they may give some protection against PID by causing the body to create thicker cervical mucus, making it harder for bacteria to reach the upper genital tract.

Any unusual discharge or pelvic pain should be checked out by a doctor. Because PID is a very serious disease that can permanently damage the reproductive organs, it is important for patients who engage in unprotected sex, or who have many partners, to have regular checkups.

penicillin   The first antibiotic to be widely used, it was developed from a type of mold first discovered by Scottish scientist Alexander Fleming. His discovery led to the development of a wide variety of antibiotics. The biggest difference between bacterial and normal cells is the thick cell wall that protects the bacterial cell membrane. Normal human cells do not have this cell wall, and so any substance that interferes only with cell wall formation could not damage a human. Penicillins and related antibiotics work by interfering with the production of the bacterial cell wall, which is why they are among the safest of drugs—they cannot harm healthy cells. Today there are more than 20 different kinds of penicillins used to treat a variety of infections. However, none of the penicillins (or any other antibiotic) will fight colds, flu, or other viral infections. By 1960 seven classes of antibiotics had been identified.

Today scientists are faced with a growing problem of bacterial resistance to many of the penicillins. Bacteria are broadly classified into two types—gram-negative and gram-positive, depending on how they respond to a particular staining technique. The gram-negative bacteria (such as *Escherichia coli* and *Pseudomonas*) are far less susceptible to the penicillin family than are the gram-positive bacteria, such as *Streptococci*. Newer forms of penicillins are much more effective against the gram-negative organisms.

Still, the bacterial ability to adapt to antibiotics seems almost limitless. As antibiotic use became common, the incidence of bacterial resistance increased to the point where some scientists consider it an overwhelming problem. Sometimes the extensive use of an antibiotic eliminates sensitive bacterial strains and favors the development of strains that possess natural resistance to antibiotics. This occurred with the proliferation of penicillin-resistant staphylococci. This resistance can be transferred from resistant bacteria to nonresistant forms, because genetic material tends to be shared and traded among bacteria.

Using inadequate doses of antibiotics encourages resistance because instead of killing the germs, it allows bacteria to adapt. Using antibiotics inappropriately has also played a significant role in the bacterial resistance problem. Physicians who prescribe certain types of broad spectrum antibiotics instead of reserving them for resistant infections curtail the drugs' useful life.

perfectionism A set of self-defeating thoughts and behaviors aimed at reaching excessively high and unrealistic goals. Many children who have trouble with writing or finishing school projects have problems with perfectionism, which may be closely related to anxiety, or to OBSESSIVE-COMPULSIVE DISORDER. Children with ATTENTION DEFICIT HYPERACTIVITY DISORDER (ADHD) often have perfectionist tendencies, particularly in areas which they feel are important.

The issue of perfectionism may seem to be linked to a failure to understand the nature of a task's requirements. However, it appears equally likely that perfectionist behavior may arise from deeper underlying factors and may best be treated with a combination of behavioral and cognitive methods.

Perfectionism is often mistakenly seen as desirable or even necessary for success, but in fact, perfectionistic attitudes actually interfere with success. The desire to be perfect can give a child a sense of personal satisfaction but cause the youngster to fail to achieve as much as those with more realistic goals.

Most perfectionists learned early in life that they were valued because of how much they achieved. As a result, they learned to value themselves only on the basis of other people's approval, so that self-esteem came to be based primarily on external

standards. This can leave people vulnerable and excessively sensitive to the opinions and criticism of others. In attempting to protect themselves from criticism, these individuals may decide that being perfect is their only defense.

A number of negative feelings, thoughts, and beliefs may be associated with perfectionism, including:

- *Fear of failure* Perfectionists often equate failure to achieve their goals with a lack of personal worth or value.

- *Fear of making mistakes* Perfectionists often equate mistakes with failure. In orienting their lives around avoiding mistakes, perfectionists miss opportunities to learn and grow.

- *Fear of disapproval* If they let others see their flaws, perfectionists often fear that they will not be accepted. Trying to be perfect is a way of trying to protect themselves from criticism, rejection, and disapproval.

- *All-or-nothing thinking* Perfectionists often think they are worthless if their accomplishments are not perfect, and they have trouble putting things in perspective. For example, a straight A student who gets a B might think he is "a total failure."

- *The "shoulds"* The lives of perfectionists are often structured by an endless list of rigid rules about how their lives should be led. With such an overemphasis on shoulds, perfectionists rarely take into account their own desires.

- *Others' success* Perfectionists tend to perceive others as achieving success with a minimum of effort, few errors, little emotional stress, and maximum self-confidence, whereas their own efforts are inadequate.

Perfectionists are often trapped in a vicious cycle in which they set unreachable goals and then fail to meet them because the goals were impossible to begin with. Failure was thus inevitable. The constant pressure to achieve perfection and the inevitable chronic failure lessen productivity and effectiveness. As perfectionists become more self-critical, their self-esteem suffers, which may also lead to anxiety and depression. At this point perfectionists may give up completely on their goals and set different unrealistic goals, but this thinking sets the entire cycle in motion again. Perfectionists need to understand that perfectionism is undesirable, and they must challenge the self-defeating thoughts and behaviors that fuel perfectionism.

peritonitis An inflammation of the membrane in the wall of the abdomen caused by bacteria that have spread into the area. In children, this most often occurs during acute APPENDICITIS which has ruptured the appendix. Symptoms include abdominal swelling, pain, nausea and vomiting, rapid heartbeat, and chills and fever. Shock and heart failure can follow. Antibiotics— and treatment of the underlying cause—can cure the inflammation.

perseveration Persistent repetition of a behavior or activity regardless of the result, or having trouble switching from one activity to another. Extreme examples of perseveration may be seen in individuals with DEVELOPMENTAL DISABILITIES or AUTISM, for whom repetitive hand motions, rocking, or other movements are common characteristics. More typical examples in childhood might involve singing a song from a video again and again.

In a school setting, perseveration can be used to describe the fixation on a specific element in a broader task, such as spending all of the time of an exam on a single essay question.

This type of behavior may be caused by inflexible strategies and problems in shifting from one task to another.

pertussis See WHOOPING COUGH.

pervasive developmental disorder (PDD) A wide spectrum of neurobiological disorders (also known as autistic spectrum disorders) characterized by delayed development of communication and social skills. The most noticeable feature of a pervasive developmental disorder (PDD) is a problem with communication, including using and understanding language. Children with these disorders can also have trouble relating to others and may play in an unusual way with toys—flicking, shaking, spinning, or lining up toys. Children with

a PDD also may lack curiosity about their environment and have difficulty with changes in routines.

Of course, all children can sometimes behave oddly or may seem shy sometimes without having a PDD. What differentiates children with PDDs is the consistency of their unusual behavior. A PDD will affect every part of a child's life, not just behavior at home or at school, with a lack of social interaction and impaired nonverbal behavior. All of these conditions, to varying degrees, inhibit normal communication skills and can affect a child's cognitive skills and behavior.

Types of PDDs include:

- *AUTISM* This condition is considered to be a PDD because it affects communication as well as cognitive and behavioral skills.

- *ASPERGER'S DISORDER* A condition that some experts believe refers to high-functioning autism in children who generally have high IQs

- *Childhood disintegrative disorder* A condition in which a child may develop fairly normally until 18 to 36 months and then begin to regress, especially in speech and social interaction

- *RETT SYNDROME*

- *PDD–Not Otherwise Specified (PDD-NOS)*

Cause

Experts do not know what causes PDDs, but they suspect it may be linked to biochemical problems in the brain that also may have a genetic component. Some studies have suggested that PDDs may be caused by many different and unrelated causes, including FOOD ALLERGIES, too much yeast in the digestive tract, and environmental toxins. Experts do know that PDDs are not caused by poor parenting or an insensitive mother.

Treatment

Although there is no cure for PDD, the earlier the treatment, the better. Treatment focuses on boosting communication with these children by using behavior modification. Medication also may be help ease problems of inattention, obsessive-compulsive behaviors, and mood swings. Some children with these disorders do well in small classes with individual attention, whereas others will benefit more from standard classrooms with support.

The goal of treatment is to enable a child with PDD to be able to be educated in a regular classroom with additional specialized programs and support, including speech and language therapy.

Facilitated communication is a type of treatment that uses another person (a "facilitator") to support the child's hand, arm, or shoulder, helping him press the keys of a computer keyboard or communication board. Although the Autism Society of America neither condones nor condemns this method, most research has found the procedure not to be valid as a treatment.

The use of gluten-free and casein-free diets has shown some positive results in treating PDDs, but more research has to be done.

pesticide poisonings   Some of the most common poisoning problems are due to the ingestion of pesticides among very young children. Alarmingly, a recent survey found that almost half of all households with children under age five store at least one pesticide in an unlocked cabinet less than four feet off the ground.

To prevent accidental poisoning, it is important to store pesticides away safely and to know how to use them properly. If a bug bomb is being used in a home with children, they should be kept out of the area for at least overnight. Areas where fumes have settled should be scrubbed. When treating a lawn with chemicals, windows should be closed and the children should be kept indoors until the treatment is over. Children should not be allowed to play on chemically treated lawns at least until the chemicals have had a chance to seep into the soil; rain or a sprinkling from a hose will speed the process.

pets and disease   Pet owners can point to many benefits from their cats and dogs, including reduced stress, higher survival rates, increased self-confidence, and improved self-esteem among children. But pets can also carry very real health risks for youngsters. The idea that pets can carry disease is not a new one. Ancient Greeks understood exactly where rabies comes from—the bite of a rabid dog. And the bubonic plagues that wiped out half the population of 15th-century Europe were understood to move from rodents to animals by way of fleas.

HOW TO BUY A HEALTHY PET

Before buying a pet, parents should make sure the animal is healthy so as to avoid passing a disease on to their children. The following tips can help prevent problems:

- Avoid animals with a dull coat, drooping feathers, lethargic behavior, weeping eyes or nose.
- Check out the animal's surroundings. Are the cages and pens clean and free of feces?
- If the pet is in a pet store, are the other animals clean and healthy?
- Ask a vet or animal welfare group if the store or breeder is reputable.
- Get a vet checkup as soon as you bring a pet home.

The list of animal-transmitted conditions is constantly changing as more and more diseases are being redefined as zoonotic conditions. Fortunately, most of these diseases are rare and almost all can be treated. The pet-related diseases include:

Cat-Scratch Disease

Known previously as "cat-scratch fever," this infection is caused by a cat bite or scratch; the responsible organism has recently been identified as *Bartonella henselae*. Three-quarters of all cases occur in children and occur more often in fall and winter. The bite wound is slow to heal and may cause other mild symptoms. The disease is rarely serious, but antibiotics can help treat it if necessary.

Lyme Disease

This disease is not in itself caused by animals, but by a tick that can be carried into the home on cat or dog and then bite a human. LYME DISEASE symptoms are many and vague but include arthritis-like joint pain. Antibiotic treatment is imperative to prevent the disease from progressing; there is now a vaccine for dogs who live in high-risk areas.

Psittacosis (Parrot Fever)

Parrot fever is a bacterial disease infecting 130 species of domestic and wild birds, most commonly ducks, turkeys, chickens, parrots, and pigeons. Children get the disease from parrots or parakeets by contact with feces and feather dust, experiencing cough, fever, chills, and vomiting. Bird symptoms may include poor eating habits or droopy feathers. Wearing a surgical or dust mask and rubber gloves while cleaning a bird's cage will help protect against this disease. A blood test can confirm the diagnosis, and antibiotics will treat the disease in both bird and human.

Rabies

Currently epidemic among certain wild animals in the northeast, rabies can be transmitted to children during a bite from an unvaccinated dog. In the northeast, canine rabies is controlled and the main source of infection is from an unvaccinated cat or from wildlife. Vaccination of pet dogs and cats is imperative to stop the spread of this deadly disease; if someone is bitten by an infected animal, the disease can be prevented if treatment with rabies shots is begun soon enough.

HOW TO PROTECT PETS AND FAMILY

Once a healthy pet has been adopted by a family, it is still possible to transmit infections to children. To help prevent problems, parents should:

- keep cages/pens scrupulously clean and free from droppings
- remove solid waste from cat litter box daily
- keep pets clean and free from ticks, fleas, and mites
- not feed pets raw meat
- not allow children to handle unfamiliar pets
- not allow children to handle a sick animal
- teach children to wash hands after handling an animal
- not adopt wild animals as pets if they are injured; call an animal rehabilitator or humane society
- not walk dogs in tick-infested areas in summer
- never use pet waste as fertilizer; this material has little value and can spread disease
- keep sandboxes covered when not in use
- check pets daily for ticks; remove any immediately

Rocky Mountain Spotted Fever

This tick-borne disease is found throughout the United States; early antibiotic treatment can head off serious complications, including a sometimes-fatal inflammation of lungs, liver, and heart.

Ringworm

Cats (especially long-haired kittens), dogs, horses, and cows can all pass on this fungal skin disease that has nothing to do with worms. Cats are the usual cause, however; the fungus infects cat hair, which passes it on to humans during petting. It causes an inflamed lesion on the skin or in the scalp; antifungal drugs and iodine-based soap cure the problem in humans.

Roundworm

This parasite is carried most often by nursing dogs and their puppies, and less often by cats. Virtually all puppies have roundworm, and because children play in the dirt they are most likely to pick up the parasite. The disease is transmitted through contact with the dog's feces or contaminated soil. So common is the presence of the dog roundworm that worm-free pups can only be produced by raising several generations in isolation, or giving high doses of worm medication to the pregnant mother dog. Both pups and children can be treated with worm medication.

Salmonellosis

Infections with the *Salmonella* bacteria can cause stomach upsets that can have serious consequences in young children. The bacteria are carried by birds and dogs, although turtles present such a risk that the sale of pet-sized turtles (less than four inches) was banned in 1975. Since a wild turtle is just as likely to have *Salmonella,* it should not be considered as a pet either.

Strep Throat

Unknown to many people, the streptococcal bacteria that causes STREP THROAT can be carried in a dog's throat and can cause repeated infections in its human family. In cases of repeated infection, the dog's throat should be checked as a possible source of infection.

Toxoplasmosis

This disease is transmitted to children most often by a parasite in cat feces or contaminated dirt. All cat breeds can become infected with the parasite; cats become infected by killing and eating small rodents. Most children contract the disease not from cats, however, but from raw meat. The meat becomes infected because sheep and cattle graze in pastures contaminated by cats. The disease, which rarely causes symptoms, can be treated with antibacterial drugs.

pharyngitis   An acute inflammation of the part of the throat between the tonsils and the larynx (the pharynx). Especially sore throats should be reported to a physician, who may take a throat culture and prescribe antibiotics.

Cause

The illness most often is caused by a viral infection, although it also may be due to a bacterial infection. It is a common symptom of a cold or INFLUENZA, of MONONUCLEOSIS or SCARLET FEVER. DIPHTHERIA is a rare cause of pharyngitis.

Symptoms

In addition to the sore throat, there may be pain when swallowing together with a slight fever, earache, and tender, swollen lymph nodes in the neck. In very severe cases the fever may be quite high, and the soft palate and throat may swell so that breathing becomes difficult. Extensive swelling and fluid buildup in the larynx can be life threatening.

Treatment

Warm salt water gargles can help ease symptoms. If the inflammation is bacterial, antibiotics can be prescribed.

phenylketonuria (PKU)   An inherited metabolic disease (one of the many possible INBORN ERRORS OF METABOLISM) that leads to MENTAL RETARDATION and other DEVELOPMENTAL DISABILITIES if untreated in infancy. In phenylketonuria (PKU), an amino acid called phenylalanine builds up in the bloodstream, causing brain damage. Infants with untreated PKU appear to develop typically for the first few months of life, but by 12 months of age most babies will have a significant developmental delay and will be diagnosed with mental retardation.

PKU is inherited as a single-gene disorder, which is a condition caused by a mutant or abnormal gene. It is an autosomal recessive disorder, which means that each parent of a child with PKU carries one defective gene for the disorder and one normal gene. In a recessive condition, an individual must have two defective genes in order to have the disorder. Individuals with only one copy of a defective gene are called "carriers," show no symptoms of having the disease, and usually remain unaware of their status until they have an affected child. In order for a child to inherit PKU, both parents must be PKU carriers. When this occurs, there is a one in four chance of their producing an affected child with each pregnancy. Boys and girls are equally at risk of inheriting this disorder.

Diagnosis

Before the 1960s, most infants born with PKU developed mental retardation and CEREBRAL PALSY. Although treatment for PKU using a low phenylalanine diet was first described in the 1950s, the inability to detect PKU early in the child's life limited effective treatment. The first newborn screening test was developed in 1959 specifically to test for PKU. This simple yet effective and economical test was developed to screen newborn infants for PKU before they leave the hospital. Today all states routinely screen newborns for PKU. The American Academy of Pediatrics recommends that infants receiving the test during the first 24 hours of life be retested at two to three weeks of age during their first postnatal pediatric visit.

To test for PKU, a few drops of blood are taken from the infant's heel and then tested in a state laboratory for abnormal amounts of phenylalanine. The normal phenylalanine level is less than two milligrams per deciliter (mg/dl). Those with phenylalanine levels of 20.0 mg/dl or higher are considered likely to have "classical" PKU. Infants with these high levels are further tested to confirm the diagnosis before treatment is started.

Some infants with slightly higher levels of phenylalanine have "mild hyperphenylalanemia." Today many clinicians believe that any child with a phenylalanine level greater than six or eight mg/dl should be treated with a modified phenylalanine restricted diet.

Treatment

Although PKU is not preventable, its symptoms can often be treated successfully through the use of a carefully regimented diet with a restricted phenylalanine content. Babies are given a special formula that contains very low phenylalanine levels; then they gradually progress to eating certain vegetables and other foods that are low in phenylalanine. Affected children must have their blood tested regularly to ensure the presence of the correct level of phenylalanine. Foods recommended for those affected by PKU contain small amounts of protein, such as fruits and vegetables, limited amounts of cereal and grain products, and special low-protein products.

High-protein foods should be avoided, including meat, fish, eggs, poultry, dairy products, nuts, peanut butter, legumes, and soy products. Artificial sugar products containing Nutrasweet also should be avoided. The food program used to treat those with PKU is quite expensive, typically costing up to $10,000 a year or more. Although health departments may pay for the formula in some states and mandated insurance coverage may cover the cost in other states, most insurance companies do not cover the cost of treatment for those with PKU because it is considered nutritional rather than medical therapy.

While phenylalanine-restricted diets have proven to be highly effective in preventing mental retardation, it is now recognized that there may still be subtle cognitive deficits. Usually the individual has a normal IQ, but the incidence of ATTENTION DEFICIT HYPERACTIVITY DISORDER (ADHD) and learning disabilities is higher compared to those children who do not have PKU.

Recent studies have found that children with PKU who stopped the diet in early childhood did not develop as rapidly as children who remained on the diet, and they also had more learning disabilities, behavioral problems, and other neurological problems. Thus, until research provides alternative treatments, everyone with PKU should remain on a restricted diet indefinitely in order to maintain a safe level of phenylalanine (believed to be in the range of two to six mg/dl).

Pregnancy and PKU

Pregnant women with PKU who are not receiving dietary therapy have high levels of phenylalanine that can damage their unborn child, causing mental retardation and other congenital defects. High levels of phenylalanine are extremely toxic to the brain of a fetus. Although the child does not have PKU, there will be brain damage from the toxic effects of phenylalanine in the womb. This is known as maternal PKU.

More than 90 percent of infants born to women with PKU who are not on a specialized diet will have mental retardation and may also have small head size, heart defects, and low birth weight. These infants cannot be treated with a special diet since they do not have PKU. Therefore, women who have PKU should be on a phenylalanine-restricted diet at least one year before pregnancy and should stay on the diet while breast-feeding to increase the chance of having a healthy child.

phobias   A pathologically strong fear that is so overwhelming that it interferes with some aspect of a child's life. Avoiding the feared thing can become so important that the child's life may be restricted. Phobias are a form of ANXIETY DISORDER that can affect children and teenagers.

There are three main groups of phobias, which include specific (simple) phobias, which are the most common and focus on specific objects; social phobia, which is an extreme anxiety in social or public situations; and agoraphobia, the fear of being alone in public places from which there is no easy escape.

Specific/Simple Phobias

Fears of animals, situations, and natural occurrences are common in childhood, especially between ages six and nine, and often go away eventually on their own. A phobia is diagnosed if the fear persists for at least six months and interferes with a child's daily routine, for example, if a child refuses to play outdoors for fear of encountering a dog. Common childhood phobias include animals, storms, heights, water, blood, the dark, or medical procedures. No one knows what causes these fears, although they seem to run in families and are slightly more common in girls.

Unlike adults with specific phobias, children do not usually recognize that their fear is irrational or out of proportion to the situation, and they may not discuss their fears. Instead, children tend to simply avoid situations or things that they fear, or endure them with anxious feelings and exhibit behaviors such as crying, tantrums, freezing, or clinging. They also may experience headaches or stomachaches.

Social Phobia

This phobia can produce fear of being humiliated or embarrassed in front of other people. This problem may also be related to feelings of inferiority and low self-esteem and can drive a child to drop out of school or avoid making friends. Although this disorder is sometimes thought to be shyness, it is not the same thing. Shy people do not experience extreme anxiety in social situations, nor do they necessarily avoid them.

In contrast, people with social phobia can be at ease with people most of the time, except in particular situations. Often social phobia is accompanied by depression or substance abuse.

Children suffering from social phobia may think small mistakes are worse than they really are, are painfully embarrassed by blushing, feel that all eyes are on them. They may fear speaking in public, dating, or talking with persons in authority, be afraid to use a public restroom or eat out, and be afraid of talking on the phone or writing in front of others.

Agoraphobia

Agoraphobia causes children to suffer anxiety about being in places or situations from which it might be difficult or embarrassing to escape, such as being in a room full of people or in an elevator. In some cases, panic attacks can become so debilitating that the child may develop agoraphobia because they fear another panic attack. In extreme cases, a person with agoraphobia may be afraid to leave their house.

Treatment

Phobias can be overcome with proper treatment, including behavioral therapy, exposure therapy, cognitive-behavioral therapy, and medication.

Behavioral therapy focuses on changing specific actions and uses different techniques to stop this behavior, such as breath control and relaxation.

Exposure therapy gradually exposes the child to the frightening object or situation and helps the patient develop coping skills.

Cognitive-behavioral therapy teaches the persons new skills in order to react differently to the situations which trigger the anxiety or panic attacks. Patients also learn to understand how their thinking patterns contribute to the symptoms and how to change their thinking to reduce or stop these symptoms.

Medications the selective serotonin reuptake inhibitors (SSRIs) such as Paxil, can be used successfully to treat social phobia.

phonics An approach to teaching reading and spelling that emphasizes symbol-sounds relationships, used especially in beginning or remedial instruction. Being able to discriminate sounds is an essential element in reading and communicating well. Phonics programs published by major educational publishers have been used to teach reading for decades. These programs offer books, workbooks, computer software, and other teaching materials that introduce letter and word patterns in a systematic and structured way.

There are two phonics approaches: synthetic and analytic. *Synthetic phonics* is a method where individuals are taught single letters and their sounds. Once the letters are mastered, individuals are taught to synthesize the letters into whole words. *Analytic phonics* teaches whole word families (cat, fat, mat, hat) and then teaches individuals to analyze the phonemic elements of the words. Traditionally, reading was taught in U.S. schools using phonics instruction with its emphasis on developing word-recognition skills.

However, the phonics approach to learning was criticized in the 1980s when many schools changed direction and embraced the whole language approach, a more holistic and content-driven approach to teaching reading. This method attempts to get students to read right away, using high-quality children's literature, and emphasizes using contextual cues to aid comprehension.

As national reading scores declined, the movement toward whole language began to change again. Studies comparing whole language and phonics showed that children who are explicitly taught phonics in a direct and systematic way achieved higher scores on reading tests.

Today, most schools use a combination of both approaches. A growing body of research suggests that contextual cues cannot replace word-recognition. Good readers do not skip words or rely on context but read virtually every word and see all letters. In fact, studies demonstrate that only poor readers rely on contextual cues for word identification. Teaching children to guess the meaning of words by context actually decreases the odds that they will learn to read well.

Children who do not understand what they read usually have poor word-recognition skills. Because these children have to devote so much attention to slowly and carefully figuring out the words, they focus less attention on what the text means. Children who recognize words more readily can focus more attention on meaning.

Many experts in education today agree that word-recognition skills as taught in phonics are the critical building blocks for reading success. Still, research also demonstrates that phonics alone is less effective than phonics combined with whole language. An average child needs to read a word four to eight times before word-recognition becomes automatic.

Therefore, the process of reading strengthens the child's ability to perceive sounds in both verbal and written language. Moreover, for practice to be most effective, children need to read stories that are at their reading level; in other words, they should be able to recognize most of the words.

photoallergy   See SUN SENSITIVITY.

physical therapist   A health professional who focuses on the neuromuscular, musculoskeletal, and cardiopulmonary systems of the human body, as these systems relate to human motion and function. Physical therapists evaluate and provide treatment for patients with health problems resulting from injury, disease, or overuse of muscles or tendons. Some physical therapists specialize in caring for children. They focus on restoring the child's mobility and function, cardiovascular endurance, muscle strength, and efficiency in the Activities of Daily Living (ADLs).

Physical therapists have an undergraduate degree in physical therapy, and many have a mas-

ter's degree. In order to practice, all graduates must be licensed by their state by passing a national certification examination. There are more than 90,000 physical therapists practicing in the United States in a variety of settings, including hospitals, rehabilitation centers, schools, sports facilities, community health centers, and private practice.

PID   See PELVIC INFLAMMATORY DISEASE.

pigeon toe   A condition of the foot in which the toes rotate inward but the heels remain straight. This common condition of infants and young children is not usually serious and is usually outgrown without treatment as children get older.

It is not clear why some children are born pigeon-toed, but it may be related to the baby's position in the womb before birth, or because of problems with the ankles, knees, or hips.

Diagnosis
Pigeon toeing is usually first noticed by parents, although sometimes a doctor will identify the problem during an office visit even before the child starts walking. The doctor may need to take X rays to assess the ankles, knees, and hips.

Treatment
A child's doctor may sometimes recommend stretching exercises to be done at home during feedings, repetitively and gently moving the foot to a straight position; this may be enough to straighten out the foot. If these exercises do not work, the doctor may recommend surgery, but this drastic step is rarely considered and not until the child is at least five or six years old. Most experts believe the best treatment is to wait and see if the child will outgrow the condition.

Special shoes and braces that had been used in the past to treat this problem have never been shown to speed up the natural, gradual improvement in this condition.

pimples   See ACNE.

pinkeye   See CONJUNCTIVITIS.

pinworms   The most common parasitic infection in the United States (known medically as enterobiasis). The human pinworm lives only in the intestine. While not technically a worm, it looks like one. The female pinworm is white, about a third of an inch long. Pinworms lay eggs in the skin around the anus. When a child scratches the area, the eggs are transferred directly by the fingers to the mouth, causing reinfestation. The eggs also may be carried on toys or blankets to other children. Once swallowed, the eggs hatch in the intestines, where they grow and reach maturity in about six weeks. Animal pinworms do not infect humans.

Symptoms
Pinworms cause tickling or itching in the anal region at night. Despite common folklore, pinworms do not cause teeth grinding, BED-WETTING, stomachaches, weight loss, poor appetite, nor APPENDICITIS. In fact, pinworms do not cause much harm, but they do itch quite a lot.

Diagnosis
A doctor can pick up some of the eggs from the patient's anal area via sticky tape; they can then be identified under a microscope.

Treatment
Ointment or carbolated petroleum jelly can relieve the itch, as can a sitz bath followed by cleaning with witch hazel around the anal area. A deworming drug (pyrantel pamoate) will kill the worm; mebendazole is the alternative for children over age two. In order to kill the newly hatched adults, it is best to repeat the treatment in two weeks. All members of the household should be treated, whether or not they have symptoms. Bed linens of the affected child should be changed daily without shaking.

Complications
In rare cases, pinworms migrate into the vagina or bladder, leading to cystitis or infection of the fallopian tubes. Severe infestations can interfere with sleep or cause a secondary bacterial infection because of constant scratching.

Prevention
In order to prevent reinfection, all family members should be treated and bathed frequently. Everyone should wear pajamas to limit the number of eggs on bed sheets, and all bed linens and clothing should be washed in hot water to kill the eggs. All sleeping areas should be vacuumed daily for a week after treatment.

PKU See PHENYLKETONURIA.

plane wart See WARTS.

plantar warts A painful WART on the sole of the foot that may appear alone or in clusters. Plantar warts tend to be hard and flat, with a rough surface and well-defined boundaries; warts are generally raised and fleshier when they appear on the top of the foot or on the toes. Plantar warts are often gray or brown, although the color may vary, with a center that appears as one or more pinpoints of black, which are clotted bits of blood.

Cause
This type of wart thrives in warm, moist environments, making infection a common occurrence in swimming pools and public showers. It is usually spread when people infected with the wart virus walk on communal shower floors, contaminating them with the papillomavirus. Plantar warts are spread by touching, scratching, or even by contact with skin shed from another wart. The wart may also bleed, which can help to spread the virus.

Symptoms
When plantar warts develop on the weight-bearing areas of the foot such as the heel or the ball, they can cause sharp, burning pain. Otherwise, they are generally painless.

Treatment
These warts can be very resistant to treatment and have a tendency to reoccur. Self-treatment is generally not advisable, since over-the-counter preparations contain acids or chemicals that destroy skin cells. It takes an expert to destroy warts without also destroying surrounding healthy tissue. Self treatment with such medications especially should be avoided by people with diabetes and those with cardiovascular or circulatory disorders.

It is far better to have a physician remove plantar warts by a simple surgical procedure, performed under local anesthetic. Lasers have become a common and effective treatment, using CO_2 laser cautery performed under local anesthesia either in a podiatrist's office or an outpatient surgery facility. The laser reduces post-treatment scarring and is a safe form for eliminating wart lesions.

Prevention

There are several ways to avoid getting plantar warts, including:

- Avoid walking barefoot, except on sandy beaches.
- Change shoes and socks daily.
- Keep feet clean and dry.
- Avoid direct contact with warts from other people or from other parts of the body.

plants, poisonous Plants are a common source of poisoning for young children who are more likely to put green plants in their mouths. While many plants can be quite toxic to young children, there are a number of other growing things that are completely safe even if the child swallows the plant.

CHILD SAFE PLANTS

African violet	lipstick plant
aluminum plant	magnolia
aspidistra	marigold
aster	nasturtium
baby's tears	Norfolk Island pine
begonia	pepperomia
bird's nest fern	petunia
Boston fern	prayer plant
bougainvillea	purple passion
California poppy	rose
camellia	sensitive plant
Christmas cactus	spider plant
coleus	Swedish ivy
creeping Charlie	tiger lily
dahlia	umbrella tree
dandelion	violet
Easter lily	wandering Jew
gardenia	wax plant
impatiens	wild strawberry
jade plant	zebra plant
kalanchoe	

NOTE: Poinsettias are NOT poisonous to children or pets. Even if a child ate an entire plant, the worst that might happen would be a bit of an upset stomach.

---

playground injuries Playgrounds and outdoor play equipment can provide lots of healthy exercise, but they also can create some safety hazards. Faulty equipment, improper surfaces, and careless behavior are just a few of the problems that send more than 200,000 American children to hospital emergency departments each year. Of these injuries, more than a third are considered severe, leading to temporary or permanent impairment. Between 15 and 20 injuries per year are fatal.

Playground Safety Guidelines

Parents can help prevent playground accidents by taking some precautions ahead of time, ensuring adult supervision, and providing equipment that is age appropriate.

Adults should always supervise their children during trips to the playground, because children cannot always gauge distances properly and are not capable of foreseeing dangerous situations. If a child is injured, adults can provide quick first aid.

Playground equipment is designed and manufactured for two age groups: two- to five-year-olds and five- to 12-year-olds. Equipment manufactured after 1994 should have a sticker indicating for which age group it is meant. Younger children must never play on equipment designed for older children because the equipment sizes and proportions would not be appropriate for small children and could lead to injury. Play areas for younger children should be separate from those meant for older children to avoid confusion about the age appropriateness of the playground equipment.

To help reduce the risk of injury from a fall, children under the age of five should not play on equipment that is taller than four feet. Equipment for five- to 12-year-olds should not be taller than eight feet. Trampolines are dangerous and are never appropriate for safe playgrounds for any age group.

Surfaces and Spacing

Other important playground safety considerations include surfaces, spacing, and maintenance.

Surfaces The surface under playground equipment, which must be soft enough to absorb the shock of falls, could include wood chips or mulch, sand, pea gravel, rubber, and rubber-like materials. Concrete, blacktop, grass, and packed-earth surfaces are unsafe. Whatever surface material is chosen, it must be at least 12 inches deep and must not be compacted. There should not be any standing water or debris on the playground surface that could trip a child, such as rocks, tree stumps, or roots. Surface materials need to cover a "fall zone" (the areas surrounding equipment), as follows:

- *Jungle gyms and climbing equipment* The fall zone should extend at least six feet in every direction.

- *Slides less than four feet tall* The fall zone should extend at least six feet from the end of the slide.

- *Slides more than four feet tall* To determine how many feet the surface should extend beyond the end of the slide, the builder should measure the height of the stairs or ladder and add four feet.

- *Swings* The fall zone should extend at least two times the height of the swing set, both in front and in back, and six feet on each side of the swing set.

Spacing To prevent overcrowding, there should be at least 12 feet between play structures, and the fall zones for equipment over two feet tall should never overlap. Swings, seesaws, and other equipment with moving parts should be located in a separate area from the rest of the playground, and a child should never have to cross directly in front of or behind the swings to reach other equipment. Each swing set should not contain more than two swings, and the swings themselves should be at least two feet apart and at least two-and-a-half feet from the edges of the swing set.

Safe equipment All equipment must be designed only for playground use. A sandbox should contain sand intended for playground purposes only; other types of sand (such as construction sand) may contain asbestos or other hazardous materials. Sandboxes should be checked for debris such as sharp sticks, broken glass, and bugs, and the box should be covered overnight to prevent contamination from animals.

Because falls are a common playground injury, all elevated surfaces must have guardrails. Equipment intended for children under age five must have guardrails on surfaces more than 20 inches tall. For older children, there must be guardrails on equipment over 30 inches.

Playground equipment should not have any pieces that protrude or that could cut or entangle a child. There should be no parts such as these:

- bolt ends extending more than two threads past the face of the nut

- hardware that forms a hook or leaves a space between parts

- open "S" hooks

- rungs that protrude outward from the sides of climbing structures

- sharp or unfinished edges on any equipment

- openings on equipment (for example, rungs on a slide and bars on monkey bars) measuring less than three-and-a-half to nine inches (this could trap a child's head)

Playground equipment with moving parts, such as seesaws and merry-go-rounds, should be checked for areas that could pinch or crush a child's finger or hand. Regardless of design, both seesaws and merry-go-rounds should be used with caution.

The following types of equipment are not appropriate for playgrounds:

- animal figure swings

- swing seats made of wood or metal

- glider swings holding more than one child at a time

- swinging ropes that could fray, unravel, or form a noose, or that are not anchored at both ends

- exercise rings (as used in gymnastics) or trapeze bars

Good repair All hardware on playground equipment should be secure, and plastic and wood should show no signs of weakening, with no splintered or rusted surfaces.

Treated Wooden Equipment

The Consumer Product Safety Commission (CPSC) stated in February 2003 that children could face an increased lifetime risk of developing lung or bladder cancer from using playground equipment treated with chromated copper arsenate. Almost all wooden playground equipment in use has been treated with a pesticide (chromated copper arsenate). The government's concern is that children can get arsenic residue from the treated wood on their hands, then put their hands in their mouths. Increasingly, advocacy groups have targeted wood preservatives containing arsenic as unsafe. Those preservatives have been commonly used in utility poles, wood decks, and playgrounds. The Safety Commission and the Environmental Protection Agency (EPA) are studying ways to coat treated wood with a sealant to prevent arsenic from seeping through.

Wood preservative manufacturers argue that treated play sets are not dangerous and say a ban is unnecessary because an agreement between the industry and the EPA stopped the chemical from being used in most consumer products by December 2003, including playground equipment, decks, fences, walkways, and landscape timbers.

The Scientific Advisory Panel (SAP), a group of independent scientists who advise the EPA on critical science issues, evaluated the agency's draft risk assessment on pressure-treated wood in December 2003. The draft assessment evaluated the potential risks to children who play on playsets and decks made with wood pressure-treated with chromated copper arsenate (CCA). However, the draft risk assessment findings are preliminary and subject to additional analysis. The panel did not yet reach conclusions about the potential for CCA-treated playsets and decks to contribute to cancer risk in children.

In addition to the SAP review, the EPA is conducting a study on whether sealants can reduce or eliminate exposure to arsenic in CCA-treated wood as a further way to help consumers make informed choices around their home. Results from this study were expected in 2004.

CPSC research released in February 2003 found that for every million children exposed to the treated wood three times a week during early childhood, two to 100 of them might develop lung or bladder cancer later in life because of the exposure. The increase is additional to other risks of getting cancer. The greatest risk factor for both kinds of cancer is smoking cigarettes. Government scientists recommend that parents and caregivers thoroughly wash children's hands with soap and water immediately after youngsters use playground equipment made of the treated wood.

Toxicology experts speaking on behalf of wood preservative manufacturers said the CPSC's research was inadequate, arguing that children are exposed to more arsenic in food and water than from treated playground equipment. They believe that the potential level of arsenic exposure does not pose a meaningful health risk to children or adults.

Safe Playground Behavior

It is also important that children know how to act responsibly at the playground, and never push or roughhouse while on jungle gyms, slides, seesaws, swings, and other equipment. A child who likes to jump off jungle gyms and other climbing toys should make certain no other children are in the way and should land on both feet with his knees slightly bent.

Children should not use equipment if it is even slightly wet, because moisture causes the surface to be slippery. Children should also be taught never to wear clothes with drawstrings or other strings at the playground, because this could pose a strangulation hazard.

Children should never run or walk in front of or in back of the swings, and never "double up," with two on a swing. Swings are only designed to safely hold one person. A child should always sit in the swing, not stand or kneel, and should hold on tightly with both hands while swinging; when finished swinging, children should stop the swing completely before getting off.

Children should avoid gliders or animal-shaped swings, because they may seriously injure a child who is hit by a moving swing. Children also should not push each other on swings, because the child pushing the swing may not be able to gauge properly how much force is necessary, and the child being pushed will not have any control if he wants to stop.

Seesaws Only one child should sit on a seesaw seat; if a child is too light to seesaw with a partner, she should find a different partner, not add another child to her side of the seesaw. Children always should sit facing one another, not turned the other way around. Children should hold on tightly with both hands while on a seesaw, not touching the ground or pushing off with the hands. Feet should be kept to the sides, out from underneath the seesaw. A child must stand back from a seesaw when it is in use, never beneath it. Because seesaws require cooperation between children, they are generally not recommended for preschoolers unless the seesaw is equipped with a spring-centering device to prevent abrupt contact with the ground.

Slides Slides can be safe if children always climb up the stairs of a slide, taking one step at a time and holding onto the handrail—never climbing up the slide itself to get to the top. The child should always slide down feet first and sitting up, never head first on back or stomach.

Only one child should be on the slide platform at a time, and children should not slide down in groups. A child should always check that the bottom of the slide is clear before sliding down; once at the bottom, the child should get off and move away from the end so it is clear for the next one. A hot metal slide can easily burn children, so on hot days, a child should feel the slide surface with a hand before climbing up to the top.

pneumococcal conjugate vaccine (PCV) A new vaccine approved in 2000 to prevent invasive pneumococcal diseases in infants and toddlers, diseases that can cause brain damage and, in rare cases, death. The pneumococcal conjugate vaccine (PCV) is not indicated for use in adults or as a substitute for other approved pneumococcal polysaccharide vaccines approved for high-risk children over age two. The previous pneumococcal vaccine (PPV) was not recommended for use in children under age two, who contract the most serious infections from this bacteria.

The new PCV vaccine (Prevnar) protects against the organism *Streptococcus pneumoniae* (also known as pneumococcus), the leading cause of PNEUMONIA, SINUSITIS, EAR INFECTION, and MENINGITIS. It has been added to the recommended schedule of childhood immunizations. It is given to infants as a series of four inoculations administered at age two, four, six, and 12 to 15 months of age. If a child cannot begin the vaccine at two months, parents should discuss alternative schedules with their doctor.

Prevnar is the first pneumococcal vaccine for children under the age of two that targets the most common seven strains of pneumococcus causing 80 percent of invasive disease in infants. For the first time, doctors have a highly effective way to prevent a major cause of meningitis and serious blood infections in the most susceptible children—those under age two. Pneumococcal infections cause about 1,400 cases of meningitis, 17,000 cases of bloodstream infections, and 71,000 cases of pneumonia every year in children under age five.

Children under the age of two are at highest risk for infection. In up to half the cases of meningitis, brain damage and hearing loss occur and about 10 percent die. There are different types of bacterial meningitis. Before the approval of the first *Haemophilus influenzae* type B (HIB) conjugate vaccine in 1990 for infants, HIB was the leading cause of bacterial meningitis, but today *Streptococcus pneumoniae* is one of the leading causes of bacterial meningitis.

Side effects in the trials were generally mild and included local injection site reactions, irritability, drowsiness, and decreased appetite. Approximately 21 percent of the children had fevers over 100.3°F.

pneumonia An infection of the lungs caused by a variety of germs including bacteria, viruses, and parasites. It is considered to be the most common infectious cause of death in the United States. There are many different types of pneumonia, classified according to what causes the condition. For example, the pneumonia may be bacterial, viral, fungal, parasitic, or mycoplasmic. If a large portion of one or more lobes of the lung is involved, the disease is called a lobar pneumonia. Bronchopneumonia (which is more common than lobar) implies that the disease process is distributed in different places in the lungs but originates in the bronchial tubes.

Risk Factors

A number of risk factors can predispose a child to developing pneumonia. Any condition that produces mucus or an obstruction (such as chronic lung disease) can make the child more likely to develop pneumonia. Also at risk are children with an impaired immune system or those confined to bed. Patients with CYSTIC FIBROSIS are prone to respiratory infection with *Pseudomonas* and

Staphylococcus. Pneumocystis carinii pneumonia has been associated with AIDS.

Bacterial Pneumonia

Streptococcus pneumoniae is the most common cause of bacterial pneumonia, occurring most often in winter and spring, when upper respiratory tract infections are most common. In addition to *S. pneumoniae*, other bacteria that can cause pneumonia include *Staphylococcus aureus, Klebsiella pneumoniae, Pseudomonas aeruginosa, Haemophilius influenzae, Legionella pneumophilia,* and *Mycoplasma pneumoniae*.

Symptoms Classic bacterial pneumonia usually begins with a sudden onset of shaking chills, a rapid rising fever (up to 105°F), and stabbing chest pain as the lungs become inflamed, made worse by coughing. The patient is severely ill and breathes with grunting and flared nostrils, leaning forward in an effort to breathe without coughing. During the most serious phase of pneumonia, the body loses fluids, which must be replaced in order to prevent shock; pus in the lungs can cause severe respiratory distress.

Diagnosis History, physical exam, chest X ray, blood culture, and sputum exam are used to diagnose this disease.

Treatment Bacterial pneumonia is usually treated with antibiotics such as penicillin G. Other effective drugs include erythromycin, clindamycin, cephalosporin, and Bactrim. Bed rest is required until the infection clears, and oxygen may be given.

Chlamydial Pneumonia

This type of pneumonia is caused by a newly recognized strain of CHLAMYDIA. Chlamydial pneumonia is the second leading cause of pneumonia in children over age five, after mycoplasma pneumonia. Most infections in children are mild, and recovery is slow but complete; the cough may last two or more weeks. Patients are infectious as long as they cough, and antibiotics do not reduce the infectious period. While one attack conveys a short-term immunity, it is possible to get chlamydial pneumonia more than once.

Cause This type of pneumonia is caused by a tiny organism *(Chlamydia pneumoniae)* similar to both viruses and bacteria that live within human cells. Because it responds to antibiotics, it is classified as a bacterium. It is related to the germ that causes the sexually transmitted disease Chlamydia.

It is transmitted by direct contact with infected individuals or by breathing in the bacteria when an infected person coughs or sneezes nearby. The disease may be passed by handling a coughing infected person's towels or sheets.

Symptoms Symptoms are similar to mycoplasma pneumonia, beginning with fatigue and weakness, sore throat, hoarseness, low fever, and cough. Some sputum may be coughed up. The incubation period after exposure varies but is usually between one and four weeks.

Diagnosis An antibody test is the best way to diagnose the disease, but many doctors diagnose it on the basis of symptoms and on tests that rule out other types of bacterial pneumonia. Chest X ray may reveal a pneumonia in the lower lobe of one lung. Throat or sputum cultures will reveal the disease, but many labs are unable to culture this.

Treatment Erythromycin or tetracycline for 10 to 21 days will cure the disease. Children should be given humidified air from a cool-mist vaporizer, clear fluids, and acetaminophen for fevers over 101°F. The child's chest should be raised while sleeping.

Mycoplasma Pneumonia

This type of pneumonia occurs primarily among children and young adults and is also known as "walking pneumonia." The infections occur sporadically throughout the year, but they are most common in late summer and early fall. There are no vaccines to prevent this type of pneumonia and no reliable methods for control.

Cause Mycoplasma pneumonia is caused by *M. pneumoniae,* a microscopic organism related to bacteria that is spread via contact with droplets from the nose and throat of infected people when they cough or sneeze. Transmission requires close contact; the contagious period is probably less than 10 days.

Symptoms After an incubation period of between nine to 25 days, symptoms of dry cough, fever, sore throat, headache, and malaise appear. Ear infections may also occur. Symptoms may last from a few days to a month or more.

Diagnosis A nonspecific blood test may help, but doctors can diagnose this condition from symptoms alone.

Treatment Antibiotics including erythromycin and tetracycline are effective.

poison control centers A network of more than 600 centers across the country can provide free poison treatment information 24 hours a day. The first center was established in 1953 in Chicago under the impetus of the American Academy of Pediatrics, which had become alarmed at the number of children's poisoning cases. A few months later, the Duke University Poison Control Center opened in North Carolina. In 1957 the U.S. Food and Drug Administration (FDA) established the National Clearinghouse for Poison Control Centers to coordinate activities across the country. The clearinghouse collected and standardized product toxicology data, reproduced this information on large file cards, and distributed them nationwide to poison control centers.

To further streamline poison emergency care, the government established a national emergency number in February 2002 so that anyone in the country can call for a poison problem. The emergency hotline—(800) 222-1222—links callers anywhere in the country to medical experts at local centers and received nearly one million calls in its first year.

Poison Control Hotline A national emergency number operated by the federal government begun in February 2002 so that anyone in the country can call for a poison problem. The emergency hotline—(800) 222-1222—links callers anywhere in the country to medical experts at local centers and received nearly one million calls in its first year.

poisoning Most accidental poisonings involving youngsters occur in children under age five; there were more than 1.1 million poisonings in children this age every year in the nineties, and about 30 of them died. Nevertheless, these figures represent a significant decrease over the past few decades, in large part because of laws passed in 1970 requiring child-resistant packaging. Still, poisoning remains a significant problem in this country, and parents and caregivers need to do more than rely on child-resistant packaging. Parents need to keep medicines and chemicals locked up. Special packaging is child-resistant, not childproof. To be legally designated as "child-resistant," a product must take

more than five minutes for 80 percent of five year olds to open. This means that 20 percent of these youngsters could get into it in less time.

For poison emergency care, the government established a national emergency number in February 2002 so that anyone in the country can call for a poison problem. The emergency hotline links callers anywhere in the country to medical experts at local centers, and it has received nearly one million calls in its first year.

To prevent poisonings, parents and caregivers should:

- keep all chemicals and medicines locked up and out of sight
- never let young children out of sight when toxic products are being used
- avoid taking medicine in front of children
- refer to medicine as "medicine," not "candy"
- keep items in original containers with their original labels and close child-resistant packaging securely after each use
- keep lamps and candles that contain lamp oil away from children, because these products can be very toxic if ingested
- always leave the light on when giving medicine; read the label before using and check the dosage every time
- clean out the medicine cabinet periodically and dispose of unneeded and outdated drugs
- keep a bottle of ipecac syrup on hand for use *only* if the poison center authorizes its administration

Substances most often swallowed by children under age five, as reported by Poison Control Centers, include:

1. plants
2. soaps, detergents, cleaners
3. perfume, cologne, toilet water
4. antihistamines, cold medications
5. vitamins and minerals
6. aspirin
7. household disinfectants or deodorizers
8. insecticides

9. miscellaneous painkillers

10. fingernail preparations

All hazardous items should be kept in cupboards or shelves out of a child's reach, or in locked drawers or cabinets. Common potentially dangerous products found in almost every home include the following:

Cleaning Products

chlorine bleach, ammonia, and detergents
toilet bowl cleaners
drain cleaners
furniture polish
floor polish and wax

Household Goods

nail polish and remover
shoe polish
rubbing alcohol
hair dye
hair spray

Medications

aspirin
acetaminophen
prescription medications
cough medicine
cold preparations

Garden Products

roach powders or baits
rat pellets
rose dust
weed killers
flower, garden, and shrub sprays
lime
treated seeds

Garage Products

antifreeze
kerosene or gasoline
paint thinners and strippers

If Poisoning Is Suspected

The most important thing to remember in a poisoning case is not to make the problem any worse. Prompt treatment is vital, and minutes can spell the difference between life and death. First aid is most effective if the parent can identify the drug or chemical that caused the poisoning.

1. Parents should call the national poison emergency hotline (800) 222-1222 that will link callers anywhere in the country to medical experts at local centers. Alternatively, the 911 operator can also help.

2. When poison control is reached, callers should provide the following information:
   a. Caller's name
   b. Child's name, age, and weight
   c. Kind of poison involved (name, ingredients, or kind of plant or creature)
   d. How much was swallowed, and when it was swallowed
   e. Child's symptoms
   f. Other medical problems (diabetes, high blood pressure, asthma, and so on)
   g. What drugs the child takes regularly
   h. Whether child has vomited
   i. What child has been given to eat or drink
   j. How long it will take you to get to the nearest emergency room

What Poison Control Will Do

The person at poison control will tell the caller whether or not to induce vomiting (certain poisons, such as acids or alkalies, should never be vomited). If the caller does not know what the child has swallowed, vomiting should not be induced.

Poison control may recommend activated charcoal, Epsom salts, or a specific product to neutralize the poison. Callers should always follow instructions given by a poison control center and NOT trust antidote information given on product labels. Callers should not use mustard or salt to induce vomiting, because these old-fashioned remedies do not work well. A child should never be forced to vomit by sticking fingers down the throat; this is especially dangerous for young children. First aid procedures differ according to the kind of poison involved and how it entered the child's body, the child's weight, how long the poison has been working, and other factors. Only medical personnel can determine the correct procedures. Treating the child without expert advice could cause further harm.

Once the Child Vomits

If possible, the child should vomit into a bucket or the sink, so some of the vomited material can be brought to the hospital to help the doctor identify the poison.

To make sure the child does not inhale the vomited material, the parent should hold small children face down over the knees; a larger child should bend over or lie down with head hanging off the bed. If the poison has spilled onto clothing, skin, or eyes, the clothing should be removed and skin or eyes flushed with water.

If the child stops breathing, cardiopulmonary resuscitation (CPR) should be performed. Shock should be treated by keeping the child quiet and lying down, with head tilted to one side. Clothing should be loosened and child covered with a blanket; no beverages or sedatives should be given.

poison ivy *(Toxicodendron radicans)* One of the most common plants in the United States that is poisonous to touch, causing a contact DERMATITIS in most people. The leaves of the poison ivy plant are glossy green, may be notched or smooth, and almost always grow in groups of three. However, according to some experts, there are exceptions; leaves may sometimes appear in fives, sevens, or even nines. In early fall, the leaves may turn bright red. Although it usually grows as a long, hairy vine (often wrapping itself around trees), it also can be found as a low shrub growing along fences or stone walls. Poison ivy has waxy yellow-green flowers and green berries that can help identify the plant in late fall, winter, and spring, before the leaves appear. Poison ivy is found throughout the United States, but it is most common in the eastern and central states.

Poisonous Parts

Poison ivy, poison oak, and poison sumac are closely related species, all three containing a colorless or slightly yellow oil called "urushiol." Skin contact with this oil causes an allergic reaction. While each of these three plants contains a slightly different type of urushiol, they are so similar that children sensitive to one type will react to all three. The entire plant contains urushiol and is therefore poisonous: leaves, berries, stalk, and roots.

Urushiol is easily transferred from the plant to an object and then to a child, so anything that touches these poison plants—clothing, gardening tools, a pet's fur, athletic equipment, sleeping bags—can be contaminated and cause poison ivy in anyone who touches the object. Urushiol remains active for up to one year, so any equipment that touches poison ivy must be washed. The smoke from burning poison ivy is especially toxic to the skin of the face, the eyes, or the lungs. It will also irritate the throat if eaten.

As the leaves die in the fall, the plant draws certain nutrients and substances (including the oil) into the stem. But the oil remains active, so that even in winter it may cause a rash if the broken stems are used as firewood, or the vines on a Christmas wreath.

Despite persistent folklore, poison ivy is NOT spread by scratching open blisters or by skin-to-skin contact. Only the oil can trigger a reaction. However, doctors recommend that a child not touch the blisters, because any remaining oil on the skin that has not been washed off could be transmitted to another part of the body. Scratching blisters also may cause infection from germs on the skin surface.

Symptoms

While not every child is allergic to poison ivy, about seven out of 10 are. Symptoms vary from one person to the next; some children exhibit only mild itching, while others experience severe reactions. Within 24 to 48 hours after exposure the skin becomes red, followed by watery blisters, peaking about five days after contamination and gradually improving over a week or two, even without treatment. Eventually the blisters break, and the oozing sores crust over and then disappear.

Treatment

The best treatment is to immediately remove jewelry and wash the affected area (within 10 minutes if possible after contact) with yellow laundry soap and *cold* water. A shower is better than bathing in a tub, since the latter could spread the oil. If a child is contaminated in a remote area, washing in a cold running stream will help remove the oil. Any clothing that may have come in contact with the oil must be washed several times.

Early application of topical steroids can minimize the severity of the skin reaction. Itching can be treated by applying cold compresses; a calamine lotion spread over the rash will help ease itching and burning. Products containing local anesthetics (such as benzocaine) or irritants (such as camphor or phenol) should be avoided.

Systemic antihistamines do not work against the rash, although their sedative action may help the child sleep. In the case of a severe reaction, a doctor may prescribe corticosteroid drugs by mouth or injection. Such systemic steroids given during the first six hours after exposure are the most effective.

Prevention

New barrier creams (bentoquatam) may offer some protection and should be applied 15 minutes before exposure is suspected, and every four hours afterward. It should not be used if a rash is already present, nor on children under age six.

Most people could be immunized against poison ivy through prescription pills, which contain gradually increasing amounts of active extract from the plants. However, this procedure can take four months to achieve a reasonable degree of hyposensitivation, and the medication must be continued over a long period of time. In addition, it often causes uncomfortable side effects such as skin problems, stomach problems, fever, and inflammation. Convulsions have occurred in children after oral doses of the plant's extract.

poison oak *(Toxicodendron diversilobum)* A plant that is poisonous to touch, closely related to POISON IVY. The leaves of poison oak occur in groups of three and are very similar to oak leaves, from which the plant gets its name. The underside of the leaves is much lighter green because of the thousands of tiny fine hairs that cover them. Berries may be green or white, although not all plants bear fruit. Poison oak usually grows as a low shrub on the west coast, from Mexico to British Columbia. (See POISON IVY for details on treatment and prevention.)

poison sumac *(Toxicodendron vernix [L.] Kuntzel [Rhus vernix L.])* This poisonous tree, a relative of POISON IVY and POISON OAK, has seven

to 13 long narrow leaves growing in pairs with a single leaf at the end of the stem. In the spring the leaves are bright orange and look something like velvet; as the season progresses, they become dark green and glossy on the upper surface and light green on the underside. In the fall the leaves turn red or orange. Poison sumac can be differentiated from nonpoisonous sumacs by its drooping clusters of green berries; nonpoisonous sumacs have red, upright clusters of berries. Poison sumac can grow to be 25 feet tall, although it is more often found between five and six feet tall. It is found in swampy areas throughout the eastern United States. (See POISON IVY for details on treatment and prevention.)

poliomyelitis (polio) A contagious viral disease that in its severe form can cause permanent paralysis and sometimes death. This extremely dangerous disease causes mild disabilities in about half of all patients; the rest may suffer permanent paralysis. However, due to modern vaccination practices, the Americas were declared polio-free in 1994, and the disease has been almost eliminated in Europe (there was an outbreak in the Netherlands in 1995). The global network of labs that track the disease reported no new cases of Type 2 polio in 2000. The last recorded cases were in India in 1999.

Still, more than 2,800 cases were confirmed in 2000 in southeast Asia, Africa, and the Mediterranean, where war, poverty, and other problems have interfered with efforts to vaccinate children.

Most American doctors have never seen an active case of polio, but in the first half of this century polio (then known as "infantile paralysis"), was called the last of the great childhood plagues.

Polio was known for hundreds of years, but the disease was not much discussed in ancient medical literature and did not occur in large epidemics until modern times. In fact, it was only in the late 18th century that the disease was first identified as polio. In ancient times, sanitation was so appallingly poor that there was plenty of opportunity for people to contract polio, which is carried in feces. The viruses infected each new generation of infants, who were protected in part by antibodies passed from their mothers. These early infections were usually mild and were rarely diagnosed as polio.

When improved sanitation and other health measures arrived (such as water purification and milk pasteurization), there was less chance for babies and young children to contract the mild form of the disease and become immune. When the disease struck older children and adults, it was more likely to paralyze. In northern Europe and the United States, small epidemics began to appear in the late 19th and early 20th centuries. It was not until the summer of 1917, when 27,000 U.S. citizens were paralyzed and 6,000 more died, that the real threat began to emerge. The northeast was especially hard hit; in New York City and its suburbs, more than 9,000 cases were reported and 2,488 people died. The 1917 epidemic set off a panic as thousand fled the city to mountain resorts. Movie theaters were closed, meetings were canceled, and public gatherings were shunned. No one understood what spread the disease, so doctors stopped performing tonsillectomies until fall and warned children not to drink from public water fountains. In some towns, New York City natives who came to visit were turned away by armed citizens who feared the spread of the disease. Yet despite these precautions, an epidemic appeared each summer after that, with the most serious outbreaks in the 1940s and 1950s. It was the 1952 epidemic that was the worst, with nearly 54,000 reported cases and 3,145 deaths.

At this point, Dr. Jonas Salk developed a vaccine tested in a 1954 field trial of 1.8 million children, proving that Salk's killed virus vaccine was very effective in preventing polio. Dr. Salk became a national hero. After the vaccine was licensed in 1955, an intense public health campaign was mounted to inoculate every American child in the country. Similar scenes were repeated in 1961, when the attenuated live virus vaccine developed by Dr. Albert Sabin was licensed. This time the vaccine was given in a sugar cube soaked in liquid vaccine. In a few short years, polio was virtually eliminated in this country, since both vaccines contain all three polio strains and prevent the disease.

The last U.S. epidemic occurred in 1979 when 10 Amish children, whose parents had refused to have them vaccinated on religious grounds, all came down with the disease.

Cause

Polio is caused by a virus with three distinct strains (types I, II, and III) that live in the nose, throat, and especially the intestinal tract of an infected person. Many people are carriers—that is, they are infected but have no symptoms—but they can spread the infection to others.

The virus is excreted in large amounts in the feces of a carrier and is probably spread through hand-to-hand or hand-to-mouth contact. Once in the body, the virus multiples in the throat and intestinal tract. In more serious cases, the virus may attack the nervous system, where it may kill or injure motor nerve cells. This can lead to extensive paralysis, including paralysis of the muscles involved in breathing—or it may be fatal. Immunity to one type of polio does not confer immunity to the other two.

Symptoms

The mild forms of polio usually begin abruptly and last just a few days. Symptoms may include fever, sore throat, nausea, headache, and stomachache. There may be pain or stiffness in the neck, back, and legs.

The more serious form—paralytic polio—begins with the same symptoms but also includes severe muscle pain. If paralysis occurs, it begins within the first week. Paralysis may affect only a small group of muscles, or it may be widespread. The legs are more often affected than the arms, but the virus may partially or completely paralyze a single limb, half the body, or all four extremities.

Those most at risk for severe neurological damage during epidemics include patients who had been recently inoculated or operated on (especially those who underwent tonsillectomies and adenoidectomies).

Treatment

There is no specific treatment for polio. The degree of recovery varies from one patient to the next.

Prevention

Mass vaccination has eliminated paralytic polio in the United States and is an essential part of every young child's preventive care. Of the two vaccines, Salk's killed virus vaccine (IPV) is currently recommended for almost all children in the United States today.

Until recently, the live oral polio vaccine (OPV) had been recommended for most children because while both vaccines provide immunity to polio, OPV was better at keeping the disease from spreading to other people. However, for a few people (about one in 2.4 million), OPV actually *causes* polio. Since there is now virtually no chance of getting polio in the United States, experts decided that using oral polio vaccine is no longer worth the chance of infecting five to 15 American children each year. The killed virus polio shot (IPV) never causes polio and is not known to cause any side effects other than minor local pain and redness.

Post-Polio Syndrome

Patients who had polio in childhood have a one in five chance of experiencing new health problems decades later. Called post-polio syndrome, the symptoms include joint and muscle pain, tiredness, and weakness. While experts are not sure what causes the problem, they do not think it represents a reactivation of the old virus. Some experts suspect the syndrome may be related to chronic overuse of muscles and joints that had appeared to be undamaged by the initial infection.

There is no known cure and no universal treatment for post-polio syndrome. Treatments may include nonstrenuous exercise, physical therapy, electrical stimulation, occupational therapy, and nonsteroidal anti-inflammatory drugs or ASPIRIN.

polio vaccine An inoculation designed to prevent POLIO. The killed virus vaccine (IPV) is currently recommended for almost all children in the United States. Until recently, the live oral polio vaccine (OPV) was recommended for most children. While both vaccines provide immunity to polio, OPV was better at keeping the disease from spreading to other people. However, for a few people (about one in 2.4 million), OPV actually caused polio. Since the risk of getting polio in the United States is now virtually gone, experts believe that using oral polio vaccine is no longer worth the slight risk. The killed virus polio shot (IPV) never causes polio.

polycystic ovary disease (PCOS) A metabolic disorder (also called Stein-Leventhal syndrome) in which cysts develop on a teenage girl's ovaries as the level of male hormones in her body increases. Many of these girls also develop insulin resistance.

Polycystic ovary disease (PCOS) was first recognized in 1935, but doctors are not sure what causes it. The condition may be related to excess insulin production, which could signal the body to release extra male hormones. PCOS seems to have a genetic component as well.

Between 6 percent and 10 percent of teenage girls have PCOS. If not treated, it can lead to infertility, excessive hair growth, ACNE, diabetes, heart disease, uterine bleeding, and cancer. Proper treatment for PCOS, however, can prevent these problems.

Cause

The cause of the syndrome is not clear, although many experts believe the underlying cause of PCOS is a hormonal imbalance that seems to be linked to the way a girl's body processes insulin, resulting in higher-than-normal levels of male hormones. PCOS also may be partially genetic.

In a girl with PCOS, the ovaries produce higher-than-normal amounts of androgens, which can interfere with egg production. The eggs that the ovaries normally produce develop into cysts. Instead of being released during ovulation as an egg would be during a normal menstrual cycle, the cysts build up in the ovaries and may become enlarged. Because the cyst production interferes with the menstrual cycle, it is common for girls with PCOS to have irregular or missed periods.

Symptoms

The long list of baffling symptoms and conditions can affect not only a girl's long-term physical health but her psychological health as well. There are many signs of PCOS caused by the increased androgen levels, which affects not only the reproductive system but also the hair and skin.

• *Missed period* A lack of ovulation can result in skipped or irregular periods. However, because it can take up to two years before menstruation becomes regular, doctors look for other symptoms that might indicate PCOS.

- *Abdominal discomfort* Severe premenstrual symptoms may appear, such as cramping, bloating, and irritability. Some doctors think the abdominal discomfort is caused by the enlarged ovaries filled with cysts.
- *Weight gain* Girls with PCOS may gain weight easily or be overweight, carrying the extra weight in the abdominal area. However, only about half of the girls with PCOS are overweight, so it is possible to be a normal weight and still have PCOS.
- *High blood pressure*
- *Hirsutism* Extra hair may appear on the face, chest, abdomen, nipples, or backs.
- *Acne* Increased acne and clogged pores
- *Pigment changes* There may be darkened skin around the neck or armpits or under the breasts.
- *Hair loss*

More potentially dangerous conditions may be related to PCOS if the syndrome is left untreated, including:

- *Uterine cancer* High levels of male hormones may mean fewer periods, which could put a girl at risk for uterine cancer if PCOS is not treated.
- *Diabetes* Some girls with PCOS have problems using their insulin, a condition known as insulin resistance, which is a risk factor for adult-onset (type-2) diabetes.
- *Heart disease* Girls with high insulin levels can also have low levels of high-density lipoprotein, (good cholesterol) and high levels of other fats. These factors can increase the risk of heart attack or stroke later in life.

Diagnosis

Early diagnosis and treatment for PCOS are important because the condition can put girls at risk for long-term problems, such as heart disease, diabetes, and breast and uterine cancer. The doctor will take a detailed medical background about menstruation and any hormonal medications. A physical and pelvic exam might be conducted.

Blood testing could reveal abnormalities in hormone levels, insulin and glucose levels, and cholesterol and triglyceride levels. An ultrasound may be used to look at the ovaries and to determine the presence of cysts, although they are not always visible.

Treatment

A combination of diet, exercise, and medication can help treat PCOS in girls before the condition causes permanent damage.

Diet and exercise Diet is one of the most important steps in managing PCOS, because losing weight will affect the high insulin state. Cutting down on carbohydrates, like breads, cereals, and pastas, and eating more fruits, grains, and vegetables also can help to regulate the insulin response. Exercise can help the body use insulin better and help drop weight.

Medications Some medications are effective in treating PCOS. Most common are birth control pills, which can help to regulate the androgen levels in the body and regulate the menstrual cycle. Birth control pills may help the symptoms of acne and excessive hair growth. Other medications used to treat PCOS include antiandrogens such as spironolactone and flutamide, which can help clear up the skin and hair problems associated with PCOS.

Metformin is a medication that stimulates insulin uptake, lowering insulin levels, and helps manage excess weight in girls with significantly high insulin levels. Some girls and women who have used metformin have experienced weight loss, lowered blood pressure, and more regular menstrual cycles. Getting treated for PCOS is also a good idea if you want to have a baby someday. PCOS often causes infertility if it is not treated, but when it is treated properly, many women with PCOS are able to have healthy babies.

Surgery Ovarian drilling is available to treat PCOS. In this procedure, a very small incision is made above or below the navel, and a small tool (laparoscope) is inserted into the abdomen. Using a small needle that carries electric current or a laser, the doctor can make punctures in the ovary, destroying a small part of the ovary. However, this surgery should not be the first fertility treatment option, because its success rate is less than 50 percent.

pools and parasites An improperly maintained pool may harbor microscopic parasites and bacteria that can make children sick. In fact, more than 15,000 swimmers became ill from swimming during the past decade. If pools are properly maintained and chlorinated, the risk of getting sick from swimming is believed to be low for germs that are killed easily by chlorine. However, over the past 10 years, more than 150 outbreaks involving thousands of people have been reported, involving pools, water parks, hot tubs, spas, lakes, and rivers. Many outbreaks are never detected.

Pools can be contaminated by germs such as *Cryptosporidium, Giardia, E. coli 0157:H7,* and *Shigella,* which are spread by accidentally swallowing water that has been contaminated with fecal matter. Swimmers share the water with everyone in the pool, so if someone with diarrhea contaminates the water, swallowing the water can make another swimmer sick.

Most often, swimming pool contamination is the result of *Cryptosporidium,* a highly infectious parasite that normally lives in the gastrointestinal tract and is found in human feces. This germ finds its way into pools most often through leaky diapers, or when a child has an "accident" in or near the pool, although older swimmers with diarrhea can unwittingly spread the bacteria as well. Because *E. coli* and *Giardia* respond fairly well to chlorine, they are more likely to be neutralized before they cause widespread gastrointestinal sickness.

However, some germs—such as *Cryptosporidium*—are resistant to chlorine and can live in pools for days. That is why even the best maintained pools can spread illness.

If swallowed by other swimmers, it can cause diarrhea, nausea, vomiting, weight loss, and dehydration. Because there is no effective treatment for this infection, it is particularly dangerous to children with weakened immune systems (such as those taking chemotherapy or steroids, or who have HIV).

According to the U.S. Centers for Disease Control and Prevention, *Cryptosporidium* outbreaks in pools peak during late summer and early fall. An outbreak in just one large public pool can quickly sicken hundreds of children.

Spotting an Unsafe Pool

Alert parents or caregivers often can spot unsanitary pool water before their children go in swimming. Pool water should be clean enough so that objects are clearly visible at the bottom of the pool, and there should be no foaming or bubbling around the sides of the pool. Murky or foamy water may indicate the presence of bacteria or other organic matter.

Anyone who spots fecal matter in a pool should immediately notify the pool attendant or lifeguard, who should ask swimmers to leave the water immediately. The pool water needs to be tested and the chlorine levels raised, depending on the policy and initial chlorine level at the pool.

Prevention

Although chlorine won't keep *Cryptosporidium* in check, it does kill other waterborne germs. Homeowners with pools should test the chlorine and pH levels once a day; heated pools and outdoor whirlpool spas may require more frequent testing and higher levels of chlorine, because bacteria and parasites thrive in warm environments. Depending on the number of swimmers, public pools should be tested at least every few hours if not more frequently.

Healthy swimming behaviors are needed to protect everyone from illness, and to help stop germs from getting in the pool in the first place. The following tips can help keep swimmers healthy:

- Anyone with diarrhea should not swim, and this is especially important for children in diapers.
- Swimmers should not swallow pool water, if possible. In fact, swimmers should try to avoid even having water get in the mouth.
- Everyone should wash hands with soap and water after using the toilet or changing diapers.
- Caregivers should take children for bathroom breaks often without waiting to hear "I have to go."
- Caregivers should change diapers in a bathroom and not at poolside, because germs can spread to surfaces and objects in and around the pool.
- Swim diapers and swim pants are unlikely to prevent diarrhea from leaking into the pool. Even though diapers or swim pants may hold in some feces, they are not leak proof and can still contaminate the pool water. Therefore, it is rec-

ommended that caregivers change a child often and make frequent trips to the toilet. Swim diapers or pants are not a substitute for frequent diaper changing.

- Caregivers should wash child thoroughly (especially the anal area) with soap and water before swimming. Invisible amounts of fecal matter in the anal area can end up in the pool. (See also SWIMMING AND DISEASE.)

port-wine stains A permanent purple-red birthmark that is present at birth and is usually found on the face. The birthmarks are usually sharply outlined and flat, although the surface may sometimes have a pebbly feel. They can range in size from a few millimeters to half the body's surface. They increase in size proportionately as the child grows, becoming darker over time. Port-wine stains may appear alone or as part of a multisystem disorder such as STURGE-WEBER SYNDROME, which also features seizures and eye abnormalities.

Cause

Recent research suggests that the blood vessels in port-wine stains have an abnormal nerve supply, which may account for their enlargement over time.

Treatment

A simple port-wine stain, when it does not occur as part of another syndrome, is still more than a cosmetic problem.

The most successful method of laser treatment is the pulsed dye device, which is popular because it has a low risk of scarring and its effectiveness is not dependent on the doctor's experience. Total clearing with pulsed dye laser treatment is uncommon, but dramatic lightening after a series of treatments is not unusual. Pulsed dye laser treatment decreases the solid color mass, thins thickened lesions, and lightens all types of port-wine stains. By treating patients early in their lives, the psychological burden is eased, the risk of darkening and thickening is reduced, and the risk of bleeding and infection during treatment is eliminated. Over the past 10 years, the pulsed dye laser has been modified several times to lengthen the wavelength and the pulse duration, two changes that have enhanced results significantly.

Until the late 1980s, the argon laser was the treatment of choice for these birthmarks. The laser works by emitting light that is absorbed by the hemoglobin in the dilated blood vessels that make up the birthmark. However, this therapy is limited because of its substantial risk of scarring (the continually delivered laser energy dissipates into the surrounding skin, causing thermal damage). Less-than-optimum treatment can result in pale, immature port-wine stains. In addition, the extent of clearing and the rate of scarring is highly dependent on the skill and experience of the doctor.

positional plagiocephaly (flattened head) A newborn's head is often slightly misshapen during the few days or weeks after birth, because the passage through the birth canal often temporarily elongates a baby's soft skull bones. However, a persistent flat spot either in the back or on one side of his head can result from being put to sleep on his back or by problems with the baby's neck muscles. Fortunately, this condition will correct itself by the time the child is one year old.

Because infants' heads are soft to allow for incredible brain growth in the first year of life, they are susceptible to being molded into a flat shape. The number of flattened head syndrome cases increased sixfold from 1992 to 1994, occurring in about 33 out of every 10,000 births, because of the "Back to Sleep" campaign begun in 1992 by the AMERICAN ACADEMY OF PEDIATRICS (AAP). The AAP recommends that babies sleep on their backs to prevent SUDDEN INFANT DEATH SYNDROME (SIDS), which has dropped by almost 40 percent in the United States since the campaign began. Experts know that the occasional side effect of this sleeping position— a flattened head—is worth preventing SIDS, especially because the condition can be corrected easily.

Premature babies are more prone to positional plagiocephaly because their skulls are softer than those of full-term babies, and they spend a great deal of time on their backs without being moved because of their extreme fragility after birth. A baby may even start to develop positional plagiocephaly before birth, if the baby's skull is pressured by the mother's pelvis or by a twin.

The deformities seen in children with flattened head syndrome should not be confused with those caused by craniosynostosis, a more serious genetic condition that occurs when skull sutures fuse too soon, causing an abnormal skull shape and possible brain damage. A child with craniosynostosis may have deformities in front of the head, a bony ridge in the skull, and a malformed ear.

Treatment

Parents must put their baby to sleep on his back to help prevent SIDS, despite the chance that he may develop a flattened head. Simply repositioning the child's head during sleep is the most common treatment for positional plagiocephaly, which successfully reshapes the child's growing skull over time. The child's direction in the crib should be repositioned (one night with head toward the top of the crib, one night toward the bottom), as well as his head position during sleep (one night with the left side of his head touching the mattress, one night with the right). Even though your child will probably move his head around throughout the night, it is still helpful to alternate sides. However, the AAP does not recommend using any devices that may restrict the movement of an infant's head.

In addition to alternating sides, parents can move the baby's crib to a different part of the room, forcing baby to look at objects in the room from a different position. Parents should also be sure to place the baby on his stomach during the day while he is awake. This not only protects the head but offers a new visual perspective to encourage learning and helps to exercise different muscles.

Doctors may prescribe a custom molding helmet or headband for infants with severe positional plagiocephaly. These work best if started between the ages of four and six months, when a child is growing fast, and are usually less helpful after 10 months of age. By applying gentle but constant pressure on a baby's growing skull, they can redirect the growth of the head. Only a small percentage of babies wear helmets.

As babies grow, they begin to reposition themselves naturally during sleep much more often than they did as newborns, and this allows their heads to be in different positions throughout the night. Most skull-flattening deformities correct themselves by the time the child is a year old; but the rare cases of persistent, severe, or cosmetically apparent deformity can be corrected with reconstructive surgery between 12 and 18 months of age. Plagiocephaly itself does not affect a child's brain or intellectual function.

post-traumatic stress disorder (PTSD) An emotional condition that often occurs after direct or indirect exposure to a terrifying event in which a child witnessed or actually experienced physical harm. Traumatic events that can cause post-traumatic stress disorder (PTSD) include violent assaults, physical or sexual abuse, shootings, natural disasters, or car accidents. One out of 13 Americans will develop PTSD during their lifetime, which is especially common among girls and women, who are about twice as likely as boys or men to develop PTSD. This may be due to the fact that girls and women tend to experience domestic violence, rape, or abuse more often.

Most children with PTSD try to avoid any reminders or thoughts of the trauma, but despite this, they often reexperience the ordeal in intense flashbacks, memories, nightmares, or frightening thoughts. Feelings of guilt from surviving an event in which friends or family died is also often a common feature of PTSD.

Any traumatic event can cause this disorder. Children under age 10 and teenagers through age 21 are more susceptible, beginning either as a sudden response to an event or a gradual development that can become chronic or persistent. Studies indicate that people who live with PTSD tend to have abnormal levels of key hormones involved in the stress response.

Symptoms

Signs usually develop within the first three months after the event, although sometimes they may not appear until months or even years have passed. These symptoms often continue for years following the trauma, or may subside and return if another event triggers memories of the trauma. Symptoms often resemble DEPRESSION, but PTSD is not the same as depression. The symptoms of PTSD include:

- sleeplessness or nightmares
- apathy
- inability to get along with others, particularly in close relationships

- paranoia and distrust
- an unwillingness to discuss the trauma
- persistent, intense fear and anxiety
- irritation or agitation
- concentration problems
- feelings of numbness or detachment
- no longer finding pleasure in previously enjoyable activities
- helplessness
- survivor guilt
- preoccupation with the event
- physical symptoms (headache, stomach distress, or dizziness)
- suicidal thoughts, plans, or gestures

Treatment

Some children can recover from PTSD without treatment, with symptoms fading away within six months. Otherwise, cognitive-behavioral therapy can help, particularly if the trauma was unusually severe or life-threatening. This type of therapy helps a child adopt new thoughts and behaviors to replace negative ones. Temporary medications may be helpful to treat depression and anxiety and can help a child cope with school and other daily living activities. Group therapy or support groups also may sometimes help.

Parents should let a child talk about the traumatic event but should not force a discussion. The child should be reassured that her feelings are normal and that she is not crazy. Parents should let a child with PTSD make simple decisions whenever appropriate, which will help her see that she has control over certain aspects of her life. Children also must be assured that the traumatic event was not their fault and should be encouraged to discuss feelings of guilt. Regressive behavior is common and should not be criticized; sleeping with the lights on or cuddling a stuffed animal is normal and soothing. (See also ANXIETY DISORDERS.)

Prader-Willi syndrome A complex genetic disorder that includes short stature, MENTAL RETARDATION or LEARNING DISABILITY, incomplete sexual development, characteristic behavior problems, low muscle tone, and an involuntary urge to eat constantly. This, coupled with a reduced need for calories, leads to obesity. The disorder is found in children of both sexes and all races and occurs in about one in 14,000 people in the United States. It is one of the 10 most common conditions seen in genetics clinics and is the most common genetic cause of obesity that has been identified.

Although Prader-Willi syndrome (PWS) is associated with an abnormality of chromosome 15, it is generally considered not to be an inherited condition but rather a spontaneous genetic birth defect that occurs at or near the time of conception. The faulty chromosome affects functioning of the hypothalamus.

Newborns with the condition have poor muscle tone and cannot suck well enough to get sufficient nutrients. Often they must be fed through a tube for several months after birth until muscle control improves. Sometime in the following years, usually by preschool age, children with PWS develop an increased interest in food and quickly gain excessive weight if calories are not restricted.

In addition to sometimes extreme attempts to obtain food, children with PWS are prone to temper outbursts, stubbornness, rigidity, argumentativeness, and repetitive thoughts and behaviors. Strategies to deal with these problems usually include structuring the person's environment, implementing behavioral management techniques, and occasionally using drug therapy.

Children with PWS can attend school, enjoy community activities, get jobs, and even move away from home, although they need a lot of help. Schoolchildren with PWS are likely to need special education and related services, such as speech and occupational therapy. In community, work, and residential settings, adolescents often need special assistance to learn and carry out responsibilities and to get along with others.

Children with PWS need around-the-clock food supervision. When they grow up, most affected individuals do best in a special group home for people with PWS, where food access can be restricted without interfering with those who do not need such restriction. Although in the past many patients died in adolescence or young adulthood, preventing obesity will allow a person with PWS to live a normal lifespan.

Diagnosis

Early diagnosis of Prader-Willi syndrome gives parents an opportunity to manage their child's diet and avoid obesity and its related problems from the start. Since infants and young children with PWS typically have developmental delays in all areas, diagnosis may facilitate a family's access to critical early intervention services and help identify areas of need or risk. Diagnosis also makes it possible for families to get information and support from professionals and other families who are dealing with the syndrome.

Many doctors will refer a suspected patient to a medical geneticist who specializes in diagnosing and testing for genetic conditions such as PWS. After taking a history and doing a physical examination, the diagnostician will arrange for specialized genetic testing to be done on a blood sample to evaluate for the genetic abnormality found in people with PWS.

Prader-Willi Syndrome Association   A nonprofit organization that provides a newsletter and other publications, an annual national conference, and chapters throughout the country to provide family support and advocacy. (For contact information, see Appendix I.)

premature babies   An infant (known as a preemie) born before the 37th week of gestation. While some premature babies can survive without special help, many need extra medical care in a neonatal intensive care unit (NICU) for their first few weeks. An NICU is designed to limit stress on the infant and meet basic needs of warmth, nutrition, and protection to assure proper growth and development.

About 9 percent of American infants are born prematurely. Babies who weigh less than three pounds five ounces at birth are most likely to develop complications; any baby weighing less than five and a half pounds needs some special help. Age in premature babies is often defined in the number of weeks after the baby was conceived until the baby is 40 weeks old, which is the average age of a full-term baby.

Cause

There are many causes of preterm delivery; usually, the cause is not within the mother's control. She could have a hormone imbalance, a physically abnormal uterus, or a chronic illness or infection. Preterm delivery also is more likely to occur if a woman is over age 35, under age 19, or carrying multiple babies. Sometimes the cause is simply unknown. Other times, the problem may have been triggered by the mother's lifestyle choices during pregnancy:

- smoking
- abusing alcohol or drugs
- poor nutrition
- not gaining enough weight
- exposure to physical stress
- poor prenatal care

Symptoms

Because they are born before development has been completed, premature infants often have problems with feeding, breathing, maintaining body temperature, and fighting infections. In general, the smaller (and more premature) the baby, the more likely and more serious the problems. Because of modern technology, more than 90 percent of premature babies who weigh a little less than two pounds survive. Those who weigh a little more than one pound have a 40 percent to 50 percent chance of survival, although their chances of complications are greater. They are prone to a number of problems, primarily because their internal organs are not completely ready to function on their own.

Hyperbilirubinemia   This common treatable condition is characterized by high levels of bilirubin, a compound formed from the natural breakdown of blood. The high level of bilirubin causes a yellow discoloration of the skin and whites of the eyes (jaundice) that at very high levels cause brain damage. Jaundiced infants are placed under lights that help the body eliminate bilirubin. Rarely, blood transfusions are used to treat severe jaundice.

Apnea   A condition in which a baby stops breathing, heart rate may drop, and skin may turn pale, purplish, or blue. Apnea is usually caused by an immature area of the brain that controls breathing. Almost all babies born at 30 weeks or less will experience apnea, which becomes less frequent with age (by 50 postconceptional weeks, apnea is rare). All premature babies are monitored for apnea; if it occurs, the baby is gently stimulated to restart breathing. If apnea occurs frequently, the infant may require medication (most commonly caffeine or theophylline) and a special nasal device that blows a steady stream of air into the airways to keep them open.

Anemia Many premature babies do not have enough red blood cells to carry sufficient oxygen throughout the body. This is easily diagnosed in the lab, which can determine the severity of anemia and the number of new red blood cells being produced. Some premature infants require red blood cell transfusions.

Low blood pressure This is a relatively common complication that may occur shortly after birth due to infection, blood loss, fluid loss, or medications given to the mother before delivery. Low blood pressure is treated by boosting fluid intake or giving medication.

Respiratory distress syndrome (RDS) Breathing problems are one of the most common and serious problems of prematurity. With respiratory distress syndrome (RDS), (formerly known as hyaline membrane disease), the infant's immature lungs do not produce enough surfactant, which normally allows the inner surface of the lungs to expand properly when the infant makes the change from the womb to breathing air after birth. RDS is treatable and many infants do quite well.

If premature delivery cannot be stopped, most pregnant women are given medication just before delivery to help prevent RDS. Immediately after birth and several times later, artificial surfactant can be given to the infant. Although most premature babies without enough surfactant will need a ventilator, the use of artificial surfactant has greatly decreased the amount of time one is necessary.

Bronchopulmonary dysplasia (BPD) A lung reaction to oxygen or a ventilator used to treat a lung infection, severe RDS, or extreme prematurity. Preemies are often treated with medication and oxygen for this condition.

Infection This is a threat to premature infants, who are less able than full-term infants to fight germs that can cause serious illness. Infections can be passed on from the mother or be acquired after birth.

Patent ductus arteriosus The ductus arteriosus is a short blood vessel that connects the aorta (main blood vessel leaving the heart) to the main blood vessel supplying the lungs. In an unborn baby, it allows blood to bypass the lungs, since oxygen comes from the mother and not from breathing air. In full-term babies, the ductus arteriosus closes shortly after birth, but it often stays open in premature babies. When this happens, too much blood flows into the lungs and can cause breathing problems and sometimes heart failure. This condition is often treated with a medication called indomethacin, which can successfully close the blood vessel in more than 80 percent of cases. If indomethacin fails, surgery may be required to close the vessel. Maintaining an open ductus is a requirement for the successful treatment of some congenital heart diseases.

Retinopathy of prematurity Abnormal growth of the blood vessels in an infant's eye. About 7 percent of very small premature babies develop retinopathy of prematurity (ROP), and the resulting damage may range from needing glasses to blindness. Experts do not know what causes ROP, but oxygen levels (either too low or too high) are only a contributing factor. Premature babies receive eye exams in the NICU to check for this condition.

Treatment

Premature babies need a great deal of special care to survive. Because they lack the body fat necessary to maintain their body temperature, even when swaddled with blankets, incubators or radiant warmers are used to keep these babies warm. Premature babies also have special nutritional needs because they grow at a faster rate than full-term babies and their digestive systems are immature.

Although breast milk is an excellent source of nutrition, preemies are too immature to feed directly from the breast or bottle until they are 32 to 34 postconceptional weeks old. Most premature infants have to be fed slowly because of the risk of developing an intestinal infection. Breast milk can be pumped by the mother and fed to the premature baby through a gastric tube directly into the stomach. The baby's blood chemicals and minerals are monitored regularly, and the baby's diet is adjusted to keep these substances within a normal range.

Because some studies have suggested that the bright, noisy environment of the NICU was not the best place for seriously ill tiny babies. Many NICUs now try to use soft lighting, a quiet environment, and provide as little disruption as possible. Health care experts and parents try to handle premature babies as slowly and carefully as possible, because they are sensitive to abrupt motions. Handling is important to their development, however, and parents are encouraged to provide skin-to-skin contact in the course of routine care.

After the NICU

After leaving the NICU, infants who were born too soon occasionally still need attention at a high-risk newborn clinic or early intervention program. In addition to the regular well-child visits and immunizations that all infants receive, premature infants also get periodic hearing and eye examinations. Careful attention is paid to the development of the nervous system, including the achievement of motor skills like smiling, sitting, and walking, as well as the positioning and tone of the muscles. Speech and behavioral development are also important in these babies; some premature infants may require speech therapy or physical therapy as they grow up. Infants who have experienced complications in the NICU may need additional care by medical specialists.

For the first few years most children who were born too soon are still small for their age, although their growth *rate* is usually normal. Although a few born prematurely may have permanent problems such as CEREBRAL PALSY, most have no serious long-term effects.

prickly heat An irritating skin rash, also known as heat rash, that is associated with obstruction of the sweat glands and accompanied by prickly feelings on the skin. The medical term for prickly heat, *miliaria rubra*, means "red millet seeds" and refers to the appearance of the rash. A milder form of the condition *(miliaria crystallina)* sometimes appears first as clear, shiny, fluid-filled blisters that dry up without treatment.

Symptoms

Numerous tiny, red itchy spots occur, covering mildly inflamed skin where the sweat collects (especially the waist, upper trunk, armpits, and insides of the elbows).

Cause

While doctors are not completely sure of the mechanism behind the development of prickly heat, it is believed to be associated with sweat that is trapped in the skin.

Treatment

Frequent cool showers and sponging the area with cool water can help ease the itch. Calamine lotion, oatmeal baths, and dusting powder also may ease the discomfort. Clothing should be clean, dry, starch-free, and loose to help sweat evaporate.

Prevention

Slow acclimation to hot weather and avoiding heavy exercise will reduce the chance of prickly heat.

progeria A rare condition characterized by an appearance of accelerated aging in children. The classic type of this disease is the Hutchinson-Gilford progeria syndrome first described in England in 1886 by Dr. Jonathan Hutchinson, and again in 1886 and 1904 by Dr. Hastings Gilford. The condition occurs in about one out of every four million newborns, in both boys and girls of all races. Since the condition was first described, more than 100 cases have been identified around the world. There is no cure or specific treatment available, although the mutant gene that causes the condition has recently been identified.

Children with progeria appear normal at birth, but by 18 months they begin to develop symptoms of accelerated aging. The skin begins to dry and wrinkle, bones become fragile, and most children are bald by the age of four. The children never grow much taller than three feet, and their internal organs also quickly age. Death is usually caused by heart disease or stroke at an average age of 13. Even as teenagers, children with progeria will weigh only 30 to 35 pounds.

Although the disease was first identified in 1886, it has been difficult to study because there are only a handful of patients alive at any one time. About one patient with progeria is born each year in the United States.

Symptoms

The general signs include dwarfism, baldness, a pinched nose, small face and jaw relative to head size, delayed tooth formation, aged skin, stiff joints, hip dislocations, generalized atherosclerosis, and cardiovascular problems. The children have a remarkably similar appearance despite racial background, and they tend to have above-average intelligence.

Cause

The condition is caused by a single misplaced DNA molecule within the human genome that contains some three billion DNA units. The gene was discovered in April 2003 by researchers at the National Human Genome Research Institute. The mutation on a gene called lamin A on chromosome 1 was found in DNA specimens from 18 of 20 progeria patients. A similar study found the gene mutation in two progeria patients. The flaw is a substitution of a single DNA base, when the amino acid guanine is switched to adenine. Lamin A, or LMNA, has already been linked to six other diseases, but the mutation and its effect are slightly different, on a molecular basis, in each of the diseases.

Brothers, sisters, and nonidentical twins are almost never affected in the same family, and the average difference in ages between father and mother is about six years as compared with the national average of about two years. Researchers now believe that progeria is not genetically inherited but develops spontaneously in each patient, although it could be that the mutant progeria gene is transferred to the embryo through a flaw in the genes of the father's sperm. Researchers are now going to study people who live to be very old see if some element of their LMNA gene makes them resistant to the diseases of aging.

Diagnosis

There is no specific lab test, so a diagnosis is based on the physical appearance of the child, usually made during the first or second year of life when skin changes and failure to gain weight become apparent.

A chemical (hyaluronic acid) can be found in much higher levels in the urine of children with Hutchinson-Gilford Progeria syndrome; the same abnormality has been found in Werner syndrome, which is sometimes called "progeria of the adult." Few other diseases are known in which elevated levels of this chemical are found, suggesting that hyaluronic acid may prove to be a useful test for progeria.

Prozac (fluoxetine)   An antidepressant medication that is the only newer drug approved to treat depressed children. Studies suggest that younger people respond to Prozac with very small doses, and that a sizable portion of young people who do not respond to other antidepressants do respond to Prozac.

Introduced in 1988, Prozac was the first of a new class of antidepressants known as selective serotonin reuptake inhibitors (SSRIs), which increase the levels of a neurotransmitter called serotonin. Many people who are depressed have low levels of this chemical and therefore improve when serotonin levels rise.

Like other pharmaceutical interventions for depression, Prozac is usually prescribed as part of a treatment plan that includes psychosocial interventions. Prozac is also approved to treat OBSESSIVE-COMPULSIVE DISORDER in children and teens and to treat major depressive disorder in adults, BULIMIA, and panic disorder. Like all antidepressants, Prozac takes one to three weeks to achieve its full effect.

Results of trials with this medication suggest that Prozac also may be helpful in treating ADHD, although the first-line therapy for ADHD is still Ritalin, Strattera, or Dexedrine (dextroamphetamine).

Side Effects

All antidepressants carry side effects, but Prozac and the other SSRIs cause fewer problems than older antidepressants. Most common side effects include (in the order of frequency) sexual problems, nausea, headache, insomnia, diarrhea, nervousness, and anxiety. Less common side effects include dry mouth, appetite loss, tremor, upper respiratory infection, and dizziness.

The government has issued a public health advisory warning to watch for suicidal thoughts in children and teens at the start of treatment with all newer antidepressants, including Prozac.

Studies suggest that younger people experience slightly different side effects, including restlessness and sweating as the most common complaints followed by drowsiness, dry mouth, and tremors.

Pseudomonas aeruginosa (P. pyocyanea) A species of gram-negative bacteria that has been isolated from wounds, burns, and infections of the urinary tract and that is noted for resistance to disinfectants and antibiotics. The bacilli cause a range of human diseases from MENINGITIS to hospital-acquired wound infections and can cause life-threatening lung infections in children with cystic fibrosis.

Also, this is a very common cause of osteomyelitis of the foot when a child steps on a nail while wearing tennis shoes.

psoriasis A chronic skin disorder affecting more than 4 million individuals, producing silvery, scaly plaques on the skin. The skin condition usually begins in adolescence and affects 2 percent of the population.

The most common type of psoriasis is called "plaque psoriasis" (or *psoriasis vulgaris*), characterized by raised, inflamed lesions with silver-white scales. Other far less common forms include pustular, guttate, inverse, and erythrodermic psoriasis.

The condition is considered to be mild if only 10 percent or less of the body is affected; 10 percent to 30 percent indicates a moderate problem, and psoriasis over more than 30 percent of the body is considered to be severe. The location of the symptoms, more than the extent, influences how disabling the condition may be. Psoriasis only on the palms and soles of the feet can be physically disabling, while psoriasis on the face can be emotionally disturbing. Typically, a person with psoriasis experiences cycles of improvement and flares; the disease can go into remission for periods ranging from one to 60 years.

Cause

The cause of psoriasis is unknown, although researchers believe that some type of biochemical stimulus triggers the abnormal cell growth in the skin. While normal skin cells take a month to mature, patients with psoriasis have skin cells that over-multiply, forcing the cells to move up to the top of the skin in only seven days. As the number of cells builds up, the skin thickens and the extra cells accumulate in raised, red, and scaly lesions. The white scales covering the red lesions are made up of dead cells that are continually shed; the inflammation is caused by the buildup of blood needed to feed the rapidly dividing cells.

Skin trauma, emotional stress, and some kinds of infection may trigger the development of psoriasis. The condition sometimes forms at the site of a surgical incision or after a drug reaction.

While anyone can develop psoriasis, there appears to be a hereditary link and a family association in one out of three cases. It is not known whether just one gene, or a collection, predisposes a person to the condition, but it is believed that one gene modified by others in combination with certain environmental factors produces psoriasis. This may be why there is not one pattern of inheritance from one generation to the next.

Both boys and girls can develop psoriasis at any age, but most patients develop lesions between ages 10 and 35, although a few may contract the disease in infancy or early childhood. Certain races seem more susceptible to developing the condition. Caucasians have the highest percentage, although East Africans are also at risk. African Americans have a low incidence of the disease.

Symptoms

The first lesions of plaque psoriasis appear as red, dotty spots that can be very small; these eruptions slowly get larger, producing a silvery white surface that is shed easily. When forcibly removed, the scales may leave tiny bleeding points. The plaques, which often appear in the same place on the right and left sides of the body, often cover large areas of skin, merging into one another. The most common sites are scalp, elbows, knees, and trunk, although they can be found anywhere on the body. Lesions vary in size and shape from one person to the next, and patches spread over wide expanses of skin can lead to intense itching, pain, dry or cracking skin, and swelling. Body movement and flexibility may be affected.

Potentially more disabling than the physical discomfort is the emotional impact of a disfiguring disease that can produce lack of self-confidence, depression, guilt, or anger.

About 10 percent of patients develop psoriatic arthritis, causing inflammation and stiffness.

Diagnosis

Psoriasis is usually diagnosed by observation. There are no blood tests for the disease, although doctors sometimes examines a skin biopsy under a microscope to confirm the diagnosis. Sometimes small pits in the fingernails, yellow discoloration of the nail, or collections of scaly skin under the nail can help diagnose the condition.

Treatment

There is no cure for psoriasis, but there are treatments that can clear plaques or significantly improve the skin's appearance. Treatment is aimed at slowing the excessive skin division, resulting in remissions lasting up to a year or more. Once the treatment is effective, it is discontinued until the psoriasis returns. Type of treatment depends on the type of psoriasis, its location and severity, patient age, and patient medical history. Dermatologists usually begin with the mildest therapy and work up to the one that is most effective in clearing up the skin problem. No single treatment works for everyone, and each patient reacts differently to the drugs.

Topical medications (emollients, steroids, vitamin D derivatives, anthralin, and coal tar preparations) are used to treat mild to moderate conditions. These may be used alone or in combination with each other, or with ultraviolet light treatments. Regular sunbathing may help clear up a case of psoriasis for some patients because of the exposure to natural ultraviolet-B light.

For more severe cases, the topical treatments above will be combined with psoralen plus UVA, chemotherapy (methotrexate), and oral retinoid medications such as Tegison. Treatments for severe psoriasis are toxic and must be weighed against their potential benefits and risks.

In a new treatment for localized psoriasis, a laser is used to target small plaques. The laser produces high-intensity UVB light at the wavelengths most effecting for clearing psoriasis. Because the light is so intense and the laser can be aimed just at the affected spot, clearing can occur in just six to eight treatments. Cleared areas may remain clear for six to eight months.

On the Horizon

More than 40 experimental drugs are being tested for the treatment of psoriasis and/or psoriatic arthritis. Some of the drugs now in testing represent attempts at improving existing therapies, but many of the innovative drugs are pursuing treatment in a new way, by targeting the immune system's role in psoriasis.

A promising drug in development is Xanelim (developed by Genentech and XOMA). This drug represents the front line of a new generation of psoriasis therapies: biologically engineered drugs that target a very specific part of the immune reaction that takes place in psoriasis. These "biologics," as they are called, hold the promise of being as effective as today's most potent psoriasis treatments but much safer and with fewer side effects. These new treatments target and block specific parts of the body's immune reaction that leads to the diseases. However, they are still under investigation and are not yet approved for psoriasis patients by the U.S. Food and Drug Administration (FDA).

Amevive (alefacept) and Raptiva have both been approved by the FDA. Amevive (alefacept), an injected medication that treats adults with moderate to severe plaque psoriasis, was approved by the FDA in January 2003. Experts believe Amevive works by simultaneously blocking and reducing the cellular component of the immune system that is thought to play a significant role in the disease process.

FDA based its approval of Amevive on the results of two studies of 1,060 adults with chronic plaque psoriasis. Both of these studies showed that a significantly higher percentage of patients receiving Amevive responded to treatment compared to those receiving placebo. In the approved labeling for Amevive, FDA is encouraging physicians to tell patients that they need regular monitoring of white blood cell counts during therapy. The approved labeling states that patients should be told that Amevive suppresses their immune system, which could increase their chances of developing an infection or malignancy. This means that patients should tell their doctor promptly if they develop any signs of an infection or malignancy during treatment.

Females of childbearing age make up a considerable segment of the patient population affected by psoriasis, but no one knows of the effect of Amevive on pregnancy and fetal development, including immune system development.

Phase III trials of the drug Xanelim were promising, but it may be several years before the drug is submitted to the FDA for approval.

puberty, precocious The onset of puberty before age seven in girls and age nine in boys. The signs of the condition include the development of breasts and pubic hair or the beginning of menstruation in girls, and pubic or facial hair, a deepening voice, or enlarged penis or testicles in boys. Acne also can occur with these other changes. Although sexual maturity does not occur at the exact same age for every person, there is a limit to how soon the signs should begin to appear. Girls are five to seven times more likely than boys to develop the condition.

One of the problems with starting puberty at an earlier age is that puberty also triggers a period of rapid growth and weight gain that stops when puberty ends. Because bone growth stops at an earlier age than normal, children with precocious puberty usually do not achieve their potential full adult height. Although they may at first seem tall compared to their classmates, they will stop growing too soon and end up at a shorter height than normal. If untreated, boys typically grow no taller than 5 feet, 4 inches and girls rarely reach 5 feet.

Reaching puberty too early also can be emotionally and socially difficult, because very young children often are not emotionally equipped to undergo the physical changes.

Cause
The onset of puberty is normally triggered by the pituitary gland. Precocious puberty may be caused by a structural problem in the brain, or a problem in the ovaries. However, in most girls, there is no underlying visible medical problem that experts can discover.

When the condition appears in boys, it may be caused by head trauma or a hormone-producing tumor in the pituitary gland or hypothalamus. The condition also may appear along with a condition such as Down's syndrome or untreated hypothy-

roidism. The condition is inherited in about five percent of boys. Precocious puberty early can be passed from father to son or from the maternal grandfather through the mother (who will be unaffected) to the son. Less than one percent of girls affected by precocious puberty have inherited the condition.

Some children develop precocious puberty as a result of exposure to estrogen in drugs or food (called "medicational precocity"). This consists primarily of breast development. Children can be exposed to estrogen if they swallow estrogen-replacement medication or birth control pills. Occasionally, reports suggest that estrogen given to livestock also can cause breast development in children.

Symptoms
The most obvious signs of the onset of precocious puberty are the development of secondary sex characteristics. In girls, the signs of precocious puberty include any of the following signs appearing before age 7:

• breast development

• pubic or underarm hair development

• onset of menstruation

• acne

• body odor

• moody and irritable behavior

In boys the signs of precocious puberty include any of the following signs before age nine:

• enlargement of the testicles or penis

• pubic, underarm, or facial hair development

• deepening voice

• acne

• body odor

• aggressiveness

• inappropriate sex drive

Partial Precocious Puberty
Many children with early signs of puberty are actually experiencing "partial" precocious puberty. Some girls, usually beginning between the ages of six months and three years, may experience breast

development that later disappears, or that may remain without other physical changes of puberty. Other girls and boys may experience early growth of pubic or underarm hair without any other changes in sexual development.

Children with partial precocious puberty may require evaluation to rule out true precocious puberty, but they generally need no treatment and usually will show the other expected signs of puberty at the usual age.

Diagnosis

The physical changes of puberty are usually obvious to a doctor during a routine physical exam. To confirm a diagnosis of precocious puberty, a child's doctor may order blood and urine tests to detect high levels of sex hormones. X rays of the wrist and hand can reveal whether the bones are maturing too rapidly. Imaging and scanning tests such as computerized tomography (CT) scans and magnetic resonance imaging (MRI) can help rule out specific causes of precocious puberty, such as a tumor in the pituitary gland, hypothalamus, brain, ovary, or testicle.

Treatment

The goal of treating precocious puberty is to halt or reverse sexual development and stop the rapid growth and bone maturation that will eventually result in adult short stature. This can be done either by treating the underlying cause of disease (such as a tumor) or normalizing hormone levels with medication to stop sexual development from progressing. Often a tumor cannot be removed, but even when removal is possible, this rarely stops precocious puberty from continuing. Treating an underactive thyroid condition with medication may be effective.

In most cases there is no underlying disease triggering the precocious puberty, so treatment usually consists of hormone therapy to stop sexual development. The currently approved hormone treatment involves synthetic drugs called LHRH analogs, which reduce the secretion of sex hormones within two weeks of administration; symptoms begin to disappear soon after this.

Dramatic results are usually seen within a year of starting treatment with an LHRH analog. In girls,

breast size may decrease and pubic hair may fall out, or there will be no further development. In boys, the penis and testicles may shrink and pubic and facial hair may decrease. A child's behavior usually becomes more age-appropriate as well.

pubic lice   See LICE.

pulse, taking a child's   A child's pulse rate is a measure of the number of times the heart beats per minute. As the heart pushes blood through the arteries, the arteries expand and contract with the flow of the blood, which can be felt in various points in the body. A child's pulse is a measure not only of the heart rate but also the heart's rhythm, and the strength of the pulse (a weak pulse could indicate heart failure, a fast heartbeat in which some beats are too weak to feel, or a low volume of blood in the circulatory system).

A child's pulse rate may fluctuate and increase with exercise, illness, injury, and emotions. Typically, girls over age 12 and women have faster heart rates than do boys and men. Athletes who do a lot of cardiovascular conditioning may have much slower heart rates.

A child's pulse is taken in the following steps:

1. The first and second fingertips are pressed firmly but gently on the arteries until a pulse is felt. Typically, the arteries can be felt either in the wrist or throat.
2. The pulse should be counted for 60 seconds (or for 15 seconds, which is then multiplied by four to calculate beats per minute).

pyloric stenosis   A malformation in the lower part of the stomach (pylorus) through which food enters the small intestine, one of the more common causes of intestinal obstruction during infancy that requires surgery. About one in every 250 babies is affected. An infant with pyloric stenosis has a thickened, stiffened, enlarged pylorus, which prevents food from emptying out of the stomach.

Risk Factors

Pyloric stenosis affects about four times as many firstborn male infants as females. There is a hereditary component; if a parent had pyloric stenosis, an infant has up to a 20 percent risk of developing the same condition. Pyloric stenosis also occurs more commonly in Caucasian infants and in those babies with blood type B or O, usually between two weeks and two months of age.

Cause

Experts suspect that the problem is not congenital, but that infants develop a progressive thickening of the pylorus after birth until it becomes so thick that the stomach can no longer empty properly. Although experts are not sure what triggers the muscle thickening, some researchers suspect that maternal hormones or allergies could be a contributing cause. Others believe that some babies lack receptors in the pyloric muscle that detect nitric oxide, a chemical that induces the pylorus muscle to relax, so that the muscle contracts almost continually, causing it to thicken over time.

Symptoms

Symptoms of pyloric stenosis generally appear around three weeks of age and include projectile vomiting, stool changes, lethargy, failure to gain weight, losing weight, and a rippling belly.

Vomiting   This is usually the first symptom of pyloric stenosis, beginning with simple spitting up that turns into projectile vomiting at the end of a feeding, although in some cases it may be delayed for hours. Rarely, the vomit may contain blood. Sometimes the vomited milk may smell curdled because it has mixed with stomach acid. A baby with pyloric stenosis is usually hungry again soon after vomiting.

Stool changes   Babies with pyloric stenosis usually have fewer, smaller stools because not much food is entering the intestines. The baby may be constipated or produce greasy stools.

Failure to thrive   Because these babies are not getting nourished properly, many babies with pyloric stenosis will stop gaining weight or even begin to lose weight. As their condition worsens, they are at risk for becoming dehydrated. An infant who is dehydrated is listless and will exhibit a sunken soft spot on their heads, sunken eyes, and softened or wrinkled skin on the belly and upper parts of the arms and legs. There may be four to six hours between wet diapers.

Belly ripples   After feeding, babies with pyloric stenosis may exhibit stomach contractions that make noticeable ripples over the infant's belly from left to right as the stomach tries to empty itself against the thickened pylorus.

Diagnosis

Detailed descriptions of a baby's feeding and vomiting patterns plus a description of the vomit can help diagnose pyloric stenosis. During a physical exam, the doctor will try to feel if there is a movable lump about the size of an olive in the infant's belly. If no lump is felt, an ultrasound of the infant's belly will usually be ordered, which can reveal an enlarged, thickened pylorus.

Treatment

Pyloric stenosis is a medical emergency that requires immediate surgical treatment with a pyloromyotomy, in which the thickened muscles of the pylorus are cut, relieving the obstruction. The surgery is performed with general anesthesia and lasts about an hour.

Any dehydration or electrolyte problems in the blood will be corrected with intravenous fluids. After surgery, most babies are able to eat normally very soon, usually feeding again three to four hours after surgery. However, because of swelling at the surgery site, the baby may still vomit a bit for a day or so after surgery. As long as there are no complications, most babies who have undergone pyloromyotomy can return to a normal feeding schedule and be sent home within 48 hours of the surgery. The condition does not usually recur after a complete pyloromyotomy.

rabies An acute viral disease of the central nervous system that is usually transmitted to humans by a bite from an infected warm-blooded animal. Untreated, the disease is a swift, deadly killer, and there is no cure; the only hope lies in giving a vaccine immediately after a bite from a rabid animal.

Although most people tend to associate rabies with dogs, in fact rabies today is more likely to be found in cats. Together with dogs and cattle, these animals make up nearly 90 percent of rabies cases in domestic animals, with horses, mules, sheep, goats, swine, and ferrets making up the rest. However, most cases of human rabies in the United States are caused by bats. Human cases have averaged just three cases a year since 1990; a total of 26 (74 percent) of the 35 human rabies deaths in the United States have been associated with bat-variant rabies viruses. Other wild animals that carry the disease include skunks and raccoons, foxes, mongooses, groundhogs, and some rodents. Rabies has been on the rise in the northeastern United States, increasing dramatically between 1990 and 1993.

Cause
Rabies is actually a form of viral ENCEPHALITIS transmitted through infected animal saliva. The virus is concentrated in the salivary glands, which is why the disease is usually spread by a bite. The virus also invades and damages muscles involved in drinking and swallowing, causing excruciating pain when swallowing liquids. Although suffering from thirst, animal and human rabies victims can be terrified by the sight of water; hence, the other name for the disease—hydrophobia.

Rabies also can be transmitted when infected saliva comes in contact with a cut or skin break. Infected bat droppings also may transmit the disease, as can transplants from patients with undiagnosed rabies.

Symptoms
The incubation period in humans may range from 10 days to more than a year, although 30 to 50 days is average. (Animals usually develop symptoms between 20 and 60 days.) The length of the incubation period seems to depend both on the location of the wound (the farther from the brain, the longer the incubation) and the dose of the virus received. Without treatment, severe bites on the head or upper body could lead to symptoms sooner than a mild scratch on the ankle.

There are two forms of the disease. "Furious" rabies primarily affects the brain and causes an infected animal to be aggressive, highly sensitive to touch, and vicious—the "mad dog" image. "Paralytic" (or "dumb") rabies primarily affects the spinal cord, weakening the animal so that it cannot raise its head or make sounds because its throat muscles are paralyzed. In the beginning stage of paralytic rabies, an animal may seem to be choking. In both forms, death may occur a few days after symptoms appear.

Symptoms in humans are mild at first and worsen over time, starting with an itching or burning at the bite site, followed by malaise, fever, headache, fatigue, and appetite loss. The child begins to grow restless, excitable, anxious, and irritable, with insomnia or depression. The child may begin to hallucinate, salivate, and have periods of intense excitement and painful muscle spasms of the throat induced by swallowing. As time goes on, other signs of nervous system damage, including disorientation or coma, follow. Four or five days later, the patient either may slip into a months-long coma ending in death, or die suddenly from respiratory or cardiac arrest.

Diagnosis

There are no tests that can detect rabies in humans at the time of a bite, and by the time symptoms appear, it is too late for treatment. The transmission of rabies by a bite can be hard to detect.

Treatment

If a child is bitten by a suspected rabid animal, the wound should be immediately washed with soap and water; the bite should be allowed to bleed to help wash out the wound. Medical help is needed at once. (If possible the animal should be trapped and confined.)

Rabies prevention no longer means a series of painful injections in the abdomen. If a child's doctor decides to begin the antirabies immunization, it will involve a monthlong series of five intramuscular injections together with human rabies immune globulin that should be started on the day of the bite. Part of rabies human immunoglobulin is usually injected near the bite area.

Unlike other vaccines, the rabies immunization is administered after exposure to the virus. This unusual technique works because the rabies virus takes a long time to induce disease. Injections of rabies vaccine may prevent the disease from developing in a person bitten by an infected animal. There are currently two vaccines licensed in the United States, both of which work the same way—triggering the immune system to produce antibodies that neutralize the virus before it causes disease. The modern vaccines are highly effective and produce few side effects. It is the only way to treat the disease in humans.

Prevention

A pre-exposure vaccine series is available that is designed for people at high risk for exposure, such as veterinarians, cave explorers, animal handlers, and those who travel to countries where rabies is common. The series is given in three shots.

rash   A temporary group of spots or red, inflamed skin that may include pimples, hives, scales, or wheals that may or may not be itchy. Only rarely does a rash in a child signify a serious underlying problem. Rashes differ so much among patients that even experienced doctors may sometimes have trouble diagnosing the exact cause. A rash from simple diaper irritation could be treated at home, but a rash that occurs together with swollen lymph nodes, fever, and other symptoms could be more serious and requires a doctor's attention.

Other common causes of a rash during childhood might include one of the following:

- *Heat or sun*   In general, children tend to have very sensitive skin that may react to overexposure to either heat or sun, causing conditions such as PRICKLY HEAT or SUNBURN.

- *Allergic reactions*   One of the most common causes of rash in children is an allergic reaction to many different substances, such as plants, nickel, food (peanuts, berries), rubber or latex, and so on. Some children react to a bite from an insect, SCABIES, or tick with a rash.

- *Drug reaction*   Many drugs (especially antibiotics) can trigger a rash in children who are sensitive to them, together with other symptoms. A child who develops a rash soon after taking medication should be taken immediately to a doctor for an assessment.

- *Disease*   Common diseases of childhood typically cause a rash in children, such as SCARLET FEVER, CHICKEN POX, or MEASLES. Other diseases that are not infectious include LYME DISEASE, RHEUMATIC FEVER, and juvenile rheumatoid arthritis.

- *Eczema*   Children who tend to have allergies or asthma may also have eczema, especially if they have sensitive skin.

- *Infestations*   Scabies is a very contagious infestation of tiny mites that tunnel into the skin, causing an intensely itchy rash.

- *Intertrigo*   During hot weather, moisture and heat can be trapped within skin folds, causing a skin rash on arms, knees, neck, diaper area, or armpits.

- *Skin infection*   Several types of rashes are caused by skin infections, including IMPETIGO, a very contagious bacterial skin infection, and RINGWORM, a contagious fungal skin rash.

Treatment

The underlying source of the rash should be treated immediately; in severe cases, a doctor may prescribe an antihistamine or corticosteroid ointment; the latter should not be used without a doctor's supervision. Home remedies can ease the itch. Remedies that may work include:

- *Cool water* Cool compresses can temporarily stop an itch almost immediately; immersion in a tepid (not too cold) oatmeal bath will also stop itching. Colloidal oatmeal bath preparations are available at most pharmacies.

- *Moisturize the skin* After bathing or to help stop the itch, a mild, unscented lotion or cream should be applied to the child's skin.

- *Humidify* During the winter a humidifier can add moisture to the air the child breathes so that the skin does not become too dry; dry skin is usually itchy skin.

- *Comfortable clothing* A child with an itchy rash should wear soft, comfortable clothes to minimize irritation of sensitive skin.

- *No irritating substances* Children with a rash should not use bubble bath or scented soaps, which can further irritate sensitive skin.

reactive airway disease See ASTHMA.

reading Students learn to read by knowing the sounds of letters and knowing the meanings of words (vocabulary), word parts, and groups of words (overall meaning, or semantics). To build this foundation, children need effective reading instruction. The two main approaches to teaching reading today are whole language and PHONICS. The whole language approach focuses on comprehension and is based on the understanding that reading is about finding the meaning in written language. Children learn meanings of words by multiple experiences with words, both written and spoken. A whole language approach to teaching reading can include teaching reading and writing throughout the day in the context of the lesson topics and emphasizing storybooks rather than work sheets. Many writing opportunities are also important in the whole language approach.

In contrast, phonics focuses on the sounds of letters and words. A phonics approach focuses instruction on learning to associate printed letters and combinations of letters with their corresponding sounds. Phonics instruction gives students strategies to unlock or decode words.

A phonics approach to teaching reading can include "sounding out" words as a way of figuring out new words. For example, in a phonics lesson, the word "hat" would be sounded out as "hh-aa-tt." Practice work sheets or exercises focus on letter sounds, matching pictures with spoken words, short vowel/long vowel, or "letter of the week."

Many schools combine both approaches because of a decade of research suggesting that there is no one best way to build students' literacy skills. A balanced approach to teaching reading combines a strong foundation in phonics with whole language methods. Only through more than one kind of instruction can students gain the skills to recognize and manipulate the sounds of letters and words and the skills to understand what they read. Since all children learn differently, only a balanced approach to teaching reading can give all children the skills they need to read well.

Students learn to read in a certain order: First they must understand that words are made up of different sounds, then associate those sounds with written words, and finally decode words and read groups of words. Students who have trouble learning to read need to be specifically taught the relationships of letters, words and sounds, since being aware of letter/sound relationships is the main tool good readers use to decode unfamiliar words.

Each child needs practice to be a fluent reader. Research at the National Institute of Health has found that phonics instruction should be taught as part of a comprehensive, literature-based reading program. Many opportunities for children to read at their own reading level help them to learn to read for meaning and enjoy reading. Highly trained teachers can help children develop good, overall literacy skills, with good vocabularies, knowledge of correct syntax and spelling, reasoning and questioning skills.

Children with language-based learning disabilities have a harder time learning to read because they have a harder time with sounds of letters and words than other children. Research indicates that because phonics instruction focuses on recognizing and manipulating sounds of letters and words, more intense phonics instruction may be helpful for children with learning disabilities.

The ability to read is a fundamental skill for success in life. Reading research has found compelling evidence that children who have a poor start in reading have trouble catching up and develop negative attitudes towards reading, have poor vocabulary growth, and have missed opportunities for development of reading comprehension strategies.

Most children who are poor readers experience early and continuing difficulties in learning how to accurately identify printed words. These students have problems with "sounding out" unfamiliar words, and with developing "sight vocabulary" of words they are able to read fluently and automatically. The ability to develop these skills is necessary for fluent reading and good reading comprehension.

Diagnostic tests can predict with a high degree of accuracy which students in kindergarten and first grade will have difficulty learning to read. These tests can distinguish, with 92 percent accuracy, those children who will read below the 20th percentile at the end of second grade. These tests take as little as ten to fifteen minutes per child, and can be administered by classroom teachers. Prediction of reading disabilities from tests given at the beginning of first grade are more accurate than those administered during the first semester of kindergarten. The results from these objective tests can be supplemented by teacher ratings of behavior and attention.

Identifying reading difficulties early means children have more time to learn to be successful readers. Since reading is learned more easily and effectively during the early years, identifying language-based learning disabilities and providing appropriate interventions will give children more time to learn to read well.

A child identified as needing help will require careful and direct instruction in reading. An effective preventive program may involve several levels of instructional intensity ranging from small groups to one-on-one teaching, depending upon

the severity of the difficulties for each child. In this way, a preventive program can be focused on the children who are most in need. Children with a reading disability/dyslexia will have a positive beginning to their education and a much greater chance for success.

Up to 90 percent of poor readers can increase their skills to "average" with prevention and intervention programs that combine instruction in phonemic awareness, phonics spelling, reading fluency, and reading comprehension strategies provided by well-trained teachers.

Early reading development follows the steps listed below:

Kindergarten

In kindergarten, children are beginning to develop the following reading skills:

- recognize some common words
- name uppercase and lowercase letters
- begin to associate letters and sounds
- recognize poetry
- distinguish reality from fantasy
- can match simple words to pictures
- are aware of whether words begin or end with same sound
- are beginning to be able to break words into syllables
- understand that reading goes from left to right, and top to bottom on the page
- are aware of time sequence in a story

First Grade

In first grade, children are beginning to develop the following reading skills:

- read long and short vowels
- read word families (hat, bat, cat)
- follow simple written directions
- have larger sight vocabulary
- are aware of author, title, and table of contents
- recognize a play
- interpret maps and globes
- identify consonants in words
- can break dictated words into individual sounds

- are aware of root words, endings, compound words, and contractions
- recognize main idea and cause/effect
- draw conclusions

Second Grade

In second grade, children are beginning to develop the following reading skills:

- sound out unfamiliar words based on individual letter sounds
- identify words from contextual clues
- vary pitch and stress when reading aloud
- recognize character, setting, and motive of story
- use library for research
- interpret graphs
- use dictionary
- master harder phonetic skills
- understand root words and endings
- are aware of syllabication

Third Grade

In third grade, children are beginning to develop the following reading skills:

- have growing sight vocabulary and word-analysis ability
- understand homophones
- have increased reading speed
- develop silent reading skills
- distinguish fiction and nonfiction, fact versus opinion
- understand synonyms and antonyms
- recognize author's purpose
- use index
- use encyclopedia
- interpret diagrams

Fourth Grade

In fourth grade, children are beginning to develop the following reading skills:

- begin to develop different reading styles for different types of reading

- expand vocabulary
- understand plot and main idea
- summarize a book or article
- organize study materials
- understand different genres (biography, folktales, science fiction, and so on)
- understand author's point of view
- can read a newspaper

reading disorder, developmental   See DYSLEXIA.

receptive language disorder   A condition in which a child may have trouble understanding certain aspects of speech, such as a toddler who does not respond to his name or the child who cannot follow simple directions. While hearing is normal, these children cannot make sense of certain sounds, words, or sentences. Because using and understanding speech are strongly related, many children with receptive language disorders also have an EXPRESSIVE LANGUAGE DISORDER. Some misuse of sounds, words, or grammar is a normal part of learning to speak. It is only when these problems persist that there is any cause for concern.

reflux, gastroesophageal (GERD)   A disorder that occurs when stomach acid moves backward from the stomach into the esophagus. Gastroesophageal reflux disease (GERD) usually occurs because the muscular valve where the esophagus joins the stomach does not close properly. When the stomach acid comes into contact with the esophagus, it causes a burning sensation. Although many people experience heartburn occasionally, GERD occurs much more often and causes serious discomfort.

Eventually, the reflux of stomach acid damages the tissue lining the esophagus, causing inflammation and pain. No one knows for sure why people get GERD, but more than one million children in the United States have the condition.

Certain foods may be linked to acid reflux, including citrus fruits, chocolate, caffeinated drinks, fatty and fried foods, garlic and onions, mint, spicy foods, and tomato-based foods.

Symptoms

The main symptoms include persistent heartburn and acid regurgitation, although some children do not experience heartburn. Instead, they may have: pain in the chest or stomach; a frequent sour taste of acid, especially when lying down; a hoarse throat; a feeling of burping acid; trouble swallowing; a feeling that food is stuck in their throat; choking feeling; dry cough; or bad breath.

Although a certain amount of reflux is normal in most people, it is sometimes overlooked in infants and children. Acid reflux can cause repeated vomiting, coughing, and other respiratory problems in children as young as newborns. When this happens, it is also called GERD. It is usually caused by an infant's immature digestive system; most infants stop having acid reflux by the time they reach their first birthday. However, some children do not outgrow acid reflux and continue having problems into adolescence.

Diagnosis

Tests may be used to rule out other possible problems besides GERD. A barium swallow radiograph uses X rays to help spot abnormalities such as a hiatal hernia, ulcer, or severe inflammation. An upper endoscopy is one of the best ways to look for esophagus and stomach damage. A doctor may perform a biopsy during the endoscopy to reveal any damage caused by acid reflux or infection and help rule out other problems. An ambulatory pH monitoring exam measures the appearance of any acid in the esophagus. This test is useful in teens with GERD symptoms but no esophageal damage. It also can detect whether the reflux triggers respiratory symptoms, such as wheezing and coughing.

Treatment

Treatment depends on the severity of symptoms, but may include lifestyle changes, medications, and surgery. Children and teens should lose excess weight, eat small meals, wear loose-fitting clothes over the midsection, and avoid food or beverages with caffeine, such as tea and some sodas. In addition, patients should not lie down for three hours after eating, nor should they eat two to three hours before bedtime. The head of the bed should be raised six to eight inches by putting wooden blocks under the bedposts (extra pillows will not help).

Antacids such as Alka-Seltzer or Maalox, which neutralize stomach acid, can help ease mild symptoms. Other medications called H2 blockers are available with and without prescription; they work by blocking the production of stomach acid. More powerful prescription drugs called proton pump inhibitors also reduce the amount of acid the stomach produces and are often recommended by doctors for severe GERD.

For some children, combinations of medications may be the best way to control symptoms. For example, children who get heartburn after eating can try taking both antacids and H2 blockers (the antacid neutralizes the acid in the stomach while the H2 blocker interferes with acid production). By the time the antacid stops working, the H2 blocker has stopped acid production.

Surgery is a last resort for people with GERD and is rarely needed in otherwise healthy children.

reportable disease   Any contagious disease that must be reported by the doctor to the public health authorities, who in turn report some of them to the U.S. Centers for Disease Control and Prevention. Examples of reportable diseases include AIDS, MALARIA, INFLUENZA, POLIO, typhus, YELLOW FEVER, SYPHILIS, GONORRHEA, CHOLERA, and bubonic plague.

respiratory syncytial virus (RSV)   A respiratory illness caused by a type of virus known as a myxovirus that commonly causes upper respiratory infections. Respiratory syncytial virus (RSV) most often attacks infants and very young children. The highest rates of RSV illness occur in infants two to six months old, with a peak at age two to three months.

RSV infections occur all over the world, most often in epidemics that can last up to five months, from late fall through early spring. Since 1990 epidemics have typically begun between late October and mid-December and peaked during January and February. Each year during these epidemic periods, about 90,000 infants and young children are hospitalized with RSV infections, and about 4,500 die. An RSV infection is often carried home by a school-age child and passed onto a younger one, especially an infant. When RSV infects a day-care center, it is not unusual to see every child come down with an RSV infection.

The first infection is the worst, but it does not confer immunity; RSV can also cause serious colds in children who have repeated infections.

Cause

The RSV is spread via contact with droplets from the nose and throat of infected patients when they cough and sneeze. RSV can spread through direct respiratory secretions on sheets, towels, and other items. This infection is a big problem for hospitalized children, who can become seriously ill with PNEUMONIA if they catch RSV.

Air pollution and smoking irritate the throat lining and can make it easier to catch RSV; people who live in areas of heavy industrial pollution or who live with smokers have more serious and longer RSV infections.

Symptoms

Symptoms can range from a mild cold to severe pneumonia and include coughing, wheezing, runny nose, and severe fatigue. Fever is unusual in young babies. Pneumonia is most likely among high-risk patients; occasionally, the infection can be fatal to infants. Symptoms occur four to six days after exposure and may persist for a few days to weeks.

In most cases, babies are not seriously ill; the virus affects infants under age three months most severely, since they have a hard time breathing. All babies except those with other medical problems should recover within a week.

Children are infectious from 24 hours before symptoms appear until two weeks after the cold starts.

Complications

RSV can cause BRONCHIOLITIS in infants, pneumonia in children under age two, or CROUP in children from six months to three years of age. Premature babies who have poorly developed lungs may be quite ill and may survive with permanent lung damage. Babies with heart problems are most at risk; some of these infants can die from an RSV infection. Infants who are not getting enough air into the lungs will have flaring nostrils and dents above and below the breastbone, or in between the ribs, as they struggle to breathe.

Diagnosis

RSV is usually diagnosed on the basis of symptoms; lab tests may be used in cases of severe illness and in special outbreak investigations. If a child has a bad cold, it is not likely that the pediatrician will test for RSV in an office visit. Children admitted to a hospital with pneumonia or bronchiolitis will be tested for RSV.

Treatment

There is no cure for this virus. Rest, high humidity, and clear fluids can help. Fever can be treated with a nonaspirin fever medicine such as acetaminophen. Aspirin should not be used in children with viral illnesses since the use of aspirin in such cases has been associated with the development of REYE'S SYNDROME, a serious ENCEPHALITIS-like illness.

The antiviral drug ribavirin will help a child recover if started in the first few days after symptoms appear. Treatment with this drug is reserved for the most serious cases because of potential side effects; an expensive medication, it is given in the hospital as a mist treatment. Most hospitalized children with RSV do not need ribavirin.

Because RSV often improves on its own, treatment of mild symptoms is not necessary for most children. Antibiotics are not effective.

In instances when children are at extremely high risk for developing RSV, there are medications, such as palivizumab (Synagis) or RSV immune globulin (RespiGam), that may be used to prevent these individuals from becoming infected with RSV.

Before birth, babies typically receive antibodies from their mothers to help fight RSV and other viruses. However, premature babies do not get enough of these virus-fighting antibodies before birth. Synagis and RespiGam provide the natural antibodies that specifically target RSV.

Synagis is recommended for prevention of serious RSV infections in infants with a chronic lung disease often seen in premature infants (bronchopulmonary dysplasia, or BPD) and infants with a history of prematurity (birth before 35 weeks gestation).

RespiGam is recommended for prevention of serious RSV infections in infants less than 24 months of age with BPD and infants with a history of prematurity.

Synagis and RespiGam are not vaccinations, but they can help protect high-risk children under age two from the most serious complications. Injections of either of these drugs are typically given once a month during the RSV season (November through May). One injection protects the baby for one month, so an injection is needed every month during the RSV season to be fully protected.

Prevention

No vaccine for RSV currently exists, although some researchers are testing various versions of a live attenuated RSV vaccine. Because RSV spreads in fluids from the nose and throat of an infected person, washing hands and avoiding touching nose or eyes after contact with someone with RSV can help prevent the spread of the disease. Since a baby is most vulnerable during the first three months of life (especially those born during the winter), it is possible to take some steps to protect the baby by:

- not smoking around the baby
- avoiding crowds
- keeping the baby away from children with obvious colds

respiratory tract infections   Any infection of the upper or lower respiratory tract. Upper respiratory tract infections include the common COLD, LARYNGITIS, PHARYNGITIS, rhinitis, SINUSITIS, or TONSILLITIS. Lower respiratory tract infections include BRONCHITIS, BRONCHIOLITIS, PNEUMONIA, TUBERCULOSIS, and so on.

Retin-A   A synthetic form of vitamin A approved as a prescription ACNE medication. Although Retin-A is in the same family as vitamin A, they are not the same. For many years, different compounds of vitamin A have been included in cosmetics (retinal, retinyl, retinylacetate, or retinyl palmitate) because the government does not consider these ingredients to be drugs. Retin-A, however, is the acid of vitamin A and has unique properties; because it is available by prescription only in the United States, it is not included in any cosmetic skin care product.

Retin-A is extremely effective in treating acne, although there is often a lag time before it is effective. Some teenagers even notice their skin condition worsens after the first two or three weeks before it gets better.

How to Apply

The higher the concentration of Retin-A, the faster and more significant the results. However, it is often irritating, and for this reason many doctors start patients with the milder forms (0.025 percent to 0.05 percent cream every other night, slowly increasing the strength and frequency of application). Higher concentrations of the product work best (0.1 percent), but these are more irritating to the skin.

Teens should first wash the skin thoroughly with a gentle cleanser, pat dry, and wait 15 minutes before spreading a tiny amount of Retin-A cream over the entire face.

Side Effects

Retin-A is a powerful drug, and side effects can include burning eyes and peeling or reddening of the skin that lasts for weeks. This reaction is most common in teens who sunburn easily and who normally have very sensitive skin. Ironically, Retin-A makes the skin more vulnerable to ultraviolet light, causing patients to sunburn more easily. Incorrect use of Retin-A can lead to extreme irritation.

Rett syndrome   A progressive neurological disorder in which children exhibit LEARNING DISABILITIES, poor muscle tone, autistic-like behavior, useless hand movements and hand wringing, lessened ability to express feelings, avoidance of eye contact, a lag in brain and head growth, walking abnormalities, and seizures. Loss of muscle tone is usually the first symptom.

The syndrome occurs in about one of every 10,000 to 15,000 live female births, with symptoms usually appearing in early childhood, between the ages of six months and 18 months. Experts believe that while boys can get Rett syndrome (RS), in boys the condition is fatal and they do not survive much past birth because of the difference in sex chromosomes. Females have two X chromosomes, but only one is active in any particular cell. That means that only about half the cells in a girl's nervous system will actually be using the defective gene. Because boys have a single X chromosome, all of their cells must use the faulty version of the gene, which presumably results in fatal defects.

Rett syndrome follows a tragic and irreversible course. Although the child develops normally for the first months of life, she begins to gradually deteriorate mentally and physically. As the damage to the nervous system worsens, she loses the ability to speak, begins to have trouble walking or crawling, and is shaken by seizures. One of the most striking symptoms is loss of conscious control of the hands, leading to continual, compulsive hand-wringing. Though rarely fatal, Rett syndrome nevertheless leaves its victims permanently impaired.

Predicting the severity of Rett syndrome in any individual is difficult, but in spite of the severe impairments that characterize this disorder, most children with Rett syndrome survive at least into their 40s. Girls and women with Rett can continue to learn and enjoy family and friends well into middle age and beyond. They experience a full range of emotions and show engaging personalities as they take part in social, educational, and recreational activities at home and in the community. However, the risk of death increases with age, and sudden, unexplained death often occurs, possibly from brain stem problems that interfere with breathing.

First described by Dr. Andreas Rett, the condition received worldwide recognition after research by Bengt Hagberg and colleagues was published in 1983.

Symptoms

The child with Rett syndrome usually shows an early period of apparently normal or near normal development until six to 18 months of life. A period of temporary stagnation or regression follows during which the child loses communication skills and purposeful use of the hands. Soon, stereotyped hand movements, gait disturbances, and slowing of the rate of head growth become apparent.

Most girls do not crawl typically but may "bottom scoot" without using their hands. Many girls begin independent walking within the normal age range, while others show significant delay or inability to walk independently. Some begin walking and lose this skill, while others continue to walk throughout life. Still others do not walk until late childhood or adolescence.

A girl's problems may include seizures, which can range from nonexistent to severe, but do tend to lessen in their intensity in later adolescence. Disorganized breathing patterns also may occur and tend to decrease with age. While scoliosis is a prominent feature of RS, it can range from mild to severe.

Apraxia (dyspraxia), the inability to program the body to perform motor movements, is the most fundamental and severely handicapping aspect of the condition. It can interfere with every body movement, including eye gaze and speech, making it difficult for the child to do what she wants to do. Due to apraxia and lack of verbal communication skills, an accurate assessment of intelligence is difficult. Most traditional testing methods require use of the hands or speech, which may be impossible for the girl with Rett. Some children start to use single words and word combinations before they lose this ability.

Cause

Most researchers now agree that Rett syndrome is a developmental disorder rather than a progressive, degenerative disorder as once thought. In October 1999 scientists discovered a genetic mutation on the X chromosome that has been linked to Rett syndrome. This mutation has been found in up to 75 percent of typical and atypical cases of Rett. Continued research will focus on other still unidentified genetic factors which contribute to the condition. Researchers agree that its severity is probably not linked to the exact location of individual mutations on the gene, but to the X inactivation patterns in each affected girl.

The gene produces part of a switch that shuts off production of as yet unidentified proteins. Experts suspect that overproduction of some proteins might cause the nervous system deterioration characteristic of the disease. Discovery of the gene will enable the unraveling of the steps of the disease process and could eventually lead to discovery of drugs to lessen the damage.

Diagnosis

Diagnosing the disorder before the child is four or five years old is often difficult. However, the discovery of the genetic mutation will lead to a genetic test to improve the accuracy of early diagnosis. If combined with an effective therapy, the test might allow doctors to forestall the drastic consequences of the disease.

The condition is most often misdiagnosed as AUTISM, CEREBRAL PALSY, or nonspecific developmental delay. While many health professionals may not be familiar with Rett syndrome, it is a relatively frequent cause of neurological dysfunction in females.

Treatment

There is no cure for Rett syndrome; however, there are several treatment options, including treatments for the learning disabilities and seizures that may occur. Some children may require special nutritional programs to maintain adequate weight.

Rett Syndrome Association, International A support group for parents of children with RETT SYNDROME founded by parents in early 1984 and dedicated to better understanding the condition. Members include parents, relatives, doctors, therapists, researchers, and friends interested in providing a better future for girls with Rett syndrome. International Rett Syndrome Association (IRSA) supports medical research to determine the cause and find a cure for Rett syndrome, increases public awareness of the condition, and provides information and support to families of affected children. (For contact information, see Appendix I.)

Rett Syndrome Research Foundation (RSRF) A nonprofit foundation created in 1999 by six parents of girls with RETT SYNDROME. It is dedicated to finding a treatment and cure. (For contact information, see Appendix I.)

Reye's syndrome A rare, potentially life-threatening condition that often follows a viral illness. Reye's syndrome appears in only about 0.1 case per 100,000 population and is still not well understood. It predominantly affects children between ages four and 16 and occurs more often when viral diseases are epidemic, such as the winter months or after an outbreak of CHICKEN POX or INFLUENZA B. The use of aspirin and other salicylates drugs during viral disease is statistically linked to the incidence of Reye's syndrome, even though there is no conclusive proof.

It was first diagnosed in 1963, when a North Carolina doctor reported an epidemic of 16 fatal cases of an ENCEPHALITIS-like illness during an influenza B outbreak. The condition, which later became known as Reye's syndrome, had been reported as early as 1929 but never before identified as a distinct entity.

The earlier the syndrome is detected, the better the chances for survival. Children who progress to the late stages of the syndrome may have continuing neurological defects.

Symptoms

Symptoms occur several days after a viral infection (either an upper respiratory tract infection, diarrhea, or chicken pox). Although many mild cases may go undetected; severe cases require aggressive care.

Symptoms include rapid breathing, nausea and vomiting, lethargy, irrational behavior, or delirium. In later stages, breathing slows down and the child falls into a coma. The liver may be enlarged, but there is usually no jaundice or fever.

Reye's syndrome can be mild and self-limiting, or (rarely) progress to death within hours. The progression of the symptoms may stop at any stage, with complete recovery in five to 10 days. Although the viral illnesses that appear to trigger Reye's syndrome are contagious, the syndrome itself is not.

Diagnosis

No single diagnostic test to detect Reye's syndrome currently is available. In the late 1960s, however, the U.S. Centers for Disease Control and Prevention developed criteria for diagnosis that included delirium or coma and a liver biopsy that showed fat accumulation in the liver (or high levels of liver enzymes and ammonia in the blood).

Prevention

Aspirin and other salicylate drugs should never be used to treat viral diseases such as chicken pox or influenza, and aspirin is not recommended in any illness contracted by children under age 12.

Treatment

Children with Reye's syndrome are usually treated in a hospital and may require intensive care. Treatment is supportive, since there is no way to "cure" the problem. The clinical care team focuses on making sure the patient maintains proper fluid and electrolyte balance, eats well, and maintains a healthy cardiorespiratory system. A respirator may be necessary if breathing becomes too slow; the body may be cooled and barbiturates given to slow metabolism and lower intracranial pressure. Small quantities of insulin may be given to increase glucose metabolism, corticosteroids to reduce brain swelling, and diuretics to increase fluid loss.

Over the years the prognosis for children with Reye's syndrome has improved; early diagnosis and better treatment have reduced the mortality rate to about 20 percent in recent years. Incidence of Reye's syndrome has fallen dramatically since its discovery.

rheumatic fever An inflammatory disease that may appear as a delayed reaction to inadequately treated strep throat, which can damage the heart. About 1 percent to 3 percent of untreated children come down with rheumatic fever from 10 days to six weeks after getting over a strep throat or SCAR-LET FEVER. Rheumatic fever usually appears in children between five and 18 and may affect the brain, joints, skin, or other tissues. Once diagnosed, the disease will tend to recur whenever the child gets a strep infection.

By the 1980s, the use of penicillin led to a dramatic drop in rheumatic fever in the United States. However, the disease has not been eradicated; today it involves a much more severe form that causes heart damage and death. Since 1985 there have been outbreaks in 24 states, especially Utah, Ohio, and Pennsylvania.

Researchers believe the resurgence can be traced to a reemergence of certain strains of bacteria (group A strep). Of the 80 different strains of group A strep, only a few can cause rheumatic fever. One of these strains of virulent bacteria killed Muppet creator Jim Henson in 1990.

Cause

Rheumatic fever is a delayed complication of group A strep infection, usually following either a strep throat or scarlet fever. It occurs because the patient's body creates antibodies to get rid of toxins produced by the strep bacteria; in the process, those antibodies mistakenly attack the host's own tissues in the joints, heart, skin, or nervous system. Scientists are not sure why some people develop rheumatic fever, but it may be a combina-

tion of the type of bacteria and the genetics of the infected person.

Symptoms

The onset of the disease is usually sudden, usually about one to eight weeks after recovery from scarlet fever or a sore throat. Early symptoms include fever, joint and muscle pain and swelling, nose bleeds, stomach pain, and vomiting. Joint pain usually affects the knees, hips, wrists, elbows, and shoulders and may move from one site to the next. Other symptoms include palpitations, chest pain, and heart failure.

Late signs of rheumatic fever are a clumsiness and awkwardness; as the symptoms progress, the child develops irregular body movements or twitching that can become severe, sometimes including the tongue and facial muscles. This group of symptoms is called "Sydenham's chorea" or "St. Vitus' Dance." Fortunately, these movements do not last long and disappear without long-term damage.

Although most symptoms disappear within weeks to months, half the time the condition damages the heart valves. The mitral valve of the heart is most often affected, although the aortic valve also may be damaged. Occasionally, the heart muscle itself and the outside covering of the heart may become inflamed. In the most severe infections, heart failure may result. This severe heart damage most often occurs in children who have several attacks of rheumatic fever, which is why it is so important to prevent future repeated attacks with prophylactic antibiotics.

Diagnosis

Rheumatic fever is hard to diagnose because it resembles so many other illnesses; lab studies, throat culture, and an electrocardiogram can help. Doctors may use a variety of criteria, including evidence of previous group A strep infection.

A diagnosis of rheumatic fever requires one (and preferably two) of the following symptoms:

- joint pain
- clumsy movements lasting from three to eight months
- inflammation of the heart muscle
- painless swellings under the skin over the joints

- rash (flat and painless)
- fever of at least 100.4°F

Treatment

Severe restriction of regular activity, together with the administration of painkillers and penicillin to eliminate any remaining strep from the previous infection. Steroids or salicylates may be used depending on the severity of the joint pain. Antibiotic treatment may be continued daily for many years to prevent recurrences of rheumatic fever, which are most likely to occur during the first three years after the initial attack. Antibiotics are usually continued until the child reaches age 18. While bed rest used to be part of treatment, it is no longer considered to be helpful.

Complications

Heart inflammation occurs in about half of all patients and can lead to congestive heart failure. It is one of the most common causes of the need for heart valve replacement.

rheumatoid arthritis, juvenile   See ARTHRITIS, JUVENILE RHEUMATOID.

rickets   A bone disease caused by a deficiency of vitamin D, or by an inherited problem in metabolizing the vitamin. Because sunlight is important in converting a substance in the skin to vitamin D, lack of sun exposure can also lead to rickets. Rickets is rare in the United States because it is usually easy to prevent.

Risk Factors

Infants who are born prematurely or who have dark skin, and babies who are breast-fed by poorly nourished mothers or who are unexposed to the sun, are all at higher risk for developing rickets.

Symptoms

The most obvious sign of advanced rickets is bone deformity, with the legs bowing or turning inward. Other skeletal problems may include enlarged ankles, knees, or wrists, curvature of the spine, and bending of the ribs. There may be pelvic pain and muscle weakness, slowed development, restless-ness and irritability, and very thin skull bones. Older infants may have flattened square skulls whose fontanels (soft spots) on the head may remain open for long periods. Other symptoms include diarrhea, bone fractures, respiratory infections, and poor tooth development.

Diagnosis

X rays, blood tests, and observation of deformities are all used to diagnose rickets in infants.

Treatment and Prevention

Vitamin D supplements in therapeutic doses is the treatment of choice. Rickets can be prevented by making sure the infant is getting enough vitamin D, which is not difficult in the United States because virtually all cow's milk and all standard infant formulas are manufactured with added vitamin D. In addition, supplements are available for premature babies, vegetarians, and others who may not otherwise get enough vitamin D. Doctors often recommend vitamin D supplements to nursing mothers who are also vegetarians and who have dark skin. Foods that are high in vitamin D include liver, some fish, cod liver oil, egg yolks, butter, and vitamin D-fortified milk, margarine, and cereal.

rickettsial infections   Diseases caused by the bite or feces of insects carrying parasitic microorganisms called rickettsia. These diseases include ROCKY MOUNTAIN SPOTTED FEVER and various forms of typhus. Most rickettsial infections cause a fever and rash, although the fatality rate differs from one variety of illness to the next.

ringworm (tinea)   A skin infection caused by a fungus that can affect a child's scalp, skin, fingers, toenails, or feet. The disease has nothing to do with either worms or rings. Scalp ringworm is the most common fungal infection in children.

Cause

Ringworm is spread by direct skin-to-skin contact with infected people or pets, or by indirect contact with items such as barber clippers, shower stalls, or floors. Children can get ringworm from playing with infected dogs or cats, or from sharing combs, brushes, headphones, towels, pillows, hats, or sofas.

Symptoms

The infection usually begins as a small pimple that gets larger and larger, leaving scaly patches of temporary baldness; infected hair is brittle and breaks off easily. Sometimes there is a yellow cuplike crusty area. The infection usually appears 10 to 14 days after contact.

Ringworm of the scalp (tinea capitis) involves scaly, temporary bad patches with dandruff-like white scales. The hair may be dull, and the infection may affect only one part of the scalp or may spread over the entire head. A severe case may include fever and swollen glands below the hairline.

Ringworm of the nails causes thick, discolored, brittle, or chalky and friable nails.

Ringworm of the body (tinea corporis) causes a flat and ring-shaped lesion; the edge is red and may be dry and scaly, or moist and crusted. The center area is clear and appears normal. Symptoms occur four to 10 days after contact. The rings can appear on face, legs, arms, or trunk.

Ringworm of the foot appears as a scaling or cracking of the skin, especially between the toes.

Diagnosis

Microscopic inspection of infected hair or skin scraping will reveal certain characteristics of the fungus. The doctor may use an ultraviolet light to diagnose ringworm.

Treatment

Antifungal medication such as griseofulvin can be given by mouth or applied to the skin. An antifungal ointment applied directly to the scalp will stop the ringworm from spreading to other areas of the head. Boggy raised areas of the scalp will require a special cream and a cotton cap to cover the scalp until the areas dry. The infected hair will need to be clipped and a special shampoo used.

Body ringworm is easier to treat; a variety of antifungal creams will work. The patient should wash well with soap and water and remove all scabs and crusts. Antifungal cream should then be rubbed into lesions.

Prevention

Children should not share towels, hats, combs, or clothing of an infected person. Good grooming and hygiene and frequent checks of a child's scalp can prevent the disease. Once an infection has been diagnosed, all contaminated articles must be cleaned to prevent further infection. Combs, brushes, hats, scarves, and bedding must be cleaned in hot soapy water.

Ritalin (methylphenidate) A medication prescribed for children with an abnormally high level of activity, or ATTENTION DEFICIT HYPERACTIVITY DISORDER (ADHD). About 3 to 5 percent of the general population has the disorder, which is characterized by agitated behavior and an inability to focus on tasks. This central nervous system stimulant has effects similar to but more potent than caffeine—but weaker than amphetamines. It has a notably calming effect on hyperactive children and a "focusing" effect on those with ADHD.

Scientists think ADHD occurs in part because certain receptors in the brain involved in focusing attention and reining in impulsiveness fail to respond to dopamine and norepinephrine, the brain's natural neurotransmitters. It is the interaction between these chemicals and the brain's receptors that helps most people stick with tedious chores, or rein in inappropriate impulses. Researchers think that drugs like Ritalin boost the level of these brain chemicals and stimulate the inhibitory receptors—which is why a stimulant drug can increase inhibition. The drugs enter the body quickly, curing nothing but helping a child focus on the important work of learning.

Although the drug clearly reduces the symptoms of ADHD, and many students have been taking the drug for years, no studies have continued long enough to see if it has a lasting effect on academic performance or social behavior. Moreover, a positive response to Ritalin does not automatically mean a child suffers from ADHD. Stimulants can temporarily sharpen almost anyone's focus.

In fact, while most experts agree that medication can help, it is not the only solution—parents and teachers need to learn new ways (such as rewards and consequences) to teach their children how to focus and sit still. First introduced in the 1940s, Ritalin is usually prescribed as a part of a treatment plan that includes educational and psychosocial interventions for children with behavior characterized by:

- moderate-to-severe distractibility
- short attention span
- hyperactivity
- impulsivity

The widespread use of Ritalin in children is not without controversy. Some experts are vehemently opposed to medicating children who are deemed to be inattentive or active for a "normal" classroom. However, there is no specific evidence that clearly establishes the mechanism by which Ritalin produces its mental and behavioral effects in children. Because a diagnosis of ADHD itself is not always straightforward, critics argue that far too many children who are simply extremely energetic are given a diagnosis of ADHD and medicated.

A doctor should prescribe Ritalin only after medical, psychological, behavioral, and educational assessments. The doctor or therapist should talk both to parents and the child and get information from teachers before prescribing stimulants.

Dosage

Closely monitored treatment with stimulants (Ritalin is one of four commonly prescribed, and its use has increased 700 percent in one decade) can erase enough symptoms of ADHD to eliminate the diagnosis for 82 to 85 percent of children. While most parents give their children a typical twice-daily dose, one recent government study suggests that three times a day works better, with a night-time dose about half the size of the first two.

It may take up to one month for the medication to achieve its maximum effect in children, and 30 minutes to take effect in adults. Medications like Ritalin are usually taken for as long as it is helpful or necessary. While there has been an increase in the number of stimulant prescriptions for children under five, there is no evidence that these drugs are safe or effective when used on young children.

Risk of Abuse

Because of its stimulant properties, however, there have been reports of Ritalin abuse by adults who turn to the drug for its stimulant effects: appetite suppression, wakefulness, increased focus and attentiveness, and euphoria. When abused, the tablets are either taken orally or crushed and snorted. Some abusers dissolve the tablets in water and inject the mixture, although this can cause problems if insoluble fillers in the tablets block small blood vessels.

Because stimulant medicines such as Ritalin have the potential for abuse, the U.S. Drug Enforcement Administration (DEA) has placed stringent, Schedule II controls on their manufacture, distribution, and prescription. For example, the DEA requires special licenses for these activities, and prescription refills are not allowed. States may impose further regulations, such as limiting the number of dosage units per prescription.

Side Effects

Common side effects include decrease or loss of appetite, nervousness, sleep problems, weight loss, and dizziness.

Contraindications

Ritalin should not be used in children with anxiety, tension, agitation, irregular heart rhythms, severe angina pectoris, or glaucoma, or in anyone with motor tics or a family history or diagnosis of TOURETTE'S SYNDROME. Although a relationship has not been established, suppression of growth (such as weight gain and/or height) has been reported with the long-term use of stimulants in children. Therefore, patients who need long-term therapy should be carefully monitored; it may be a good idea to withhold the drug on weekends and during school holidays.

Rocky Mountain spotted fever A rare infectious disease caused by the parasite rickettsia (similar to bacteria) and characterized by a spotted rash. The disease is transmitted from ticks to rabbits and other small mammals, most often in wooded areas along the Atlantic coast. The rickettsia are carried by the dog tick in the eastern United States and by the wood tick in the Rocky Mountain states; the lone star tick is sometimes a carrier in the West.

The disease gets its name from its discovery in the Rocky Mountain lab, but its incidence of the disease has been rising steadily since 1980; there are more than 1,000 cases reported each year all over the country.

Diagnosis

Diagnosis may be difficult because the disease resembles several other infections. The diagnosis can be confirmed by taking at least two different blood samples several weeks apart and identifying antibodies against the infection. Because it usually takes many days for these tests to show positive results, treatment generally begins before test results are available.

Symptoms

Mild fever, loss of appetite, and slight headache may develop slowly about a week after a tick bite. However, sometimes symptoms appear suddenly—high fever, prostration, aching, tender muscles, severe headache, nausea, and vomiting. Two to six days after symptoms appear, small spots appear on wrists and ankles, spreading centrally over the rest of the body. As the infection progresses, the original red spots may begin to look more like bruises or bloody patches under the skin. The illness subsides after about two weeks, but untreated cases with very high fever may be fatal as a result of PNEUMONIA or heart failure.

Treatment

Before antibiotic treatment was available, between 20 percent and 30 percent of patients would die. Today, drugs such as tetracycline or chloramphenicol usually cure the disease. Treatment in an intensive care unit may also be necessary for children with abnormal bleeding or for complications that affect the brain, heart, lungs, liver, or kidneys.

Prevention

People in tick-infested areas should use insect repellent and examine themselves daily for ticks.

Ronald McDonald Houses A group of special houses around the world which provide a "home away from home" for families who need a place to stay while a sick child in the family is cared for at a nearby hospital. To date, more than 10 million families with sick children have stayed at a Ronald McDonald House, saving more than $120 million in housing and meal costs.

Dedicated administrative and volunteer staff focus on the family so the family can focus on the needs of their sick child. Families support and coach each other, and children, often self-conscious and embarrassed about their illnesses, feel at home in the warm and nurturing environment.

The first Ronald McDonald House opened in Philadelphia in 1974 with the efforts of Fred Hill, a Philadelphia Eagles football player. When his daughter Kim was diagnosed with leukemia, Hill and his wife camped out on hospital chairs and benches, eating food from vending machines. They noticed other families, many who had traveled great distances, suffering the same fate.

Hill was introduced to Dr. Audrey Evans, a pediatric oncologist at Children's Hospital in Philadelphia who had dreamed of providing temporary housing for families like the Hills. Along with considerable help from local McDonald's franchisees and Hill's Eagle teammates, Hill and Dr. Evans founded the first Ronald McDonald House.

roseola (exanthem subitum) A common infectious disease of early childhood that primarily affects youngsters aged six months to two years. Only about a third of children with the infection have any symptoms, and all children recover completely.

Cause

The source of this infection was not known until 1986, when scientists discovered that the cause was human HERPES virus-6 (HHV6). Still, its etiology is not fully understood. Because scientists have found HHV6 in the saliva of healthy children, it is believed that the virus may be spread through contact with saliva of family members or other children who carry the virus but do not have symptoms.

Research suggests that after an active infection, HHV6 can become latent, hiding in the body to reappear later to cause other illnesses. Some scientists suspect it may be linked to the development of chronic fatigue syndrome.

Symptoms

Most cases of roseola occur in spring and summer. It is characterized by the abrupt onset of irritability and fever, which may climb as high as 105°F. By the fourth or fifth day, the fever breaks, dropping to normal. At about the same time, a rash appears on the body, often spreading quickly to the face, neck, and limbs, and then fading away after a day or two. Other symptoms may include a sore throat, enlarged lymph nodes, and occasionally a febrile seizure.

Diagnosis

Roseola is usually diagnosed by noting symptoms and ruling out other causes of high fever. Tests have been developed to look for both the virus and its antibodies, but these are available only for research purposes.

Treatment

Because this is not a serious disease at all and will fade away on its own, there is no specific treatment other than acetaminophen for fever, rest, and fluids.

rotavirus The common name for a family of viruses that share several features. The group A rotaviruses are the most common cause of severe diarrhea in children, striking 130 million people a year. It causes a diarrhea so severe that 870,000 children die from this virus around the world every year.

While few U.S. children die, the disease still sends 50,000 of them to the hospital every year. If an infant or toddler develops diarrhea in the winter, there is a good chance that a rotavirus is the culprit.

By age four, most people have been infected and developed antibodies to the virus. While the disease is not particularly deadly in the United States among children with healthy immune systems, rotavirus in the developing world is often fatal because the children are already malnourished when they become infected. In the United States, the chance a child will be hospitalized with rotavirus is one in 40, and one in every 800 hospitalized children will die.

The rotavirus season begins in late fall and ends in the spring.

Cause

Rotavirus invades the cells of the small bowel, preventing the absorption of liquids and causing a severe diarrhea. While the rotavirus also infects animals, scientists do not believe it is passed from pets to humans. The virus is thought instead to be spread by the fecal-oral route. The virus must be swallowed in order for it to infect the digestive tract. Children who are infected once can be infected again.

Symptoms

Symptoms develop quickly; most babies begin with vomiting and a low fever followed by watery diarrhea lasting from three to eight days. The child is infectious until the diarrhea stops. It is not unusual for a child to experience as many as 20 vomiting and 20 diarrhea episodes a day.

Diagnosis

Physicians can diagnose rotavirus from symptoms alone, noting the age of the child and time of year. A new test of stool samples can detect rotavirus in 15 minutes.

Treatment

There is no cure for rotavirus infection. Nonprescription antidiarrhea medicine should not be given to infants and young children. Infants with severe dehydration and vomiting require intravenous-fluid replacement.

Prevention

Although a vaccine for rotavirus was approved by the U.S. Food and Drug Administration (FDA) in August 1998, it was abruptly withdrawn in 1999 after seven months of use because nine infants developed bowel obstruction after being vaccinated. This was more than double the cases reported in the previous seven years. Within the first 14 days after vaccination, the risk of obstruction was 10 times higher than normal, according to research, and within the first seven days after vaccination, the risk was 14 times higher than normal.

The AMERICAN ACADEMY OF PEDIATRICS had recommended routine use of the vaccine in November 1998, and the Centers for Disease Control (CDC) included it in the schedule of routine vaccinations for children in January 1999. But on October 22, 1999, the Advisory Committee on Immunization Practices (ACIP), after a review of scientific data from several sources, concluded that bowel obstruction occurs with significantly increased frequency in the first one to two weeks after the rotavirus vaccine is given, particularly following the first dose. Therefore, vaccination of infants is no longer recommended. Children who received rotavirus vaccine and remain well are not now at increased risk for bowel obstruction.

roundworms A class of elongated, cylindrical worms also known as nematodes that include half a dozen types that affect humans. The most common type affecting children are PINWORMS. In many cases, the adult worms live in the human intestines without causing symptoms unless there are many worms present. Most infestations are treated relatively easily with ANTIHELMINTHIC DRUGS.

rubella See GERMAN MEASLES.

rubeola See MEASLES.

Sabin vaccine   See POLIO VACCINE.

salicylic acid   A drug used to treat a variety of skin disorders, including DERMATITIS, ECZEMA, PSORIASIS, ICHTHYOSIS, ACNE, and WARTS. The drug is also sometimes used for fungal infections. For the treatment of warts, salicylic acid pads can be very effective; it is important not to cut too large a square to place over the wart at the risk of irritating the surrounding skin. The perimeter of the wart should be lightly coated with petroleum jelly to protect the adjacent skin.

Side Effects

This drug may cause inflammation and skin ulcers if used for a long period of time or if applied to a large area of skin.

Salk vaccine   See POLIO VACCINE.

salmonella poisoning   Known medically as salmonellosis, this major type of food poisoning is caused by bacteria that multiply rapidly at room temperatures. Every year about four million cases of salmonellosis are reported in the United States. Children are the most likely to get salmonellosis, and young children are among those most likely to have severe infections. Experts estimate that about 600 people die each year with acute salmonellosis.

Salmonellosis is very common in this country; bonemeal, fertilizer, and pet foods all may be implicated in the spread of the disease. In particular, recent outbreaks have been linked to chickens and eggs; it is estimated that 35 percent of all chickens in processing plants harbor the bacteria.

The largest outbreak ever recorded occurred in 1994 and involved more than 200,000 Americans. In this case, commercially pasteurized ice cream premix was contaminated by bacteria during transport to a Minnesota ice cream plant in tanker trailers that had previously carried nonpasteurized liquid eggs. The outbreak ended only after sales of the ice cream were stopped.

Unfortunately, salmonella resistant to standard antibiotics used to treat infection in children are emerging across the country. Between 1996 and 1998 doctors recorded 13 cases of salmonella infection resistant to the antibiotic ceftriaxone. Another possible 28 cases occurred in 1999. Because there are several million salmonella infections each year, researchers believe this means that several thousand are probably caused by the ceftriaxone-resistant strain.

Cause

Salmonellosis is caused by infection with the *Salmonella* bacteria; even extremely small amounts can cause food poisoning. The incidence of salmonellosis appears to be spreading in epidemic proportions. Bacteria are now commonly found in eggs and poultry. It is also found in raw meat, fish, raw milk, bonemeal, fertilizer, and pet foods as well as carried by small pet turtles and in marijuana. It also can be transferred to food from the excrement of infected animals or people. One type of the bacterium (*S. enteritidis*) has been found in the eggs of chickens with the disease.

Symptoms

While tiny amounts of the bacteria can be ingested without harm in otherwise healthy children, a minimal amount can cause symptoms within 12 to 72 hours. Symptoms vary, depending on the amount of bacteria ingested, but include headache, nausea and vomiting, fever, stomach cramps, and diarrhea. The illness usually lasts four to seven days, and most children recover without treatment. However, some may have such severe diarrhea that hospitalization is required. In these children, the *Salmonella* infection may spread from the intestines to the bloodstream and then to other body sites; it can be fatal unless the child is treated promptly with antibiotics, especially in infants or children with compromised immune systems.

Diagnosis

Because many different kinds of illnesses can cause diarrhea, fever, or abdominal cramps, determining that *Salmonella* is the cause of symptoms depends on lab tests to identify the germ in the stool of an infected child. Once *Salmonella* has been identified, further testing can determine its specific type, and which antibiotics could be used to treat it.

Treatment

As with most types of food poisoning, there is no specific treatment for mild cases. Children should eat a bland diet and drink plenty of fluids to prevent dehydration. Antibiotics should be given only in cases of severe infection, or if there is an indication of bacteria in the blood.

Prevention

Proper handling and cooking of contaminated food will kill the bacteria, and proper refrigeration and cooking methods for meat and eggs should be observed at all times. Eggs should be refrigerated and not used raw (such as in eggnog); children should not be allowed to lick batter that contains raw eggs. Raw chicken should never touch other foods or utensils during preparation, and cooks should wash hands after touching raw chicken.

Researchers have developed a bacteria mixture that, when sprayed on newly hatched chicks, blocks the growth of salmonella in their intestines. Industry and health officials hope it will cut down on the amount of salmonella found in raw chicken and lessen the threat of food poisoning from undercooked chicken. The product (Preempt) is made up of 29 healthy, nonharmful bacteria naturally present in adult birds. Newly hatched chicks sprayed with the mixture peck at their wet feathers and ingest the solution. The culture then grows inside the chicken and eliminates other microbes,

preventing salmonella bacteria from attaching to the chicken's intestines. In tests of 80,000 chickens, seven percent of the untreated birds developed salmonella—but none of the treated birds became infected. Farmers who use Preempt must not feed their birds preventive antibiotics that could kill the beneficial microbes. United States Dairy Administration (USDA) researchers say lab tests show the mixture also looks promising in the fight against other germs that infect chicken, including CAMPYLOBACTER, listeria, and ESCHERICHIA COLI.

salmonellosis   See SALMONELLA POISONING.

SARS   See SEVERE ACUTE RESPIRATORY SYNDROME.

scabies   A fairly common skin infestation caused by the mite *Sarcoptes scabiei,* which burrows into the skin and lays its eggs. Scabies infect children from all socioeconomic levels. Clusters of outbreaks are sometimes seen in schools or child-care centers.

Cause

Scabies mites are passed by direct skin-to-skin contact; indirect transfer from underwear or sheets can occur only if these have been contaminated right beforehand by infected people. Hatched mites can pass from one individual to another simply by direct contact. A child can continue to spread scabies until the mites and their eggs have been destroyed.

Symptoms

The most common symptom is an intense itch (especially at night). Tiny gray, itchy swellings appear on the skin, between the fingers, on wrists and genitals, waist, thighs, nipples, breasts, lower buttocks, and in the armpits. Reddish lumps may later appear on arms, legs, or trunk.

Symptoms may appear from two to six weeks in people who have not been previously exposed to scabies. Those who have had cases in the past may show symptoms within one to four days after a reexposure.

Treatment

Insecticide lotion such as prescription permethrin or crotamiton should be applied to all skin below the child's head to kill the mites. Itching may continue for up to two weeks longer, but this is not necessarily a failure of treatment or a reinfestation. All members of the family should be treated at the same time.

Those with symptoms should be treated with a second course of lotion seven to 10 days later, followed by a cleansing bath eight hours after application, and a change of clothing.

Prevention

Scabies can be prevented by avoiding physical contact with an infested person or contaminated belongings.

scalded skin syndrome   First recognized as a distinct condition in the mid-1800s, this disease has been incorrectly called by many different names, including Ritter's disease or toxic epidermal necrolysis. Only recently was its cause discovered to be a toxin-producing strain of *Staphylococcus aureus.*

This syndrome is primarily found in newborns and young children, where it has a fatality rate of less than 4 percent. Epidemics have occurred in contaminated nurseries, and the strain of bacteria may be transmitted by a carrier with no symptoms.

Symptoms

First symptoms usually include evidence of a primary staphylococcal infection, such as IMPETIGO, CONJUNCTIVITIS, EAR INFECTION, or sore throat with fever. The center of the face gets tender and the skin around the mouth becomes red, weeping, and crusting. The trunk also may be affected. In some patients the rash stabilizes, while in other cases flaccid blisters begin to develop all over the skin within 24 to 48 hours. Large areas of skin slough off, and hair or nails may be lost.

Treatment

Prompt administration of antibiotics is usually given in the hospital, since children often appear very ill with low fluid levels and risk of secondary infections. The skin is treated with wet dressings for crusted sites and antibiotic ointments. Patients usually heal without scarring within a week.

scalding   Scalding is one of the most common, and potentially serious, injuries to occur in the home. One in every 200 children is likely to have been scalded severely enough to require hospital admission by the age of five. Children under the age of four are three times more susceptible to scald injury than the rest of the population. Scalds account for 75 percent of all burns to young children, and they are the second leading cause of accidental death to children under the age of four.

Thousands of children are hospitalized each year for scald burns, which are among the most painful and disfiguring injuries. Severe scalds can require skin grafts and may leave severe scars.

Microwave ovens are usually perceived by many families as "safer" than conventional ovens and stoves, and many families allow children to use the microwave but not other heating appliances. In fact, microwave ovens are more dangerous because they heat foods and liquids unevenly and to very high temperatures that can lead to burns from spills, splashes, and release of steam. Microwaved foods and liquids can reach temperatures hotter than boiling without the appearance of bubbling.

Scalding hot tap water, bath, or shower water; overly hot foods or drinks; microwaved food and stovetop cooking steam can all cause a severe scalding burn within seconds. Scalding formula can not only injure an infant's mouth at the site of initial contact, it can continue to burn delicate throat tissue as the hot liquid passes down the baby's throat.

Prevention

To lower the risk of an accident, families should lower the temperature setting of the water heater and install scald-prevention devices (such as faucet covers) for the water systems in the home. Water heaters usually come from U.S. factories set at 140°F or above—a temperature that can scald a child within two seconds. The simplest method of protecting against scalds throughout the house is to reduce the temperature setting to between 120° and 125°F. If that is not possible, installing scald-protection devices can help.

scaling disorders of infancy   It is completely normal for newborns to shed their skin, especially those babies who have gone beyond full term.

However, excessive scaling may indicate one of a group of disorders known as ichthyoses, featuring dry, rough, and scaly skin. These are caused by a defect in the process by which skin cells move upward toward the outer layer of skin (keratinization). The ichthyosis disorders are caused by a genetic defect causing the skin's natural shedding process to slow down (in some forms of ichthyosis, the production of skin cells is too fast).

There are at least 20 varieties of ICHTHYOSIS. Of the four main types, three are very rare: X-linked ichthyosis, lamellar ichthyosis, and epidermolytic hyperkeratosis. The most common type is ichthyosis vulgaris, affecting one out of every 250 children. All types of ichthyosis occur at conception, although in some cases symptoms do not become apparent until sometime during or after the first year of a child's life; in other instances, it is obvious at birth that something is wrong with the baby's skin.

As yet, there is no cure for ichthyosis. Doctors try to care for ichthyosis by moisturizing the skin, holding in the moisture, and keeping the scale thickness to a minimum.

Other scaling conditions found in infancy include ECZEMA, seborrheic dermatitis, and PSORIASIS. See also DERMATITIS, SEBORRHEIC.

scarlatina An older term for SCARLET FEVER.

scarlet fever An infectious bacterial childhood disease characterized by a skin rash, sore throat, and fever. It is much less common and dangerous than it once was. No longer a reportable disease, no one knows for sure how many cases occur today in the United States, although it is believed that the disease has been on the increase in the past few years. In the past the disease was associated with poor living conditions that once swept through large cities, killing large numbers of children. Inexplicably, by the 1920s the death rate of the disease dropped to 5 percent, for reasons that are still not completely understood. It is believed that the bacteria underwent a natural mutation that made it less deadly. The introduction of penicillin reduced the death rate even more.

Today most cases occur in middle-class suburbs, not in inner cities. Because it is possible to get strep infection and scarlet fever more than once, and because the incidence of all strep infections is rising, prompt medical attention is important when strep is suspected. A child with a sore throat or skin rash should see a doctor.

Cause

Scarlet fever is caused by an infection with *group A Streptococcus*. Scarlet fever strains of the bacteria produce toxins that are released in the skin, causing a bright red rash that feels a bit like sandpaper. The disease is spread in droplets during coughing or breathing, or by sharing food and drink. When bacteria particles are released into the air, they can be picked up by others close by. For this reason, some experts advise children to avoid drinking fountains.

Symptoms

After an incubation period of two to four days, the first signs of illness are usually a fever of 103°F and a severe sore throat. This is followed by fatigue, facial flushing, and a white tongue coating with red spots. Twelve to 18 hours after the fever appears, a rash appears as a mass of rapidly spreading tiny red spots on the neck and upper trunk. Other common symptoms include headache, chills, vomiting, tiny white lines around the mouth, fine red striations in the creases of the elbows and groin. After a few days, the tongue coating peels off, followed by a drop in fever and fading rash. Skin on the hands and feet often peel as well.

Complications

As with other types of sore throat caused by the strep bacteria, untreated infection carries the risk of rheumatic fever or kidney inflammation.

Treatment

A 10-day course of antibiotics with rest, liquids, and acetaminophen is used to treat scarlet fever. Children are contagious for a day or two after they begin antibiotic treatment, but after that they can return to school. Alternative treatment is a shot of long-acting penicillin, which slowly releases the antibiotic over several weeks. Anyone can develop scarlet fever, but most cases occur among children aged four to eight.

schizophrenia A mental illness that causes strange thinking, abnormal feelings, and unusual behavior. It is an uncommon psychiatric illness in children under age 12, and it is hard to recognize in its early phases in children. Schizophrenia is far more common in adolescence, when it occurs in about three out of every 1,000 teens.

Symptoms

The behavior of children and teens with schizophrenia may differ from that of adults with this illness. Most schizophrenic children show delays in language and other functions long before their symptoms of hallucinations, delusions, and disordered thinking appear. In the first years of life, about 30 percent of these children have transient symptoms of a PERVASIVE DEVELOPMENTAL DISORDER, such as rocking or arm flapping. There may be uneven motor development, such as unusual crawling.

The early warning signs of schizophrenia in children include:

- trouble telling the difference between dreams and reality
- visual or auditory hallucinations
- confused thinking
- vivid and bizarre thoughts and ideas
- extreme moodiness
- peculiar behavior
- feeling of persecution
- immature behavior
- severe anxiety and fearfulness
- confusing TV or movies with reality
- severe problems in making and keeping friends

However, the behavior of children with this illness may change over time. Schizophrenic psychosis develops gradually in children, without the sudden psychotic break that sometimes occurs in adolescents and adults. Children may begin talking about strange fears and ideas, clinging to parents, or saying things that do not make sense. Those who used to enjoy relationships with others may become more shy or withdrawn.

Treatment

Early diagnosis and medical treatment are important. Children with the symptoms listed above may need a combination of medication and individual therapy, family therapy, and specialized programs.

Psychiatric medication can be helpful for many of the symptoms. Clozapine was helpful for half of the children who do not respond to other medications, treating all the symptoms and avoiding the movement side effects, but it posed a risk of a potentially fatal blood illness. Children appeared to be even more susceptible to adults to the toxic effects of clozapine; about a third of them had to stop taking the drug because of side effects.

The challenge was to develop better drugs that avoided the side effects of both standard therapy and clozapine. The first, Risperdal, hit the market in 1994. It was followed by olanzapine (Zyprexa), which affects even more areas of the brain than Risperdal and does not pose a risk of the fatal blood illness. Zyprexa is approved for schizophrenic patients who do not respond to existing medicines. Chemically similar to clozapine, it appears to have the benefits of clozapine without the side effects, although the risk of movement problems did rise once patients reached the recommended daily dose of 10 milligrams. Olanzapine can cause sedation, dizziness and weight gain.

In 2002, the U.S. Food and Drug Administration approved Geodon (ziprasidone mesylate) for injection to rapidly control agitated behavior and psychotic symptoms such as hallucinations and delusions in patients with acute exacerbations of schizophrenia. Geodon for Injection is the first atypical antipsychotic medicine approved in the United States for intramuscular (IM) use.

It is the first in a batch of similar new drugs, by such makers as Abbott, Pfizer and Sandoz, that are now in the pipeline.

scoliosis   A condition in which the spine curves abnormally from side to side. Unlike poor posture, these curves cannot be corrected simply by learning to stand up straight. On an X ray, the spine of a child with scoliosis looks more like an "S" or a "C" than a straight line. Sometimes the spinal bones in a child with scoliosis may rotate slightly, making the child's waist or shoulders appear uneven.

Scoliosis affects about two percent of the population and tends to run in families. If someone in a family has scoliosis, the likelihood of another child having the condition is about 20 percent. The primary age of onset for this condition is between 10 and 15 years of age, occurring more often in girls.

Fortunately, four out of five children with scoliosis have curves of less than 20 degrees, which are barely noticeable to the untrained eye and are no cause for concern, provided they show no sign of further progression. However, in growing children and adolescents, mild curvatures can worsen quite rapidly (10 degrees or more in a few months). Therefore, for this age group, frequent checkups are important.

Cause

Most cases of childhood scoliosis are "idiopathic," which means the cause is unknown. Scoliosis usually develops in middle or late childhood, before puberty, and is seen more often in girls than boys. Although scoliosis can occur in children with diseases such as CEREBRAL PALSY, MUSCULAR DYSTROPHY, or SPINA BIFIDA, most scoliosis is found in otherwise healthy youngsters.

Symptoms

Scoliosis can go unnoticed in a child because it is rarely painful in the early years. Symptoms begin to appear when a child is about eight years of age and include:

- uneven shoulders
- prominent shoulder blade or shoulder blades
- uneven waist
- elevated hips
- leaning to one side

Treatment

Treatment is different for every child and depends on a variety of factors, including the history of scoliosis in the family, the age at which the curve began, the curve's location, and its severity. Most spine curves in children with scoliosis remain small and need only to be watched by a doctor for any sign of worsening. If a curve does worsen, a brace can be used to prevent it from getting worse. Children undergoing treatment with braces can continue to participate in the full range of physical and social activities.

Electrical muscle stimulation, exercise programs, and manipulation have not been found to improve scoliosis. If a curve is severe when first diagnosed or if treatment with a brace does not control the curve, surgery may be necessary. In these cases, surgery has been found to be a highly effective and safe treatment.

scooter safety Scooters are associated with an increased risk of injury, particularly in young children, which is why children under age eight should not use them without adult supervision, according to the American Academy of Pediatrics (AAP). Young children do not have the developmental skills required for safe scooter riding, including balance, coordination, good judgment, and a realistic sense of their own dexterity and strength.

Scooter-related injuries (primarily fractures or head injuries) accounted for more than 84,400 emergency room visits in 2001—more than double the number of injuries from the previous year. Most injuries were caused when riders fell from the scooter. Fractures and dislocations accounted for 29 percent of the injuries and 85 percent of the injuries occur in children less than 15 years old. Most fractures and dislocations involved the upper extremities.

To reduce the risk of injury, the AAP suggests that children who ride scooters should:

- always wear helmets that meet safety standards, as well as knee pads, elbow pads, and wrist guards
- never ride in the street or anywhere near traffic
- never ride at night
- never ride on wet pavement or surfaces that have sand, gravel, or dirt
- avoid steep hills, slippery/uneven surfaces, and crowded walkways/streets
- obey traffic signs
- wear sturdy shoes and never wear sandals or flimsy footwear
- be familiar with the steering, handling, and brake system

The AAP also recommends that children younger than 10 not use skateboards unsupervised, and children younger than five not use them at all. The AAP also reminds parents never to let their kids hitch a ride onto the back of a car while riding a skateboard. Whenever possible, children should ride in community skateboard parks, which are more likely to have safer surfaces and ramps.

seasickness See MOTION SICKNESS.

seborrhea A condition in which excess sebum is secreted, causing increased facial oiliness and a greasy scalp. While the exact cause of this excess production is not understood, male sex hormones (androgens) do play a role in the problem. Not surprisingly, therefore, the problem is most common in adolescent boys. Seborrhea usually disappears by adulthood without treatment, but people with seborrhea are also more likely to have other skin problems such as ACNE vulgaris and seborrheic dermatitis.

secondhand smoke Exposure to secondhand smoke puts children (even older children) at risk for ASTHMA, wheezing, and decreased lung function. Researchers found that children aged four to 16 with the highest levels of a blood chemical called cotinine (which increases with exposure to tobacco smoke) were more likely to have asthma or wheezing and miss days from school. Cotinine is considered to be an excellent marker for recent smoke exposure; children exposed to tobacco smoke typically have cotinine levels more than 10 times higher than levels in children without smoke exposure. Children aged four to six with high blood levels of the chemical were more than five times as likely to have had asthma symptoms as those with the lowest levels of cotinine.

Tobacco smoke exposure, both before and after birth, is associated with adverse health effects in children. Other studies have found that secondhand tobacco smoke is linked to the risk of tooth decay in children. In 1993 the Environmental Protection Agency classified secondhand smoke as a cancer-causing toxin to humans. It also has been shown that children of smokers incur a higher risk for blood vessel damage.

Other research has found that passive smoke lowers vitamin C levels in children, depriving children of an important vitamin that may protect against heart disease and is needed for growth and development. In one study of nearly 3,000 children, those who were exposed to the most cigarette smoke had the lowest levels of vitamin C in their blood, regardless of how much vitamin C they took in food and multivitamins. Since vitamin C protects against metabolic changes that can lead to heart disease, the report highlights the dangers of passive or secondhand smoke to children.

seizures Abnormal electrical discharges in the brain that may trigger unusual sensations, uncontrollable muscle spasms, and loss of consciousness. Seizures may be caused by low blood sugar, an infection, a head injury, accidental poisoning, or drug overdose. Alternatively, a seizure can be caused by a brain tumor or other problem in the central nervous system. In addition, anything that interferes with the oxygen flow to the brain can cause a seizure. Most often, the cause of the seizure is never known. Recurring seizures may be caused by EPILEPSY.

Febrile seizures are relatively common in children younger than five with a high fever, usually with the temperature spiking beyond 102°F. While terrifying to parents, these seizures are usually brief and rarely cause any problems, unless the fever is associated with a serious infection (such as MENINGITIS). A child who has a febrile seizure is not more likely to develop epilepsy.

First Aid

During a seizure, the child should be placed on the ground or floor away from other objects. Clothing around the head or neck should be loosened, but nothing should be placed into the child's mouth or between the teeth, nor should the child's movements be restricted in any way. Once the seizure ends, roll the child onto his side.

Immediate emergency medical care should be obtained if the child:

- has trouble breathing
- turns blue
- has sustained a head injury
- seems sick

- has a heart condition
- may have swallowed poisons or medications

If the child is breathing normally and the seizure lasts just a few minutes, a doctor can be consulted after the seizure is over. However, if the child has never had a seizure before, parents should seek help right away. For children prone to seizures, parents should call emergency services if the seizure lasts more than five minutes, or if the seizure differs from normal occurrences.

After the seizure, it is normal for a child to fall into a deep sleep. Parents should not wake the child nor try to give food or drink until the child is awake and alert. Children who get febrile seizures may be given fever-reducing medicine (such as ibuprofen) to control the fever and prevent seizures from recurring. A doctor may also recommend sponging the child with lukewarm water.

sensorimotor stage   A developmental stage in which a child has little ability with language or the use of symbols but experiences the world through sensation and movement. The first of four stages in child psychiatrist Jean Piaget's theory of cognitive development, the sensorimotor stage lasts from birth to about age two.

Infants are normally born with a range of reflexes that ensure their survival, such as sucking and grasping. As the infant adapts these reflexes over time, the child can begin to interact with the environment with greater efficiency. By the end of this stage, the child is able to solve simple problems, such as looking for a lost toy or communicating simple needs to a parent or another child. It is also during this stage that the infant develops a sense of object permanence—the awareness that things and people continue to exist even when they cannot be perceived.

For example, before the age of two if a parent hides a toy under a pillow in front of the child, the child will not understand that the toy still exists under the pillow. Once a sense of object permanence is developed, the child will understand that the toy hidden under the pillow still exists and will lift up the pillow to retrieve the toy.

Modern technology was not available in Piaget's time, so he often used motor tasks to test the cognitive understanding of an infant. With the avail-ability of more advanced techniques that can track an infant's eye movements or rate of sucking in response to stimuli, researchers now know that infants reach cognitive milestones such as object permanence at a younger age than Piaget had suspected. However, Piaget's view of the infant as a "little scientist" who comes to understand the world through trial and error experiments remains consistent with recent findings.

sensory integration   The process of taking in sensory information, organizing this information in the central nervous system, and using the information to function smoothly in daily life. Sensory integration is a continual process: As children become more competent, their sensory integration improves, so that the more children do, the more they can do. Sensory experiences include touch, movement, body awareness, sight, sound, and the pull of gravity; as the brain organizes and interprets this information, it provides a crucial foundation for later, more complex learning and behavior. This critical function of the brain is responsible for producing a composite picture of a child's existence, so that the child can understand who he is physically, where he is, and what is going on in the environment around him.

For most children, effective sensory integration occurs automatically and unconsciously, without effort, in the course of ordinary childhood activities. But for some children, sensory integration does not develop as efficiently as it should. When the process breaks down, a number of problems in learning, development, or behavior may develop.

The concept of sensory integration comes from a body of work developed by occupational therapist A. Jean Ayres, Ph.D., who was interested in the way in which sensory processing and motor planning disorders interfere with daily life function and learning. This theory has been developed and refined by the research of Dr. Ayres, as well as other occupational and physical therapists. In addition, literature from the fields of neuropsychology, neurology, physiology, child development, and psychology has contributed to theory development and treatment strategies.

Children with sensory integration problems may be bright, but they may have trouble using a pencil, playing with toys, or taking care of personal tasks, such as getting dressed. Some children with this problem are so afraid of movement that ordinary swings, slides, or jungle gyms trigger fear and insecurity. On the other hand, some children whose problems lie at the opposite extreme are uninhibited and overly active, often falling and running headlong into dangerous situations. In each of these cases, a sensory integrative problem may be an underlying factor. Its far-reaching effects can interfere with academic learning, social skills, even self-esteem.

Research clearly identifies sensory integrative problems in children with developmental or learning difficulties, and independent research shows that a sensory integrative problem can be found in some children who are considered learning disabled by schools. However, sensory integrative problems are not limited to children with learning disabilities; they can affect all ages, intellectual levels, and socioeconomic groups.

A number of situations can trigger sensory integration problems:

Prematurity As more premature infants survive today, they enter the world with easily overstimulated nervous systems and multiple medical problems. Parents need to learn how to give their premature infant the sensory nourishment their child requires for optimal development, and how to avoid harmful overstimulation.

Developmental disorders Severe problems with sensory processing is a hallmark of AUTISM. Autistic children seek out unusual amounts of certain types of sensations but are extremely hypersensitive to others. Similar traits are often seen in other children with developmental disorders. Improving sensory processing will help these children develop more productive contacts with people and environments.

Learning disabilities As many as 30 percent of school-age children may have learning disabilities. While most of these children have normal intelligence, many are likely to have sensory integrative problems. These children are also more likely than their peers to have been born prematurely, to have had early developmental problems, and to have poor motor coordination. Early intervention can improve sensory integration in these children, minimizing the possibility of school failure before it occurs.

Many studies indicate that children with learning disabilities are at risk for later delinquency, criminal behavior, alcoholism, and drug abuse because of repeated failure in school. By interrupting the vicious cycle of failure, intervention to help children with sensory integration and learning problems may also prevent serious social problems later in life.

Brain injury Trauma to the brain as a result of accidents and strokes can have profound effects on sensory functioning. Children who suffer from these effects deserve treatment that will lead to the best possible recovery. In order for this to occur, their sensory deficits must be addressed. (See also SENSORY INTEGRATION DYSFUNCTION.)

sensory integration dysfunction (SID) The inefficient brain processing of information received through the senses. A child with sensory integration dysfunction (SID) has trouble detecting, discriminating, or integrating sensations. This complex neurological problem leads to either sensory seeking or sensory avoiding patterns, or a motor planning problem called DYSPRAXIA.

Sensory Seekers

These children have nervous systems that do not always process sensory input that is sent to the brain. As a result, they respond too strongly to sensations. Children who are under-responsive to sensation seek out more intense or longer duration sensory experiences. They may:

- be hyperactive as they seek more and more movement input
- be unaware of touch or pain, or touching others too often or too hard (may seem aggressive)
- engage in unsafe behaviors, such as climbing too high
- enjoy sounds that are too loud, such as TV or radio volume

Sensory Avoiders

At the other end of the spectrum of this disorder are those children who have nervous systems that feel sensation too easily or too much so that they are overly responsive to sensation. As a result, they may have "fight or flight" responses to sensation, a condition called "sensory defensiveness." They may:

- respond to being touched with aggression or withdrawal
- be afraid of, or become sick with, movement and heights
- be very cautious and unwilling to take risks or try new things
- be uncomfortable in loud or busy environments such as sports events or malls
- be very picky eaters or overly sensitive to food smells

Dyspraxia

These children are clumsy and awkward. They have particular problems with new motor skills and activities. They may have:

- very poor fine motor skills such as handwriting
- very poor gross motor skills such as kicking, catching, or throwing balls
- trouble imitating movements such as "Simon Says"
- trouble with balance, sequences of movements, and bilateral coordination

Treatment

Sensory integration dysfunction is a neurological problem that affects behavior and learning. Medicine cannot cure the problem, but occupational therapy can address the child's underlying problems in processing sensations. A good sensory treatment plan may be a major component in treating the child with SID.

If a child is suspected of having a sensory integrative disorder, a qualified occupational or physical therapist can conduct an evaluation. Evaluation usually consists of both standardized testing and structured observations of responses to sensory stimulation, posture, balance, coordination, and eye movements. After carefully analyzing test results and other assessment data along with information from other professionals and parents, the therapist will recommend appropriate treatment.

If therapy is recommended, the child will be guided through activities that challenge the ability to respond appropriately to sensory input by making a successful, organized response. Training of specific skills is not usually the focus of this kind of therapy. Instead, adaptive physical education, movement education, and gymnastics are examples of services that typically focus on specific motor skills training. Such services are important, but they are not the same as therapy using a sensory integrative approach.

The motivation of the child plays a crucial role in the selection of the activities in a sensory integrative approach. Most children tend to seek out activities that provide the best sensory experiences at that particular point in their development. It is this active involvement and exploration that enables the child to become a more mature, efficient organizer of sensory information.

The most important step in promoting sensory integration in children is to recognize that it exists and that it plays an important role in the development of a child. By learning more about sensory integration, parents, educators, and caregivers can provide an enriched environment that will foster healthy growth and maturation.

The goal of occupational therapy is to enable children to take part in the normal "job" of childhood, such as playing, enjoying school, eating, dressing, and sleeping—activities that are often a problem for children with SID. Each child is provided with an individualized treatment plan that directly involves parents.

Occupational therapy usually takes place in a large, sensory-enriched gym with lots of swinging, spinning, tactile, visual, auditory, and taste opportunities.

separation anxiety disorder An intense anxiety about being away from home or caregivers that affects a child's ability to function socially and academically. These children have a great need to stay at home or be close to their parents, worrying excessively about their parents when they are apart. When they are together, the child may cling to parents, refuse to go to school, or be afraid to sleep alone. Repeated nightmares about separation and physical symptoms such as stomachaches and headaches are also common in children with separation anxiety disorder. (See also ANXIETY DISORDERS.)

septicemia   The medical name for blood poisoning, a potentially lethal blood infection characterized by the rapid multiplication of bacteria and the presence of their toxins. Septicemia is the body's response to severe infection, mediated through the immune system and involving nearly every other system in the body. The condition may produce harmful effects in other organs, leading to very high death rates.

Cause

Septicemia can occur when certain forms of bacteria enter the bloodstream. These bacteria give off poisonous toxins that remain even after the bacteria disintegrate, and that can lead to a dramatic drop in blood pressure (SEPTIC SHOCK), with rapid heartbeat and breathing.

Symptoms

Septicemia is characterized by sudden onset of fever, chills, rapid breathing, headache, nausea or diarrhea, and clouding of consciousness. Skin rashes and jaundice may occur, and the hands may be particularly warm. If large amounts of toxins are produced by the bacteria the patient may fall into a state of septic shock.

Treatment

Until recently, there was no way to treat sepsis other than to give patients antibiotics to try to minimize the severity of their symptoms. Xigris, the first drug ever found to directly attack sepsis, was approved by the FDA in 2001. However, it has not yet been approved for all children (Xigris is only available under an experimental study protocol for children younger than 18 years). Because no one yet knows if Xigris will help children with sepsis, drug manufacturer Eli Lilly agreed to FDA requests to study Xigris in children.

The FDA also warned that Xigris is to be used only for the sepsis patients deemed least likely to survive. When given to such people, the drug can cut the chances of death 13 percent. In lower-risk patients, the drug seemed to make no difference. When the initial drug results were released, the drug was referred to as a "landmark" in critical-care treatment. It was only after the study was completed, however, that the FDA did an analysis concluding that the beneficial effect was concentrated in high-risk patients.

Because Xigris works by interfering with blood clotting, it can cause severe bleeding, including strokes, the FDA warned. In clinical trials, serious bleeding occurred in 2.4 percent of patients. This means the drug should never be used for patients with active internal bleeding or who are at high risk of bleeding because of a recent stroke or head or spinal injury.

The drug is a genetically engineered version of a naturally occurring human protein (activated protein C) that interferes with some of the body's harmful responses to severe infection, including blood clots that can lead to organ failure and death. While not everyone will benefit from this treatment, experts believe the approval of Xigris is an important advance for the treatment of this often-deadly disease. Because sepsis is a life-threatening condition and because treatment with Xigris comes with potentially serious risks, the benefits and risks of treatment with Xigris must be carefully weighed for each individual patient.

septic shock   A type of shock that occurs in SEPTICEMIA (blood poisoning) when poisons are released from bacteria in the bloodstream, triggering a drop in blood pressure. Fever, rapid heartbeat and breathing, and confusion or coma may occur.

This type of shock usually follows signs of severe infection (often in the stomach or intestines, or urinary tract). It is usually treated with fluids and antibiotics. TOXIC SHOCK SYNDROME is one type of septic shock.

severe acute respiratory syndrome (SARS)   A severe respiratory illness that was first reported in 2002 in China, and quickly spread throughout Asia, North America, and Europe. Most of the U.S. cases of severe acute respiratory syndrome (SARS) occurred among travelers returning to the United States from other parts of the world with SARS. There have been very few cases as a result of spread to close contacts such as family members and health-care workers. Currently, there is no evidence that SARS is spreading more widely in the United States.

Researchers at Chinese University in Hong Kong have released preliminary findings that suggest SARS is much milder in children and teens than in adults. Scientists found that while teens had symptoms similar to those of adults (muscle aches and chills) younger children tended to have milder symptoms, such as coughs and runny noses, and recovered sooner.

The first case of SARS was diagnosed in November 2002 in southern China's Guangdong province, and within one month the province reported 300 cases. The disease quickly spread to 20 other countries, including parts of Asia, Europe, and North America; by April 2003 there were 3,000 cases of SARS reported and more than 100 deaths worldwide. To put things in perspective, however, flu-related complications kill more than 36,000 people every year in the United States alone. The SARS epidemic had faded away by the end of summer 2003. A few new cases appeared in 2004.

Cause

SARS is caused by a previously unrecognized coronavirus; these viruses are a common cause of mild-to-moderate upper respiratory illness in humans; they also are associated with respiratory, gastrointestinal, liver, and neurological disease in animals.

The primary way that SARS appears to spread is by close person-to-person contact. Most cases of SARS have involved people who cared for or lived with someone with SARS, or had direct contact with infectious material (for example, respiratory secretions) from a person who had SARS. Potential ways in which SARS can be spread include touching the skin of other people or objects that are contaminated with infectious droplets and then touching the eyes, nose, or mouth. This can happen when someone who is sick with SARS coughs or sneezes droplets onto themselves, other people, or nearby surfaces. It also is possible that SARS can be spread more broadly through the air or by other ways that are currently not known.

Most SARS cases occur among those who have come into direct contact with an infected person (either those living with someone infected with SARS or health-care workers who did not use infection control procedures while taking care of a patient with SARS). Those in the United States infected with the disease had traveled to and from a SARS hotbed region.

Diagnosis

Several laboratory tests can be used to detect the SARS-associated coronavirus in blood, stool, and nasal secretions. Testing also can detect SARS-CoV antibodies produced after infection. Finally, viral culture has been used to detect SARS-CoV.

Symptoms

SARS typically begins with a fever above 100.4°F, together with flu-like symptoms including headache, an overall feeling of discomfort, chills, and body aches. Some people also experience mild respiratory symptoms. After two to seven days, SARS patients may develop a dry cough and have trouble breathing. Although the vast majority of patients survive, it can be fatal in about 8 percent of cases. Although its very name (severe acute respiratory syndrome) suggests a focus on severe cases, there may be milder forms of the infection that are not yet being diagnosed.

Prevention

Scientists have identified the genetic makeup of the virus, which may help speed up the development of an effective immunization, although this is likely to take some time.

The American Academy of Pediatrics (AAP) emphasizes that children do not need to restrict their activities, except as they relate to official travel alerts. Likewise, youngsters who have been exposed to someone who is not ill but has traveled to an area affected by SARS do not need to be isolated.

sexually transmitted diseases (STDs)   Contagious diseases usually transmitted during genital contact. In the United States the most commonly reported infections are sexually transmitted, and the incidence has risen over the past 20 years despite improved methods of diagnosis and treatment. Once known as "venereal diseases," these conditions are sometimes acquired in childhood as a result of child abuse. Some of the major sexually transmitted diseases (STDs) are also transmitted by blood.

STDs affect boys and girls of all backgrounds and economic levels and are most common among teenagers and young adults. Nearly two-thirds of all STDs occur in people younger than age 25. The incidence of STDs is rising in part because in the last few decades, young people have become sexually active younger but are marrying later. As a result, sexually active teenagers today are more likely to have multiple sex partners.

STDs include GONORRHEA, SYPHILIS, chancroid, SCABIES, HERPES, genital WARTS, pubic LICE, trichomoniasis, genital candidiasis, HEPATITIS B, nonspecific URETHRITIS, CHLAMYDIA, CYTOMEGALOVIRUS, and AIDS.

Symptoms

Most of the time STDs cause no symptoms, especially in women. If symptoms do develop, they may be confused with other diseases that are not transmitted sexually. Even if an STD does not cause symptoms, however, a teenager who is infected may be able to pass the disease on to a sex partner. This is why many doctors recommend periodic testing or screening for teens who have more than one sex partner.

Health problems caused by STDs tend to be more severe and more common among girls and women, partly because girls may not have symptoms and thus do not seek care until serious problems occur. Some STDs can spread into the uterus and fallopian tubes, causing PELVIC INFLAMMATORY DISEASE, which in turn is a major cause of infertility and tubal pregnancy. STDs in girls and woman also may be eventually associated with cervical cancer. For example, human papillomavirus infection causes genital warts and cervical cancer.

In addition, STDs can be passed from a mother to her child before, during, or immediately after birth; some of these infections in the newborn can be cured easily, but others may cause a baby to be permanently disabled or die.

Treatment

When diagnosed and treated early, many STDs can be treated effectively, although some infections have become resistant to the drugs used to treat them and now require newer types of antibiotics. When being treated, patients should notify all recent sex partners, complete the full course of medication, and take a follow-up test to make sure the infection has been cured. Patients also should avoid all sexual activity while being treated for an STD.

Prevention

The best way to prevent STDs is to avoid sexual contact with others. To reduce the risk of developing an STD, teens who are sexually active should:

- have only one partner
- correctly and consistently use a condom
- prevent and control other STDs to decrease susceptibility to HIV infection
- delay having sex, because the younger a person is having sex for the first time, the more vulnerable to an STD
- have regular checkups for STDs even in the absence of symptoms, especially if having sex with a new partner
- avoid having sex during menstruation—HIV-infected women are more infectious, and HIV-uninfected women are more susceptible to becoming infected during this time
- avoid anal intercourse, but if practiced, use a condom
- avoid douching, because this removes some of the normal protective bacteria in the vagina and increases the risk of getting some STDs

shaken baby syndrome Forceful shaking of an infant or young child by the arms, legs, chest, or shoulders can cause brain damage leading to MENTAL RETARDATION, speech and LEARNING DISABILITIES, paralysis, SEIZURES, hearing loss, and death. It may cause bleeding around the brain and eyes, resulting in blindness. A baby's head and neck are especially vulnerable to injury because the head is so large and the neck muscles are still weak. In addition, the baby's brain and blood vessels are very fragile and are easily damaged by whiplash motions such as shaking, jerking, and jolting.

About 50,000 cases of shaken baby syndrome occur each year in the United States; one shaken baby in four dies as a result of this abuse. Head trauma is the most frequent cause of permanent damage or death among abused infants and children, and shaking accounts for a significant number of those cases. Some studies estimate that 15 percent of children's deaths are due to battering or shaking and an additional 15 percent are possible cases of shaking. The victims of shaken baby syndrome range in age from a few days to five years, with an average age of six to eight months.

While shaken baby abuse is not limited to any special group of people, in 65 percent to 90 percent of cases the shakers are men. In the United States adult males in their early 20s who are the baby's father or the mother's boyfriend are typically the shaker. Females who injure babies by shaking them are more likely to be babysitters or child-care providers than mothers.

Severe shaking often begins in response to frustration over a baby's crying or toileting problems. The adult shaker also may be jealous of the attention which the child receives from a partner. Shaken baby syndrome is also known as abusive head trauma, shaken brain trauma, pediatric traumatic brain injury, whiplash, shaken infant syndrome, and shaken impact syndrome.

Diagnosis

Shaken baby syndrome is difficult to diagnose unless someone accurately describes what happens. Physicians often report that a child with possible shaken baby syndrome is brought for medical attention due to falls, difficulty breathing, seizures, vomiting, altered consciousness, or choking. The caregiver may report that the child was shaken to try to resuscitate it. Babies with severe or lethal shaken baby syndrome are typically brought to the hospital unconscious with a closed head injury.

To diagnose shaken baby syndrome, physicians look for bleeding in the retina of the eyes, blood in the brain, or increased head size indicating buildup of fluid in the tissues of the brain. Damage to the spinal cord and broken ribs from the baby being grasped too hard are other signs of shaken baby syndrome. Computerized tomography (CT) and magnetic resonance imaging (MRI) scans can reveal injuries in the brain but are not regularly used because of their expense.

A milder form of this syndrome may be missed or misdiagnosed. Subtle symptoms which may be the result of shaken baby syndrome are often attributed to mild viral illnesses, feeding dysfunction, or infant colic. These include a history of poor feeding, vomiting, or flu-like symptoms with no accompanying fever or diarrhea, lethargy, and irritability over a period of time. Without early medical intervention, the child may be at risk for further damage or even death, depending on the continued occurrences of shaking.

Treatment

The treatment of babies who survive can be divided into three major categories: medical, behavioral, and educational. In addition to medical care, children may need speech and language therapy, vision therapy, physical therapy, occupational therapy, and special education services. Some may need the assistance of feeding experts and behavioral consultants.

Prognosis

Immediate medical attention can help reduce the impact of shaking, but many children are left with permanent damage. Fewer than 10 to 15 percent of shaken babies recover completely; the rest have a variety of disabilities, including partial or complete loss of vision, hearing problems, seizure disorders, CEREBRAL PALSY, sucking and swallowing disorders, DEVELOPMENTAL DISABILITIES, AUTISM, cognitive or behavior problems, or a permanent vegetative state.

shellfish poisoning   Eating shellfish has been linked to a number of illnesses, including those caused by bacteria, a variety of viruses, and toxins. This is because shellfish are highly susceptible to bacterial and viral contamination, since they live close to the shore where pollution tends to be worse. While shellfish by themselves are not poisonous, they can become contaminated by their environment, passing infection on up the food chain until they are eaten by humans.

Oysters, clams, and mussels are particularly prone to becoming contaminated because of their metabolic systems, which pump water across gills to isolate plankton; this makes them vulnerable to bacteria, viruses, and contaminants. Lobsters and other crustacean shellfish only rarely become contaminated.

Most cases of shellfish poisoning have occurred when people ate raw or undercooked shellfish; raw shellfish have been linked to nearly 1,000 cases of HEPATITIS a year. This is why doctors recommend that no one eat raw shellfish. Another common viral contamination in shellfish is caused by the NORWALK AGENT VIRUS, which leads to food poisoning when raw or improperly cooked food comes in contact with water contaminated by human excrement.

Red Tide

Gonyaulax catanella (popularly known as red tide) is a species of plankton that produces a toxin ingested by shellfish along the North American coasts. Anyone eating shellfish contaminated with red tide can become sick. The type of shellfish poisoning caused by these toxic forms of red tide comes in three forms: *neurotoxic shellfish poisoning, erythematous shellfish poisoning,* and *paralytic shellfish poisoning (PSP).* Each has quite different etiology, symptoms and prognosis for recovery, but of the three, PSP is by far the most serious. There is no known antidote for these types of shellfish poisoning; administration of prostigmine may be effective, together with artificial respiration and oxygen as needed.

Prevention

The shellfish industry and government regulators try to control the problem by seeing that shellfish are harvested from unpolluted beds not tainted by sewage. Unfortunately, these efforts cannot guarantee that shellfish from unapproved beds do not reach the market.

shigellosis A diarrheal disease caused by any of a group of four different species of bacteria known as *Shigella.* Two-thirds of cases occur in children between six months and 10 years of age, although the disease is rare in infants under age six months. The highest rate of infection occurs in child-care centers, large camps, and institutions.

Shigella were discovered more than 100 years ago by Japanese scientist Kiyoshi Shiga, who first described the bacterial origin of dysentery caused by this bacteria. The group includes *Shigella sonnei* (group D *Shigella*) that account for more than two-thirds of the shigellosis in the United States. A second type, *S. flexneri* (group B *Shigella*), accounts for almost all of the rest. Other types of *Shigella* are rare in the United States, though they continue to be important causes of disease in the developing world.

Cause

The bacteria are found in milk and dairy products, poultry, and mixed salads, although they can develop in any moist food that is not thoroughly cooked. The bacteria multiply rapidly at or above room temperature. A person gets sick after ingesting bacteria, and it only takes a few organisms to cause illness. The bacteria also may be found in contaminated bodies of water, or in food that has been left out in the open where flies can contaminate it. Dogs who eat infected human feces can spread the infection to humans (especially children), and the disease also can be spread sexually with anal-oral contact.

Symptoms

Symptoms usually appear eight hours to eight days after ingestion, beginning with nausea and vomiting, water or bloody explosive diarrhea and stomach cramps, weakness, vision problems, headache, and problems swallowing. Young children and those with weakened immune systems may have more serious diarrhea and may take longer to recover. Those children who are already malnourished or weak will be much sicker.

Diagnosis

The infection can be diagnosed by culturing the stool, which will reveal the type of bacteria.

Treatment

Most children with the infection will recover on their own; some may need fluids to prevent dehydration. To treat severe cases, antibiotics will help stop the diarrhea, although *Shigella* has become resistant to some drugs. Antidiarrheal medications should not be given. Diluted drinks high in sugar and bland foods high in carbohydrates are tolerated best by the patient.

Prevention

Confirmed cases must be reported to the health department, which will begin an investigation and control measures to prevent large-scale outbreaks. Although several vaccines have been tested, none has yet been licensed for use in preventing the disease. The single most important way to prevent the spread of this infection is to carefully wash hands after using the toilet, since *Shigella* is passed in feces.

shingles A painful red blistering viral infection of the nerves that supply certain areas of the skin, caused by reactivation of the CHICKEN POX virus (varicella-zoster virus). After causing chicken pox, the virus stays dormant in the child's body. In some children it can become reactivated and cause shingles.

Symptoms

The main symptom of shingles is a rash on one side of the body that begins as a cluster of red bumps, eventually changing into small blisters that crust over. The child may also feel itchy but will otherwise be well. The rash usually continues to develop for a few days and then completely crusts over and goes away in about seven to 10 days without treatment. Because the nerves have been damaged after the virus attack, after the blisters heal the nerves tend to continue to produce strong pain impulses that may last for weeks or months. This is less likely in younger children, however.

Cause

Although most typically the virus lies dormant in sensory nerves along the spine for many years, if a child's immune system is weakened the virus can reemerge and migrate along the sensory nerve, breaking out at the receptor ends in the skin. Shingles also may appear in children with LEUKEMIA, those who are undergoing chemotherapy, or children who have had an organ transplant.

Because shingles is caused by the chicken pox virus, children with shingles are contagious and can transmit chicken pox to others who are not immune. Direct contact with the rash is necessary for it to be contagious, so the child does not need to stay home from school if the rash is completely covered.

Treatment

There is little that can be done for the rash or the pain afterward, but prompt use of antiviral drugs such as acyclovir, famcyclovir, or valacyclovir can shorten the rash stage and lessen the chance of pain later. This is why the child should see a doctor as soon as the signs of shingles appear. While the antiviral drugs can shorten the course of the infection, it cannot completely prevent nerve pain following an attack.

Some experts maintain that steroid drugs such as prednisone can prevent this pain. Other treatments include antidepressants and anticonvulsants (these drugs affect chemicals in the body related to pain).

An over-the-counter product called Zostrix or Valtrex (active ingredient: capsaicin, a red pepper derivative) may help relieve the pain. It should only be used once all the blisters have disappeared and should *never* be applied to active blisters. As a counterirritant Zostrix is designed to be used on unbroken skin.

Complications

Parents should call the pediatrician if the rash involves the child's eyes, becomes red and drains pus, or lasts more than two weeks.

Prevention

Some research suggests that the chicken pox vaccine may reduce the risk of later developing shingles.

sibling rivalry The natural feelings of competition among siblings that can flare into squabbles and bickering are completely normal and can help children learn valuable lessons in getting along with others and settling differences. However, sibling rivalry can become a problem if the rivalry escalates unchecked into severe physical violence, verbal abuse and harassment, or if parents expect their children to get along together perfectly at all times or if parents consistently take sides against one child.

Learning to cope with disagreements and disputes with brothers and sisters can help to promote several important skills, such as how to compromise and negotiate and control aggressive feelings. However, while some degree of sibling conflict can help teach life skills, parents must keep conflict under control.

Conflict among siblings is influenced by the personalities of all the children in the family, especially those who lack skills in language or social interaction. Recent research suggests that the family dynamics also can affect sibling conflict, and it is less likely to be a problem if parents model ways to solve problems and disagreements in ways that are respectful, productive, and not aggressive. Keeping sibling rivalry to a minimum is also easier if the family clearly forbids physical aggression and name-calling and instead spends time together in enjoyable activities.

Research also shows that exposure to violent TV and movie images increases the risk of aggressive behavior among children, and that children's shows that portray significant sibling conflict and disrespect can increase sibling rivalry at home. This is why it is important for parents to teach critical viewing skills and to help their children understand the consequences of violence and disrespect.

Most experts agree that parents should get involved in their children's disputes if there is a risk of physical harm; otherwise, children should be encouraged to resolve the problems themselves. If parents must intervene, they should separate the children and ask them to come up with at least one idea about how their conflict could have been avoided or resolved. It is far more effective to allow children to solve their own problems than to punish them for not getting along. At the same time, parents should try not to figure out which child is to blame but simply assume that since it takes two to fight, everyone involved is partly responsible.

Severe sibling rivalry may best be handled during weekly family meetings in which parents remind their children of family rules about fighting and name-calling and review ways to settle conflicts.

In a few families, the conflict between siblings is so severe that the help of a mental health professional may be required. Signs that a family may need outside help in solving the problem include conflict that is causing marital problems, creates a real danger of physical harm, or that is hurting a child's self-esteem or psychological well-being.

sickle-cell disease   An inherited blood disorder that affects red blood cells. Children with sickle-cell disease have red blood cells that contain mostly "hemoglobin S," an abnormal type of hemoglobin (the main substance in red blood cells that helps carry oxygen from the air in the lungs to the rest of the body). In sickle-cell disease, these red blood cells become abnormally shaped into a sickle, or crescent, which makes it difficult for them to pass through small blood vessels.

When sickle-shaped cells block small blood vessels, this interferes with the flow of blood to that part of the body, eventually damaging the tissue. This is what causes the complications of sickle-cell disease.

Cause

Normal red blood cells contain hemoglobin A; hemoglobin S and hemoglobin C are abnormal types of hemoglobin. Normal red blood cells are soft and round and can squeeze through tiny blood vessels and typically live for about 120 days before new ones replace them.

Children with sickle-cell conditions produce a different form of hemoglobin A, called hemoglobin S ("S" stands for *sickle*). Red blood cells containing hemoglobin S live only about 16 days, becoming stiff and distorted until they cannot pass through the body's small blood vessels. When sickle-shaped cells block small blood vessels, less blood can reach that part of the body. Tissue that does not receive a normal blood flow eventually becomes damaged. This is what causes the complications of sickle-cell disease.

Types of Sickle-Cell Disease

There are several types of sickle-cell disease, but the most common are sickle-cell anemia (SS), sickle-hemoglobin C disease (SC), sickle beta-plus thalassemia, and sickle beta-zero thalassemia.

Sickle-cell trait (AS) is an inherited condition in which both hemoglobin A and S are produced in the red blood cells, although there is always more A than S. Sickle-cell trait is not a type of sickle-cell disease. People with sickle-cell trait are generally healthy.

Heredity

Sickle-cell conditions are inherited diseases. The types of hemoglobin a child produces depends on what hemoglobin genes the child inherited from both parents. Like most genes, hemoglobin genes are inherited in two sets—one from each parent. For example, if one parent has sickle-cell anemia and the other is normal, all of the children will have sickle-cell trait. If one parent has sickle-cell anemia and the other has sickle-cell trait, there is a 50 percent chance of having a baby with either sickle-cell disease or sickle-cell trait with each pregnancy. When both parents have sickle-cell trait, they have a 25 percent chance (one of four) of having a baby with sickle-cell disease with each pregnancy.

Diagnosis

A simple blood test followed by a lab technique called hemoglobin electrophoresis can determine the type of hemoglobin a child has. This technique differentiates between normal hemoglobin (A), sickle hemoglobin (S), and other different kinds of hemoglobin (such as C, D, or E).

Complications

Sickle cells are destroyed rapidly in the bodies of people with the disease causing anemia, jaundice, and gallstones. The sickle cells also block the flow of blood through vessels, resulting in lung tissue damage, pain episodes, STROKE, and priapism (painful prolonged erection). It also causes damage to most organs, including the spleen, kidneys, and liver. Damage to the spleen causes sickle-cell disease patients, (especially young children) to be easily overwhelmed by certain bacterial infections.

Treatment

Health maintenance for patients with sickle-cell disease starts with early diagnosis, preferably in the newborn period, and includes penicillin prophylaxis, vaccination against pneumococcus bacteria, and folic acid supplementation. Treatment of complications often includes antibiotics, pain management, intravenous fluids, blood transfusion, and surgery, all backed by psychosocial support. Like all patients with chronic disease patients are best managed in a comprehensive multidisciplinary program of care.

In search for a substance that can prevent red blood cells from sickling without causing harm to other parts of the body, Hydroxyurea was found to reduce the frequency of severe pain, acute chest syndrome, and the need for blood transfusions in adult patients with sickle-cell disease. Droxia, the prescription form of hydroxyurea, was approved by the Federal Drug Administration (FDA) in 1998 and is now available for adult patients with sickle-cell anemia. Studies are being conducted to determine the proper dosage for children.

sick school syndrome   Many of the nation's schools have poor ventilation and significant sources of pollution inside the buildings, which can be a serious problem for children with asthma; in particular, indoor pollutants can be a problem. When a building has indoor air problems, it is known as a "sick building." When a school is deemed sick, it means that the people inside experience health problems that have no other obvious cause and that these symptoms or problems disappear or improve when they leave the building. According to a 1995 federal government survey, half of all schools in the country were sick schools.

Diagnosis

There are no strict criteria for diagnosing sick school syndrome; health experts make a diagnosis by examining the child and assessing whether the symptoms seem related to being in school. Sick school syndrome is often wrongly blamed for several illnesses and disorders ranging from INFLUENZA to ATTENTION DEFICIT HYPERACTIVITY DISORDER. Therefore, it is important for health experts to look for other explanations for a child's symptoms before attributing them to the school environment.

The most frequent contributing factor to sick school syndrome is poor indoor air quality, usually because of poor ventilation. Without ventilation, too much moisture leads to mold and bacteria. Buildings are more tightly sealed today than they were 50 years ago because of energy concerns, and this can result in poorer air quality indoors. In addition, synthetic building materials and furnishings and pesticides add to indoor chemical pollution.

In new buildings the combination of the tight seal and the presence of chemical materials are often at fault. With older buildings ventilation systems may have been turned off or allowed to fall into disrepair. Moisture can also contribute to the development of a sick building. If a roof leaks and carpets are damp, they can harbor bacteria, mold, and fungi that can make children sick. Housekeeping supplies such as copy machine chemicals and pesticides can add to the problem.

Symptoms

The most common symptoms of sick school syndrome are headache, fatigue, and shortness of breath, plus sinus congestion, sneezing, coughing, and nausea, as well as eye, nose, throat, and skin irritation, and dizziness. Because the symptoms of sick school syndrome are similar to those of many other illnesses, it can be difficult to pinpoint indoor air pollutants as the cause. Children with asthma are particularly susceptible to indoor pollutants.

Treatment

The best way to treat the illnesses triggered by indoor air pollutants is to fix the environmental problem. The six basic methods for getting rid of indoor air pollution are removal or relocation of the source of pollution, providing exhaust systems in rooms where there are pollutants (such as science labs or copy machine rooms), improving ventilation, using chemicals when children are not in school (such as waxing floors on the weekends), using clean air filters in ventilation systems, and making sure the school staff is familiar with the importance of clean indoor air.

SIDS   See SUDDEN INFANT DEATH SYNDROME.

sinusitis   An inflammation of one or more of the sinuses, often as a complication of an upper respiratory infection or dental infection. It also may be caused by allergies, air travel, or underwater swimming. Sinusitis is extremely common and afflicts some people with every bout of the common cold. In many children, once a tendency toward sinusitis develops, the condition recurs with each viral infection.

Cause

Sinusitis is often caused by an infection spreading from the nose along the narrow passages that drain mucus from the sinuses into the nose. As the nasal mucous membranes swell, the openings from the sinuses to the nose may become blocked. This leads to a buildup of sinus secretions, often teeming with bacteria. The disorder is usually caused by a bacterial infection that develops as a complication of a viral infection.

Symptoms

Pressure, throbbing headache, fever, and local tenderness, together with a feeling of fullness or tension. It also may cause a stuffy nose and loss of the ability to smell.

Complications

Often sinusitis leads to the formation of pus in the affected sinuses, causing pain and a nasal discharge. More severe complications include MENINGITIS.

Diagnosis

CT scans are the best way to diagnose the disease. X rays may be taken to determine the location and extent of the disorder, and a culture may be grown from a swab of the sinus to identify the bacteria.

Treatment

Steam inhalations, nasal decongestants, painkillers, and antibiotics can help. Surgery to improve drainage may be performed for chronic problems.

sixth disease   See ROSEOLA.

skin, care of   Skin must be cleansed daily to remove the dirt and grease, bacteria, and odor. Soaps are the products used for these purposes. There are differences in the types of soaps that may be used on the skin, and they differ in outward appearance, fragrance, cost, and composition.

For example, superfatted soaps contain excess fatty material and leave an oil residue on the skin, which is designed to improve mildness. Transparent soaps contain glycerin and varied amounts of vegetable fats. Other soaps may be produced for specific purposes, such as oatmeal soap for skin that tends to break out. The choice of a proper soap demands on the child's age, skin texture, skin problems, and personal needs. All soaps are good at cleansing, but because of age, heredity, climate, and skin texture, there are many different methods of proper skin cleansing.

Infancy

In infancy the skin's oil glands are not very active, although the sweat glands are quite active. Tepid water is recommended for bathing, and a mild soap may be used sparingly to remove skin oil. The diaper area requires special attention: Soiled diapers should be changed frequently to avoid the harsh irritants of urine and feces. Removal of fecal material may require gentle rubbing with a cotton ball soaked in an oily solution. Avoid using soap if an irritating rash appears—in fact, a great deal of soap is not required at this early age.

The child's skin should be examined regularly, while diapering, bathing, and dressing. Any change (mole, growth, spot, or sore) should be pointed out to the baby's doctor. While it is normal for toddlers to develop new moles and other brown spots, those that continue to change should be checked by a doctor. Some medications make skin ultrasensitive; when parents get a new prescription for their child, they should ask the physician if the sun should be avoided.

Because it make take several years for an infant's melanin production to be fully developed, its skin is especially vulnerable to the sun—even in those with darker skin. Because a baby's skin constitutes a larger percentage of total body mass than adults, they are especially vulnerable to anything affecting the skin. A bad sunburn can cause serious fluid and electrolyte loss, fever, faintness, delirium, shock, low blood pressure, and irregular heartbeat.

Infants under age six months should not be given sunscreen and should be kept out of the sun entirely by using carriage hoods, canopies, and tightly woven umbrellas, along with a lightweight but tightly woven hat. Time in the sun should be limited to short trips, and babies should be kept in the shade as much as possible. Since sand, concrete, snow, and water reflect ultraviolet radiation, it is better to park the carriage on grass instead of a patio. When at the beach, the baby should stay away from the water. Even on overcast days, as much as 80 percent of the sun's harmful radiation can still penetrate the clouds.

Babies over age six months should avoid the hours from 10 A.M. to 3 P.M. when the sun is most intense; at other times, the baby should be covered up with tightly woven hats and clothes (a broad-brimmed hat will shade ears, nose, and lips and may reduce the baby's chance of cataracts in later life). However, the sun can penetrate some fabric, including cotton undershirts, which only have a sun protection factor (SPF) of about 8, so parents should not rely on clothes alone for protection. Parents also should limit time spent in the sun with babies this age, regardless of hour or season.

After a baby reaches six months of age, experts agree on the importance of using sunscreen especially made for children. Most of these do not contain PABA, which can be irritating to the skin.

Unscented sunscreens are a better choice because they do not attract insects. The product's SPF should be at least 15, manufactured by a major drug company and purchased at a store with a large turnover. Look for an expiration date (lack of one probably indicates that there are no ingredients that could deteriorate).

No matter how safe and effective the product seems, it is a good idea to test it on a child's skin before using. A small amount placed on arm or abdomen will reveal if redness or irritation appear; if it does, parents should select another product. Normally, creamy products work best on youngsters because they do not dry the skin and they can be easily seen.

Sunscreen should be applied to all exposed areas, and under thin clothing, 15 to 30 minutes before exposure (it takes that long for the ingredients to penetrate the skin).

Childhood

As the child gets older, the need for soap increases, but if a rash appears then the soap should be discontinued. It may be particularly difficult to use soap on a child who has atopic dermatitis, an inherited dry, scaly condition of the skin. Preteens have a greater need for daily soap and bathing, as the sweat and oil glands are now functioning with more efficiency and can withstand repeated use of soap.

Teenagers

During puberty (age 13 to 19 years) the oil glands function at peak capacity, especially on the scalp, forehead, face, and upper chest. Some degree of acne and an oily complexion are quite common, and routine showering or bathing should become a habit. While frequent washing may appear to decrease oiliness, it will not alleviate acne by itself.

skin infections Skin infections can range from a local superficial problem, such as IMPETIGO, to a widespread and more serious infection. Examples of bacterial skin infections include ECTHYMA, folliculitis, BOILS, CARBUNCLES, SCARLET FEVER, CELLULITIS, and so on. Viral infections with skin symptoms include HERPES, CHICKEN POX, SHINGLES, WARTS, MEASLES, GERMAN MEASLES, FIFTH DISEASE, and AIDS.

skin rash See RASH.

skull fracture   See HEAD INJURY.

sleep apnea   See APNEA.

smallpox   A highly infectious, serious viral disease causing a skin rash and flu-like symptoms that has been totally eradicated throughout the world since 1980. The last naturally acquired case of smallpox occurred in Somalia in 1977, and the last cases of smallpox (from lab exposure) occurred in 1978. In May 1980 the World Health Assembly certified that the world was free of naturally occurring smallpox. However, the threat of smallpox has reemerged as a potential terroristic threat since the attack on the World Trade Center in New York City on September 11, 2001.

In the United States vaccination programs and quarantine regulations meant that by the 1960s the risk for importing smallpox had been reduced. As a result, recommendations for routine smallpox vaccination were rescinded in 1971. In 1976 the recommendation for routine smallpox vaccination of health-care workers was also discontinued. In 1982 the only active licensed producer of vaccinia vaccine in the United States discontinued production for general use, and in 1983 distribution to the civilian population was discontinued. Since January 1982 smallpox vaccination has not been required for international travelers, and International Certificates of Vaccination forms no longer include a space to record smallpox vaccination.

In the United States routine vaccination against smallpox ended in 1972. The level of immunity among vaccinated Americans is uncertain, so these people are assumed to be susceptible. Most estimates suggest immunity from the vaccination lasts only three to five years, which means that nearly the entire U.S. population has only partial immunity at best. Approximately half of the U.S. population has never been vaccinated.

In 1992 the government formed volunteer Smallpox Response Teams who can provide critical services to citizens in the event of a smallpox attack. To ensure that the teams can mobilize immediately in an emergency, health-care workers and other critical personnel were asked to volunteer to receive the smallpox vaccine. Although the United States currently has enough vaccine to vaccinate every single person in the country in an emergency, the federal government does not recommend vaccination for the general public because of both the possibility of side effects and the low level of threat. However, the Department of Defense vaccinates certain military and civilian personnel deployed in high threat areas, along with some personnel assigned to certain overseas embassies.

In addition, the government is preparing to make unlicensed vaccine available to those adult members of the general public without medical contraindications who insist on being vaccinated. Immunity can be boosted effectively with a single revaccination, and prior infection with the disease grants lifelong immunity.

The U.S. Centers for Disease Control (CDC) maintains an emergency supply of vaccine that can be released if necessary, since post-exposure vaccination is also effective in preventing the disease. In 2000 the CDC awarded a contract to a vaccine manufacturer to produce additional doses of smallpox vaccine in case of a bioterrorism attack. In the event of an outbreak, the CDC has clear guidelines to provide vaccine swiftly to people exposed to this disease. The vaccine is securely stored for use in the case of an outbreak.

Symptoms

The incubation period before symptoms appear ranges between seven and 17 days after exposure. Initial symptoms include high fever, fatigue, and head and back aches. A characteristic rash of flat red lesions, most prominent on the face, arms, and legs, follows in two to three days. Lesions become filled with pus after a few days, and then begin to crust early in the second week. Scabs develop, separate, and then fall off after about three to four weeks. Most patients with smallpox recover, but death may occur in up to 30 percent of cases.

In most cases, smallpox is spread from one person to another by infected saliva droplets that expose a susceptible person having face-to-face contact with the ill person. People with smallpox are most infectious during the first week of illness, because that is when the largest amount of virus is present in saliva. However, some risk of transmission lasts until all scabs have fallen off. Contaminated clothing or bed linen could also spread the virus. Special precautions need to be taken to ensure that all bedding and clothing of patients are cleaned appropriately with bleach and hot water. Disinfectants such as bleach and quaternary ammonia can be used for cleaning contaminated surfaces.

Vaccine

Smallpox vaccine does not contain smallpox virus but another live virus called vaccinia virus, which is related to smallpox. Vaccination provides immunity against infection from smallpox virus. If the vaccine is given within four days after exposure to smallpox, it can lessen the severity of illness or even prevent it. In addition to the stock of smallpox vaccine in the United States, an additional 50 million to 100 million doses are estimated to exist worldwide, and the World Health Organization (WHO) recommends that countries with stocks of smallpox vaccine maintain these stocks.

Side Effects

Side effects from successful vaccination include tenderness, redness, swelling, and a lesion at the vaccination site. In addition, the vaccination may cause fever for a few days and the lymph nodes in the vaccinated arm may become enlarged and tender. These symptoms are more common in those receiving their first dose of vaccine than in those being revaccinated. The overall risks of serious complications of smallpox vaccination are low and occur more frequently in those receiving their first dose of vaccine and among young children.

The most frequent serious complications are encephalitis, progressive destruction of skin and other tissues at the vaccination site, and severe and destructive infection of skin affected already by eczema or other chronic skin disorder. Encephalitis occurs in about one in 300,000 doses in children.

Who Should Not Be Vaccinated

The vaccine is not recommended for those who have abnormalities of the immune system because the complication of progressive destruction of skin and other tissues at the vaccination site has occurred only among recipients in this group. The vaccine is also not recommended for recipients who have eczema or other chronic skin disorders because the complication of severe and destructive infection of skin has occurred only among these patients.

Treatment

There is no proven treatment for smallpox, but researchers are studying new antiviral drugs. Patients with smallpox are given supportive treatment including intravenous fluids, medicine to control fever or pain, and antibiotics for secondary bacterial infections.

smoking and children   Every day, almost 5,000 children and teens try smoking for the first time. Cigarettes and smokeless tobacco kill hundreds of thousands of Americans every year. The nicotine and the other poisonous chemicals in tobacco cause heart problems and cancer. Some of these illnesses take years to develop, but others can show up right away; smokers are much more likely to get infections such as colds and pneumonia.

The problem is particularly serious in adolescence, since teenagers can become addicted to cigarettes in as little as a few weeks by taking just a few draws on a cigarette every other day, according to research from the University of Massachusetts. Research also shows that smoking is particularly dangerous for teens because their bodies are still developing and the 4,000 chemicals (including 200 known poisons) in cigarette smoke can adversely affect this process.

Most people start using tobacco before they finish high school. This means that if a teen stays smoke-free in school, he or she will probably never smoke.

social phobia   An ANXIETY DISORDER characterized by a constant fear of social or performance situations such as speaking in class or eating in public. This fear is often accompanied by physical symptoms such as sweating, blushing, heart palpitations, shortness of breath, or muscle tenseness. Social phobia usually emerges in the mid-teens and typically does not affect young children.

Teens with this disorder typically respond to these feelings by avoiding the feared situation. For example, they may stay home from school or avoid parties. Young people with social phobia are often overly sensitive to criticism, have trouble being assertive, and suffer from low self-esteem. Moreover, social phobia can be limited to specific situations, so the adolescent may fear dating and recreational events but be confident in academic and work situations.

solar warning index   A daily warning index forecasting the ultraviolet light radiation exposure for major cities in the United States designed to help people avoid skin cancer. The index is issued daily to forecast the amount of dangerous ultraviolet light that will reach the Earth's surface at noon the next day. The scale is one to 10 in most areas, rising to one to 15 in regions that receive stronger solar radiation. The higher the number, the greater the danger.

The goal of the warnings, which are issued by the National Weather Service, is to remind people of the danger to their skin so they will use sunscreens and sunglasses and reduce exposure to themselves and their children. Damage from sun exposure accumulates over time, and much of the injury occurs during childhood. The general categories of hazard are:

Minimal (Index of 0–2)
Fair-skinned people may burn in 30 minutes; those with darker skins may be safe up to two hours.

Low (3–4)
Fair-skinned people may burn in 15 to 20 minutes; others may be safe from 75 to 90 minutes.

Moderate (5–6)
Fair people may burn in 10 to 12 minutes; others may be safe for 50 to 60 minutes.

High (7–9)
Fair people may burn in 7 to $8\frac{1}{2}$ minutes; others may be safe for 33 to 40 minutes.

Very High (10 and Up)
Fair people may burn in 4 to 6 minutes; others may be safe for 20 to 30 minutes.

sore throat   A scratchy, painful throat known medically as PHARYNGITIS, that often accompanies a cold or other infection caused by a variety of organisms. Although a sore throat in itself is not serious, it may indicate a bacterial infection such as STREP THROAT.

Symptoms
Strep throat may cause swollen/tender lymph nodes in the neck, fever for more than two days, and pain with swallowing. Any of the following signs indicate the onset of EPIGLOTTITIS, which is much more serious than a sore throat and requires immediate medical attention:

- sudden severe pain in throat
- refusal to swallow
- uncontrolled drooling
- breathing problems
- harsh sound when inhaling

southern tick-associated rash illness (STARI)
An infection causing a rash similar to that produced by LYME DISEASE affecting residents in southeastern and south central United States. Southern tick-associated rash illness (STARI) is associated with the bite of the lone star tick *(Amblyomma americanum)*. These ticks are found through the southeast and south central states. Even though spirochetes have been seen in *A. americanum* ticks, attempts to culture them in the laboratory have consistently failed. However, a spirochete has been detected in *A. americanum* by DNA analysis and was given the name *Borrelia lonestari*.

Symptoms
People who live or travel in the south and who develop a red, expanding rash with central clearing after the bite of a lone star tick should see a doctor. The Centers for Disease Control and Prevention is interested in obtaining samples from such patients under an Institutional Review Board-approved investigational protocol. In 2001 one patient with evidence of *B. lonestari* infection was reported in the medical literature. This patient had been exposed to ticks in Maryland and North Carolina and had developed a typical Lyme disease rash. DNA analysis indicated the presence of *B. lonestari* in a skin biopsy taken at the leading edge of the rash and in the tick removed by the doctor. Testing for Lyme disease was negative. The patient was treated with an oral antibiotic and recovered.

Lone star ticks can be found from central Texas and Oklahoma eastward across the southern states and along the Atlantic coast as far north as Maine. Although several studies have demonstrated that between 1 percent and 3 percent of these ticks are infected with a spirochete, a thorough assessment of risk of infection has not been conducted.

Treatment/Prevention

As with Lyme disease, prompt treatment with antibiotics cures the infection. Prevention measures similar to those for Lyme disease will reduce the exposure to infected ticks.

Spanish flu   See INFLUENZA.

spatial-material organizational disorder   A problem with organizing materials so that the child constantly struggles for survival within an ordered environment. A child with this problem has a hard time organizing information on paper. Margins are missing, spacings between words and letters are incorrect, centering is difficult, and the overall appearance of the work is messy. Teachers often have trouble reading the child's work. A child with this problem often forgets assignments or books needed to complete assignments. Assignments themselves may be incomplete, or the child cannot find completed assignments.

In addition, a child with this problem is often disorganized and has problems following routines or completing tasks. Desk and home environment are usually quite messy and disorganized, although the child may appear to have his own system of organization in his own space.

special education   Educational services and programs for students with abilities ranging from giftedness to MENTAL RETARDATION, and including various physical, emotional, or learning differences.

Although the history of special education can be traced at least as far back as Plato's recommendation that children with extraordinary intellectual ability should be provided special leadership training, in more modern times special education was practiced in the 16th century when Pedro Ponce de León taught deaf Spanish children to speak, read, and write. In the 18th century Jean-Marc-Gaspard Itard developed special education techniques with Victor, the so-called Wild Boy of Aveyron. During the late 18th and early 19th centuries, special education procedures for teaching some school skills to pupils with sensory handicaps were supported by Thomas Hopkins Gallaudet. For example, individuals with profound hearing loss were taught meanings for printed words by repeated simultaneous presentations of a printed word and a picture of what the word represented.

About the same time, attempts to educate individuals with mental retardation or with emotional or behavioral disorders increased in number and success, as exemplified in the work of the American educator Samuel Gridley Howe. Successful attempts to educate the deaf and blind led to scientific methods to teach the mentally retarded in Europe. For example, Maria Montessori, a pediatrician and innovative educator, used multisensory methods to teach mentally retarded and culturally deprived children in Rome in the late 19th century.

In the 20th century, the enactment and implementation of compulsory education laws led to an increasing need for special education services. In the latter half of the 20th century, great gains have been made in special education. In most developed countries, addressing the educational needs of the disabled has become universal. However, it was not until the mid-1970s, with the passage of the Education for All Handicapped Children Act of 1975 (PL 94-142), that the education of disabled children carried the force of law in the United States. This revolutionary legislation, guaranteeing a free and appropriate education for all children, paved the way for a rapid expansion of the field of special education that continues to this day.

Public Law 94-142, renamed Individuals with Disabilities Education Act (IDEA) in 1990, requires students with disabilities to be placed in the least restrictive environment (LRE) available in order to avoid segregating students with disabilities.

Schools that comply with the laws receive more money from the federal government to offset part of the costs of providing special education services. The federal government also requires that schools report the number of special education students they serve. During the 1989–90 school year, more than four-and-a-half million children received such services. About 85 percent of these children were between the ages of six and 17.

Special equipment is used extensively with students who have problems with vision or hearing. Such equipment might include computers to convert printed materials into synthetic speech. Special desks, chairs, writing devices, and school buses may help students with physical handicaps. Special ramps and wide doors, swimming pools, and schoolrooms specially equipped with hearing aid transmitting equipment are all part of special education.

Special services for exceptional individuals include speech training, physical and occupational therapies, counseling, and vocational training for students with mental retardation. The most common elements of special education are the specialized instructional techniques, such as:

- sign language
- programmed instruction procedures designed to present information in small steps
- behavior modification techniques such as token economies

While most special education takes place in regular public schools, some classes are provided in special public or private day or residential schools, public or private hospitals, and, in some cases, the homes of individuals whose disabilities prevent them from attending school. Most individuals with disabilities do not require an entire program of services apart from conventional instruction but rather only a modification of features.

When children are considered able to benefit from participation with other children, they are usually taught in the normal school program. This process, known as mainstreaming, was believed to be consistent with the legal mandate for education in the least-restrictive environment. More than two-thirds of students with disabilities receive most of their education in regular education classes.

If a child's handicap is not severe, a special education teacher works with the regular classroom teacher to develop skills. In other cases, an assistant teacher may be able to care for a student's specific needs. For individuals with more serious problems, special education may be provided in a separate classroom for part of the school day; students with severe learning and behavioral problems may remain in a separate special education room all day. The ratio of students to teachers is usually much lower in a special education classroom than in an ordinary classroom.

With the development of assistive technologies, the field of special education continues to evolve, although its goal remains the same as it was from the beginning—to educate and integrate individuals with disabilities into society.

speech-language problems A problem or delay in verbal, gestural, or speaking skills including articulation (pronunciation), voice quality, fluency, or language that interferes with learning, social adjustment, or communication. Some problem with speech affects one out of every 10 American children.

Cause
Hearing problems, low intelligence, or lack of verbal stimulation at home all may interfere with the development of speech. Children with older siblings or one child in a set of twins may not talk because others talk for them.

Diagnosis
Early detection is critically important if the child is to develop normal speech patterns and prevent the problem from interfering with learning in other areas. Problems with hearing or speech and language development can create barriers to social interaction and emotional well-being at a very young age and make it difficult for a child to progress in school.

Parents who suspect a speech problem should take the child to a speech and language specialist as soon as possible for an evaluation, which will include a full speech workup and a hearing test.

Treatment
Many speech problems can be corrected with short-term treatment, especially if the problem is diagnosed before first grade.

If a child needs therapy, some of the speech therapy options could include individual speech therapy. If the speech-language pathologist thinks the child may not need therapy right away, she may give parents some suggestions for techniques to use at home and check back with the family in a few months to check progress.

Warning Signs

All children develop at different rates, but there are some obvious signs that a child may be developing speech problems. Parents should consult their pediatrician or a speech therapist If the child:

- is not babbling or using language by 15 to 18 months of age
- by age three is using mostly vowels or omitting the beginning sounds in words, or if other people cannot understand what the child is saying
- has not mastered all speech sounds by age eight.

At certain ages, certain speech problems are normal. For example, stuttering is common between ages three and four years, but most children grow out of the habit of repeating sounds and hesitating between words. However, if this is happening for longer than two or three months and interferes with communication, the child may be developing a stuttering problem. Parents should ignore stuttering and not correct the child, but children with a severe stuttering problem should receive speech therapy to avoid a long-term problem.

Nodules on the vocal cords can cause hoarseness; a child should be seen by a doctor if he breathes through the nose while speaking and is hoarse.

Babbling that stops after a brief period may be a sign of a hearing disorder. Frequent ear infections can affect hearing and delay speech.

By the time a child is four years old she should be able to tell a story, and by age five should be able to listen to a story and answer questions.

What Parents Can Do

Parents can encourage speech development by talking and reading to the child, singing songs to the baby. Vocabulary and sentence length should be adjusted for the child's level. Reading together out loud also helps to improve vocabulary, sequencing, and attention span.

spider bite   While most of the more than 50,000 species of spider found in the United States actually possess poison glands connected to their fangs, only a very few are capable of piercing human skin. Those that can include the black widow *(Latrodectus)*, brown recluse spider *(Loxosceles)*, jumping spider *(Phidippus)*, and tarantula (a common name given to many large spiders). Two species of spider are responsible for most of the serious spider bites in the United States; widow spiders and the brown recluse.

In general, most spider attacks occur when someone disturbs a spider's nest while working outdoors or making house repairs. While tarantulas rarely cause problems, their bite is painful because of their size of their fangs. Brown recluse spiders are most often found in dark places like outhouses.

spina bifida   The most common permanently disabling birth defect that affects about one out of every 1,000 newborns in the United States. Spina bifida, the most common NEURAL TUBE DEFECT, is one of the most devastating of all birth defects.

Cause

Spina bifida occurs when the spine does not close properly during the first month of pregnancy. In severe cases, the spinal cord protrudes through the child's back and may be covered by skin or a thin membrane. Surgery to close a newborn's back is generally performed within 24 hours after birth to minimize the risk of infection and to preserve existing function in the spinal cord.

Many things can affect a pregnancy, including family genes and things women may come in contact with during pregnancy. However, recent studies have shown that folic acid is one factor that may reduce the risk of having a baby with a neural tube defect such as spina bifida.

Symptoms

Because of paralysis resulting from the damage to the spinal cord, children born with spina bifida may need surgery and other extensive medical care. The condition also can cause bowel and bladder complications.

In addition, many children born with spina bifida also have an accumulation of fluid in the brain (HYDROCEPHALUS), which can be controlled by a surgical procedure called "shunting" to relieve the fluid by redirecting it into the abdominal area.

Most children born with spina bifida live well into adulthood as a result of today's sophisticated medical techniques.

Some children with spina bifida also experience learning problems. They may have difficulty with paying attention, expressing or understanding language, organizing, sequencing, and grasping reading and math.

Other conditions associated with spina bifida include LATEX ALLERGY, tendonitis, OBESITY, skin breakdown, stomach problems, DEPRESSION, and social and sexual issues.

Treatment

Children with spina bifida need to learn how to walk with crutches, braces, or wheelchairs. With new techniques, children also can become independent in managing their bowel and bladder problems. To promote personal growth, parents should encourage children (within the limits of safety and health) to be independent, to participate in activities with their nondisabled peers, and to assume responsibility for their own care.

Early intervention can help to prepare children with spina bifida and learning disabilities for school, with normal day-to-day activities. It often helps to have a psychological evaluation, which tests the child's intelligence, academic levels, and basic learning abilities (visual perception, receptive and expressive language skills).

Prevention

While taking folic acid cannot guarantee a healthy baby, it can help. Taking folic acid before and during early pregnancy reduces the risk of spina bifida and other neural tube defects. All women should take a daily vitamin including 400 micrograms (mcg)—the same as 0.4 milligrams (mg)—of folic acid every day.

A woman thinking about getting pregnant, who already has a child with spina bifida, who has spina bifida herself, or who has had a history of pregnancy affected by a neural tube defect, needs a higher dose of folic acid. These women should take 4,000 micrograms (mcg) of folic acid by prescription for one to three months before becoming pregnant. Taking this amount of folic acid by prescription may reduce the chance of a neural tube defect like spina bifida in future pregnancies.

However, any woman taking this extra folic acid should not get this amount by taking more multivitamins, because too much of some of the other vitamins could harm either mother or child. A doctor should prescribe the extra folic acid supplement.

Before the next pregnancy, a woman with any of the above risk factors should speak with her health care provider about her personal risk of having a baby with a neural tube defect. She may need to get a prescription for folic acid before trying to become pregnant.

Folic acid is a common water-soluble B vitamin that is essential for the functioning of the human body. During periods of rapid growth (such as pregnancy and fetal development) the body's requirement for this vitamin increases. Folic acid can be found in multivitamins, fortified breakfast cereals, dark green leafy vegetables such as broccoli and spinach, egg yolks, and some fruits and fruit juices. However, the average American diet does not supply the recommended level of folic acid.

Spina Bifida Association of America A nonprofit organization dedicated to publicizing developments in medicine, education, and legislation; supporting research, promoting treatment; and encouraging the training of competent professionals. The Spina Bifida Association of America (SBAA) publishes brochures, reports, and educational videotape programs for parents and health professionals, plus a 35-mm slide presentation on the abilities and potential of people with spina bifida. (For contact information, see Appendix I.)

spinal meningitis See MENINGITIS.

spinal tap The common name for a lumbar puncture, a procedure in which cerebrospinal fluid is removed by using a hollow needle inserted into the lower back, usually between the third and fourth lumbar vertebrae. The fluid is checked for appearance, white blood cells, sugar, and protein in a lab and is also sent for culture, which can help determine what sort of germ is causing symptoms.

While some children fear the thought of a spinal tap, in fact the procedure is not terribly painful. It is a safe procedure when done in a large hospital emergency room or in an experienced pediatrician's office. A spinal tap must be done whenever there is a suspicion of MENINGITIS.

sports injuries Football, basketball, baseball, soccer, hockey, gymnastics, and volleyball are the top six sports that cause the most injuries in children. Although these activities help develop muscles and coordination, they can also result in injury, especially in children, whose bones, muscles, tendons, and ligaments are still growing.

An estimated 3.5 million children's fractures, dislocations, and soft-tissue injuries related to these recreation activities were treated at U.S. hospital emergency rooms, doctor's offices, and clinics each year.

Basketball leads the list of most dangerous sport, with 574,000 injuries reported in 2001, followed closely by football, with 448,200 injuries. Children playing baseball received 252,665 injuries; those playing soccer included 227,100 injuries. Hockey, which many consider to be a violent sport, was fifth on the list, with 80,700 injuries, followed by gymnastics at 75,000, and volleyball at 50,100.

Other non-team sports can also lead to a considerable number of injuries. For example, biking causes a very high number of fractures, dislocations, strains/sprains, and abrasions; among children ages five to 14, there were 415,000 injuries a year to arms, legs, and trunk. Roller sports caused more than 297,000 injuries, and trampolines caused 135,000 injuries. Scooter-related injuries increase each year (including sprains and strains, cuts and bruises, fractures, and dislocations); more than 84,400 injuries were severe enough to go to the emergency room in 2001 for treatment.

Prevent Injuries

Coaches and parents can prevent injuries by promoting an atmosphere of healthy competition emphasizing self-reliance, confidence, cooperation, and a positive self-image, rather than just winning. Young athletes need proper training before participating in a sport; they should not expect the sport itself to get them into shape. Injuries can be prevented if children participate in a regular conditioning program designed by a coach. It is also important that parents make sure their child's coaches are qualified to supervise a particular sport, provide well-maintained safety equipment, and help with proper conditioning.

Alarmingly, experts estimate that at least 500,000 young athletes use black-market anabolic steroids to improve their athletic performance. Although these types of steroids can increase muscle mass, they also cause serious and potentially life-threatening complications.

Children playing sports should follow these guidelines to reduce injuries:

- Follow the rules of the sport.
- Wear appropriate protective gear (for example, shin guards for soccer, a hard-shell helmet when facing a baseball pitcher, a helmet for bike riding).
- Check equipment first and know how to use athletic equipment (breakaway bases have dramatically reduced leg injuries in children).
- Always warm up before playing.
- Avoid playing when very tired or in pain.

sprain An overstretched and partly torn ligament, which holds bones together. It is more serious than a strain, which is simply an overstretching of any part of the musculature. Sprains and strains usually cause swelling, pain, and bruises around the injured area. After medical evaluation, most sprains can be treated at home.

If a sprain involves a child's neck or back, he should not be moved unless the child is in imminent danger. Movement can cause serious nerve damage. If the child must be moved, the neck and back must be completely immobilized first and the head, neck, and back aligned.

Sprain vs. Break

It is sometimes difficult to tell the difference between a sprain and a broken bone. If there is any doubt, the child should be taken to the nearest hospital emergency department, where an X ray can identify a broken bone. A strain typically involves simple swelling, bruising, and pain. A possible broken bone should be suspected if a child heard or felt a bone snap, if the child cannot move the injured part, or if the injured part moves in an unnatural way or is very painful.

Treatment

First aid for sprains and strains includes rest, ice, compression, and elevation (known as RICE). As the injured part of the body is rested, ice packs or cold compresses should be applied for up to 10 or 15 minutes at a time every few hours for the first two days to prevent swelling. Wearing an elastic compression bandage (such as an ACE bandage) for at least two days also will help reduce swelling. Keeping the injured part above the level of the heart as much as possible is another good way to reduce swelling. Heat should not be applied in any form for at least 24 hours, because heat will increase swelling and pain.

A doctor may recommend an over-the-counter pain reliever such as acetaminophen (Tylenol) or ibuprofen (Motrin or Advil).

staphylococcal infection Infections caused by staphylococci bacteria and characterized by the formation of abscesses in the skin or other organs. Staphylococci, which grow in grapelike clusters, are a common cause of skin infections, but they also can cause serious internal disorders.

Staphylococcal bacteria are normally found on the skin of most people, but if the bacteria get trapped within the skin by blocked sweat or sebaceous glands, they can cause a wide variety of skin infections including pustules, boils, styes, or carbuncles. The bacteria also can cause a severe blistering rash in newborn babies called SCALDED SKIN SYNDROME.

The bacteria is found in the throats and nose in most people; when mucus is not cleared from the lungs (such as after a viral infection), organisms can multiply in the lungs and cause PNEUMONIA.

Staphylococcal infections are among the most common infections in surgical patients, and the number of hospital-acquired staph infections that are resistant to antibiotics has been steadily rising.

STD See SEXUALLY TRANSMITTED DISEASES.

stimulant medications Stimulants are often used in the treatment of ATTENTION DEFICIT HYPERACTIVITY DISORDER (ADHD). RITALIN (methylphenidate) is most commonly prescribed. Other stimulant medications that are frequently prescribed include Dexedrine (dextroamphetamine), Adderall (amphetamine and dextroamphetamine), and Cylert (pemoline).

For more than 50 years, these drugs have been used to treat the behavior of children with hyperactive symptoms; as many as 80 percent of students with ADHD respond to these drugs. Exactly what makes these medications effective against ADHD is unknown, although experts suspect they affect the rate and balance of specific neurotransmitters in certain areas of the brain. This results in a greater ability to pay attention and stay focused, and a decrease in hyperactivity. Since these children also tend to become less impulsive, aggressive, and destructive, the drugs also help improve social acceptance. These medications are often used in combination with behavioral and educational interventions.

Children who respond to stimulant medications generally show improvement in their academic work and in their interactions with others right away. (However, there is a lag before Cylert achieves its maximum effect in children.) Several studies have found that after students with ADHD started taking stimulants, their test scores and accuracy and speed in completing homework improved. The long-term gains are less clear.

Because most stimulant medications are metabolized quickly, often several doses a day are necessary. Stimulant medications are taken for as long a period of time as is helpful or necessary. Some children find that in adolescence the medication is no longer necessary; others find the medication less necessary as their situation changes, for example a change in environment or academic demands. Many find that they face the frustrations of ADHD through adolescence and adulthood and some of these individuals may benefit from using stimulant medication on a long-term basis.

Successful treatment with stimulants lies in finding the right drug at the right dosage. It is important to remember that the child with ADHD will still remain impulsive and energetic even while taking stimulants, but their ability to pay attention should improve.

Treatment with stimulants for ADHD is a long-term therapy; the government estimates that 80 percent of those who need medication for ADHD in childhood will still need drugs as teenagers, and 50 percent will be helped by stimulants as adults.

Side Effects

The most common side effects include weight loss and appetite loss, together with problems in falling asleep, although these problems may fade away as a student becomes used to the drug. Some studies have found that a child's growth begins to lag, although this usually rebounds after the first year in those who are on low or moderate doses. Children taking Dexedrine or high doses of Ritalin may experience prolonged growth lag as long as they remain on the medication, but once the drug is stopped growth begins again. For this reason, some experts recommend "drug holidays" during vacation to allow a child's growth to catch up.

Less common side effects include stomach problems, headaches, lethargy, irritability, nausea, euphoria, depression, nightmares, dry mouth, constipation, anxiety, hallucinations, nervous tics, and tremors. In children at risk for TIC disorders such as TOURETTE'S SYNDROME the medication may trigger the condition. Because individual reactions and needs change, it is very important that the use and result of the medication be monitored.

Addiction

While some stimulants can be addictive if abused, low doses seem to be safe for children, who do not become addicted nor become likely to be addicts when they are older. On the other hand, some studies suggest that untreated students with ADHD are at higher risk for developing substance abuse in adolescence.

St. Louis encephalitis See ENCEPHALITIS.

stork bite A harmless small flat pink skin blemish (also called "salmon patch") found in up to 50 percent of newborn babies. These blemishes found around the eyes usually disappear within the first year; those around the nape of the neck may persist indefinitely.

strabismus See LAZY EYE.

Strattera (atomoxetine) The first nonstimulant medication approved for the treatment of ADHD (ATTENTION DEFICIT HYPERACTIVITY DISORDER) in children, adolescents, and adults. The U.S. Food and Drug Administration (FDA) approved Strattera, November 26, 2002, judging it safe and effective for the treatment of ADHD. Strattera is a selective norepinephrine reuptake inhibitor—a class of drugs that works differently from the other ADHD medications available. Strattera works by selectively blocking the reuptake of norepinephrine, a chemical neurotransmitter, by certain nerve cells in the brain. This action increases the availability of norepinephrine, which experts believe is essential in regulating impulse control, organization, and attention. The precise mechanism by which Strattera works on ADHD is not known.

Because Strattera does not appear to have a potential for abuse, it is not classified as a controlled substance and is therefore simpler to obtain, although it is still a prescription drug. Strattera is an oral capsule and can be taken once or twice a day to provide full-day relief from ADHD symptoms. Strattera was studied in children, adolescents, and adults. The drug's safety and effectiveness were established in six double-blind placebo-controlled studies in patients who met specific diagnostic criteria. The clinical studies demonstrated that Strattera significantly improves patient's symptoms compared to placebo, without side effects such as insomnia common in stimulant drugs such as RITALIN.

While parents may notice improvements in ADHD symptoms by the first week, it may take up to a month to see the full therapeutic benefit of the effect as the child adjusts to the new medication.

Because Strattera works differently than other ADHD medications, children who previously took a stimulant (such as Ritalin) might notice a difference in the way the drugs work. Stimulants tend to produce an immediate impact when they take effect, and children usually can tell when they stop working. Because Strattera is a different type of medication, children will not experience this. Instead, parents should watch for behavior patterns to help assess how Strattera works, such as sitting through dinner time, settling at bedtime, getting off to school in the morning, or participating in group activities.

Side Effects

Side effects of the drug include decreased appetite, upset stomach, nausea or vomiting, and fatigue.

strawberry birthmark Also called strawberry nevus, this is a bright red BIRTHMARK that usually appears shortly after birth, when it enters a rapid growth phase during the first several months. Growth then gradually slows down and stops, beginning to regress by age one. Most of these birthmarks will have disappeared completely by age seven.

Treatment

Because these birthmarks eventually disappear on their own, treatment is not often recommended. Treatment is indicated when the mark grows rapidly, interfering with function or vital organs. In most cases, a limited course of oral corticosteroids will cause the marks to regress.

strep throat The common term for streptococcal pharyngitis, a bacterial throat infection caused by group A *beta-hemolytic Streptococcus*, a bacterium also known as *S. pyogenes*. Only group-A strep causes the infection known as strep throat; most kinds of sore throats are not strep infections.

Strep throat usually affects school-age children in the winter and spring in temperate zones of North America. Some children have a tendency toward developing multiple strep throat infections, while others rarely come down with the disease. It is rare in children under age three.

Because there are many types of group-A strep bacteria, one bout of strep throat does not confer long-term immunity; children can therefore come down with repeated episodes.

Cause

Some children carry group A strep in their throats and nasal passages and remain healthy, but these "carriers" can spread the infection to others, as can those who are actively ill. A sneeze or a cough can project the organisms up to two feet, so it spreads easily in schools and group living situations. Some epidemics have been traced to infected health-care workers in operating rooms and to infected food handlers; other outbreaks have been caused by eating contaminated food.

Children are most infectious in the beginning of the illness; untreated, a child is infectious for 10 days to three weeks. Carriers are infectious for two to three weeks, although the bacteria may be carried in nose and throat for several months. Those who receive antibiotics are no longer infectious after 24 hours. This means that children with strep throat can go back to school or child care one or two days after receiving an antibiotic, if they feel well and have no fever.

Symptoms

Up to half of all children with strep throat have no symptoms but are considered healthy carriers. If symptoms do appear, they show up one to three days after the initial infection. Young children often have high fevers and red, swollen throats, but their throats are usually less painful than those of adults with the same infection. A few children (one in 10) become quite ill, with extremely high fevers, nausea, and vomiting. Most children simply have a sore throat, fever, and pain in swallowing.

A strep throat is different from the sore throat caused by a common cold or the flu. With strep throat, there is no runny nose or cough, and symptoms appear abruptly, with a fever as high as 104°F, headache, stomachache, and a red, swollen throat. By the second day, the throat and tonsils may be covered with white or yellow patches that spread together to cover the entire throat. However, it is also possible to have strep throat without these telltale white patches, or even without a fever.

Most children with strep throat also have swollen lymph glands in the front of the neck just below the point where the ear and jawbone meet. These glands may remain swollen for up to a month after recovery from the infection.

**WARNING SIGNS OF
STREP THROAT COMPLICATIONS**

The doctor should be notified immediately for any of the following signs:

- breathing problems
- dark, murky urine
- drooling in older child
- extreme problems in swallowing
- fever that goes away and then returns
- headache
- high fever above 105°F
- joint pain
- less urine than normal
- no improvement in two days
- rash
- seal-bark cough
- swelling
- vision changes

Diagnosis

Because almost all of the symptoms of strep throat also can occur with viral infections, lab tests are needed to confirm the diagnosis. Anyone with a suspected strep throat should be seen by a doctor for a throat culture or rapid strep test. A throat culture is the best, most accurate test, but rapid strep tests are also widely used in doctors' offices and can give results within three minutes.

Treatment

A positive strep test requires antibiotic treatment to prevent complications. Antibiotics given seven to nine days after the illness starts will prevent RHEU-MATIC FEVER. High temperatures may be treated with fever reducers; easy-to-swallow food or cold food (ice cream, mashed cold bananas, or frozen juice bars) are good choices. Fluids are very important in the treatment of strep throat.

Complications

The risk of severe complications is the primary concern with strep throat and the reason why it is so important to be properly diagnosed and treated. One of the most serious complications is rheumatic fever, a disease that affects up to 3 percent of children with untreated strep infection. Rheumatic fever can lead to rheumatic heart disease.

Kidney inflammation is another possible complication of strep throat, which can appear from 10 days to six weeks after the throat infection. In this case, the bacteria do not directly infect the kidneys; instead, the body's immune system response damages the kidney's filtering mechanism. Warning signs of impending kidney problems include swelling hands, face, and feet; dark or bloody urine; headaches; vision problems; and decreased urinary output. Children usually recover, albeit slowly.

SCARLET FEVER is an uncommon strep infection that may follow untreated strep throat within two days, producing a fever and a red rash over the upper body. With antibiotics, recovery is complete within two weeks, although skin may peel on fingers and toes afterward. A severe form of scarlet fever can cause serious illness.

Prevention

People should avoid any child with strep throat who has not received antibiotics. Children should not return to school until they have taken antibiotics for 24 hours, or if there is still a fever and sore throat. (See also STREPTOCOCCAL INFECTIONS.)

streptococcal infections A group of infections caused by bacteria of the Streptococcus family, which are among the most common bacteria in humans. These infections are responsible for a wide range of health problems, including SCARLET FEVER or wound infections. Different groups of Strep bacteria are separated according to letters, from Group A through T. Some types of strep exist harmlessly in the throat; if the bacteria gets in the bloodstream, they are usually destroyed, unless the child has a heart condition, which may lead to bacterial endocarditis. Other types of strep bacteria can lead to sore throats, TONSILLITIS, EAR INFECTIONS, STREP THROAT, or PNEUMONIA. These same bacteria may lead to RHEUMATIC FEVER.

Common throughout the world among school-aged children, incidence of infection has decreased since the beginning of the 21st century. The dangers of resistance to antibiotics were of little concern with these infections until the 1970s, when penicillin-resistant strains of strep bacteria began to crop up. In addition, various types of strep bacteria continue to mutate, some becoming less virulent and others becoming more so. For example, as strep A infections became less worrisome, strep B infections became more virulent. Then in the 1980s strep A became more dangerous again; a much stronger *S. pneumoniae* is part of this resurging tide of infection.

Group A Strep

Group A strep (GAS) is responsible for most cases of strep illness. Syndromes caused by group A strep include strep throat, skin infections such as CELLULITIS and IMPETIGO, and PNEUMONIA. Occasionally, group A strep can cause much more severe diseases, such as flesh-eating disease (necrotizing fasciitis) and streptococcal TOXIC SHOCK SYNDROME.

Invasive GAS disease is a severe, sometimes lifethreatening infection, in which the bacteria have spread to other parts of the body, such as the blood, muscle and fat tissue, or the lungs. Two of the most severe (but least common) forms are necrotizing fasciitis (infection of muscle and fat tissue) and toxic shock syndrome. About 20 percent of patients with necrotizing fasciitis and 60 percent of those with streptococcal toxic shock syndrome (STSS) will die; only 10 to 15 percent of those with other forms of invasive group A strep die.

About 10,000 to 15,000 cases of invasive GAS occur in the United States each year, causing more than 2,000 deaths. The Centers for Disease Control estimates between 500 and 1,500 cases of necrotizing fasciitis and 2,000 to 3,000 cases of STSS each year in the United States; on the other hand, there are several million cases of strep throat and impetigo each year.

In 2001 scientists cracked the genetic code of the bacteria, which may lead to better treatments for the illnesses it causes. Now that the bacteria's complete DNA sequences have been determined, scientists hope they can develop other antibiotics or vaccinations for the organism.

Invasive GAS disease occurs when the bacteria gets past the body's immune defenses. The germs are spread by direct contact with nose and throat discharge, or by touching infected skin lesions. The risk is greatest when the child is ill or has an infected wound. Health conditions that impair the immune system make infection with GAS more likely. In addition, there are some strains of GAS that are more likely to cause serious disease.

Most children who come in contact with a virulent strain of GAS still will not develop invasive disease; most will have a simple throat or skin infection. Some may not have any symptoms at all. While it is possible for a healthy child to contract invasive GAS, those with chronic conditions such as cancer, diabetes, or kidney problems, or who use steroid medications, are at highest risk.

There have been no reports of casual contacts (such as classmates) developing invasive GAS disease after contact with a patient. However, occasionally close family contacts *have* developed severe disease. There are no current recommendations regarding whether close family contacts should be tested and treated for disease if a family member becomes ill.

Treatment Group A strep bacteria can be treated with common antibiotics; penicillin is the drug of choice for both mild and severe disease. In addition to antibiotics, supportive care in an intensive care unit and sometimes surgery is needed. Early treatment can reduce the threat of death, although even the best therapy may not prevent death in every case.

Prevention Hand-washing may help stop the spread of all types of group A strep infections, especially after coughing or sneezing and before preparing food. Those with a strep throat should stay home from work or school or day care until 24 hours after taking an antibiotic. Wounds should be cleansed and watched for signs of possible infection.

Early signs and symptoms of necrotizing fasciitis include fever, severe pain and swelling, and redness at wound site. Early signs of STSS include fever, dizziness, confusion, rash, and abdominal pain.

Group B Strep

Group B strep (GBS) causes most of the strep infections in newborns and mothers who have just delivered. Each year there are more than 50,000 cases in pregnant women. It is the most common cause of blood infections (sepsis), MENINGITIS, and pneumonia in newborns. About 15,000 to 18,000 infants are infected in the United States each year, and up to 15 percent of these die. Those who survive may have hearing or vision problems or developmental disabilities. While many people carry group B strep in their bodies, most do not get sick. Other common diseases caused by GBS include blood infections, skin or soft tissue infections, and pneumonia.

Symptoms About 2 percent of infants infected with GBS develop symptoms, most appearing during the first week of life—usually within a few hours after birth. It is also possible for infants to contract GBS several months after birth; meningitis is more common with this type of late-onset disease.

Diagnosis GBS can be diagnosed by growing bacteria in spinal fluid or blood cultures, which can take a few days to complete.

Treatment Antibiotics (penicillin or ampicillin) are the treatment of choice.

Prevention Since one-third of pregnant women carry GBS bacteria, all pregnant women should be screened for the bacteria at 35 to 37 weeks of pregnancy. Most GBS among newborns can be prevented by giving infected pregnant women antibiotics through the vein during labor. Any pregnant woman who has had a baby with GBS disease, or who has GBS infection should receive antibiotics during labor. Women who have been diagnosed with GBS infection at labor are at higher risk if they have fever during labor, rupture of membranes 18 hours or more before delivery, are black, are under age 20, or have labor or rupture of membranes before 37 weeks. Women who have GBS but do not have these risk factors have a relatively low risk of delivering a baby with GBS disease. Unfortunately, some babies still get GBS in spite of testing and antibiotics. Vaccines to prevent GBS disease are being developed, but are still years away.

stroke Sudden interrupted flow of blood to the brain that can cause symptoms that vary in severity from a temporary weakness to profound paralysis, coma, and death. A stroke occurs when the blood supply to any part of the brain is interrupted, resulting in tissue death and loss of brain function. If blood flow in any of the arteries that lead to the brain is interrupted for longer than a few seconds, brain cells can die, causing permanent damage. There are two types of stroke: hemorrhagic stroke, caused by blood leaking from blood vessels into the brain, or ischemic stroke, caused by a blockage. Although childhood strokes are far less common than adult strokes, they, too, can kill or leave survivors disabled.

Between 1979 and 1998 there were an average of 244 deaths a year due to childhood stroke in the United States. Overall, stroke deaths declined by 58 percent in the 20-year period, but the reduction in deaths varied by type of stroke. Although deaths from stroke in children have declined sharply, black children still have higher stroke death rates than other youngsters.

Recent declines in stroke deaths may be related to better detection methods and to the fact that children now survive previously fatal conditions that can cause strokes, such as prematurity, congenital heart disease, and leukemia.

Perinatal Stroke

Perinatal (or "prenatal") stroke includes strokes that occur between the 28 weeks of gestation and the 28 days after birth. Stroke occurs more frequently in the perinatal and prenatal age group than in older children.

Some perinatal strokes are caused by inherited clotting disorders or coagulation abnormalities that make the infant more likely to have a blood clot. Congenital heart disease and sickle-cell disease are common causes of stroke in children. No cause can be detected in about a fifth of the children with ischemic stroke, but many of these children seem to recover well after birth.

Cause

Up to one-third of all strokes in children occur for unknown reasons. The most common cause of stroke in children is a heart disorder often related to a developmental defect in the structure of the heart. Disorders of the blood such as SICKLE-CELL DISEASE, blood clotting problems, and genetic disorders, are the next most common causes. Following these, there are a whole variety of causes including infections, abnormal arterial-venous connections in the brain, chicken pox virus, and trauma to the head.

Risk Factors

Childhood stroke deaths are poorly understood, since it is not possible to take the risk factors important for strokes in adults (such as high blood pressure, poor diet, or diabetes) and apply them to children. Experts suspect an unknown genetic predisposition may play a role in these deaths. Hormonal differences may be a factor in the higher stroke rates in boys.

Known risk factors for childhood strokes caused by bleeding include brain tumors or vascular malformations, HEMOPHILIA, cancer, and sickle-cell disease. Childhood strokes caused by blockages (ischemic strokes) have also been linked to sickle-cell disease and cancer. Risk factors that contribute to ischemic strokes include MENINGITIS, ENCEPHALITIS, congenital heart disease, and certain blood clotting disorders.

Hemorrhagic strokes showed the steepest drop in death rates in the past 20 years: Childhood stroke deaths from subarachnoid hemorrhagic strokes (bleeding into the space between the brain and the skull) dropped by 79 percent, while strokes from intracerebral hemorrhages (bursting of a defective brain vessel) declined by 54 percent.

The declines were not as dramatic for deaths from ischemic stroke, which results from a blood clot that blocks blood flow to the brain. Ischemic stroke deaths declined 19 percent in the same time period.

Unfortunately, black children and boys have much higher risks for dying of strokes for some unknown reason. Black children were more than twice as likely to die from strokes caused by intracerebral hemorrhage, and about 75 percent more likely to die from ischemic strokes or subarachnoid hemorrhage. No factors (such as sickle-cell disease, which is more common in blacks than whites) fully accounted for excess stroke deaths. Boys of all races were also 30 percent more likely to die from subarachnoid hemorrhage and 21 percent more likely to die from intracerebral hemorrhage than girls.

Symptoms

The stroke-related symptoms depend on the area of the brain affected, the extent of the damage, and the cause of the stroke. In infants and very young children, stroke symptoms include seizures, coma, and paralysis of one side of the body; the signs of a stroke may not appear until months, perhaps even years, later so that the child cannot use one hand as agilely as the other or the child may have a slight limp. When stroke occurs in older children, symptoms include a sudden paralysis of one side of the body, difficulty with vision, and/or difficulty with swallowing.

Diagnosis

The sooner a stroke in children is diagnosed and treated, the better the chance they will have to recover. In a child where the brain is still developing, the developing brain may be able to take over for the functions that have been lost as a result of the stroke. A physician can use a variety of tests and scans to learn what type of stroke has occurred, such as a clot or other occlusion in the blood vessel; bleeding into the brain; bleeding around the brain.

Brain scans   Magnetic resonance imaging (MRI) or computerized tomography (CT) scans can identify the affected area of the brain and reveal the status of the blood vessels. Younger children may need to be sedated for an MRI.

Blood tests   A number of blood tests can be used to check for any chemical problems, infection, or blood clotting that may have caused the stroke. Some of the clotting tests may need to be repeated later on as they may be inaccurate if they are carried out too soon after the stroke.

Echocardiogram   This ultrasound scan reveals the structure of the heart to check whether the stroke was caused by a clot moving from the heart to the brain. If traditional scans on the chest do not provide enough information, a more detailed scan can be done using a scanner placed in the child's throat while under general anesthesia.

Spinal tap   In this test, a sample of cerebrospinal fluid is taken from the space around the spine to reveal if there is an infection or chemical imbalance in the body, as a cause or a result of the stroke.

Angiogram   This test gives detailed information about the blood vessels in the brain and is usually done only if less invasive scans have not provided answers. For this test a child is given general anesthesia. A fine tube is inserted into a blood vessel at the top of the leg and dye is injected through this into the brain; X-ray pictures are then taken of the blood vessels in the brain.

Treatment

There are several treatments for children who have had a stroke, depending on the different needs of the individual child. Medications include aspirin, heparin, or warfarin, all of which thin the blood and make it less likely to clot. A child given heparin or warfarin needs regular blood tests to monitor the effects. Aspirin is much milder and does not require regular blood monitoring.

Prognosis

The outcome after a stroke is better for children than for adults. Children often have less permanent disability and often only minor delays in the development of coordinated movement or in cognitive functioning. Early diagnosis is important in order to prevent a second stroke and to start treatment to help the child recover fully.

Sturge-Weber syndrome A rare condition that affects the skin and the brain, caused by a spontaneous genetic mutation. How often it occurs in babies is not known, and because it is not often diagnosed, it is difficult to estimate how many children currently have the disease. The most obvious symptom of the disease is a PORT-WINE STAIN birthmark, typically involving at least one upper eyelid and the forehead. However, every case of Sturge-Weber is unique, and symptoms and skin abnormalities vary.

Neurological problems include unusual blood vessel growths on the brain called angiomas, which usually cause seizures beginning before one year of age and may get worse as the child grows. Seizures usually appear on the side of the body opposite the port-wine stain and vary in severity. About 30 percent of children with Sturge-Weber also develop glaucoma (increased pressure inside the eye that impairs vision). Glaucoma is usually restricted to the eye that is affected by the port-wine stain. This eye may also become enlarged. In some cases, strokes can occur.

Treatment

Children as young as one month old who have Sturge-Weber may undergo laser treatment to reduce or remove port-wine stains. Anticonvulsant medication may be used to control seizures associated with the disorder, and surgery is available to control glaucoma and vision problems.

stuttering A communication disorder in which the flow of speech is broken by repetitions, prolongations, or abnormal stoppages of sounds and syllables. There may also be unusual facial and body movements associated with the effort to speak. Stuttering affects more than three million Americans, and four times as many boys as girls. About 20 percent of all children go through a stage of development during which they encounter stuttering problems severe enough to be a concern to their parents.

Cause

Despite decades of research, scientists still are not sure what causes stuttering, although a variety of factors contribute to its development, including genetics, neurophysiology, child development, and family dynamics. Stuttering may occur when a combination of factors occur and may have different causes in different people. Experts believe that what causes stuttering is not the same thing as the reasons for the problem to continue or get worse.

Children and adults who stutter are no more likely to have psychological or emotional problems than children and adults who do not. There is no reason to believe that emotional trauma causes stuttering.

Prevention/Treatment

The best way to prevent stuttering is to treat problems early. If the stuttering lasts longer than three to six months or is particularly severe, parents may need to consult a speech-language pathologist who specializes in stuttering. There are a variety of successful approaches for treating children who stutter, although treatment is not an overnight process. However, a qualified clinician can help children and teenagers make significant progress toward fluency. (See also STUTTERING FOUNDATION OF AMERICA.)

Stuttering Foundation of America The first and largest nonprofit organization in the world working toward the prevention and improved treatment of STUTTERING, reaching more than one million people annually. The foundation offers extensive educational programs for professionals and provides free online resources, services, and support to those who stutter and their families, as well as support for research into the causes of stuttering.

stye A small pus-filed abscess near the eyelashes caused by a bacterial infection (usually a staphylococcal organism). If the stye is painful, a warm compress may help eliminate the pain. Prescription antibiotic ointments designed for the eyes can prevent a recurrence.

sudden infant death syndrome (SIDS) The sudden and unexplained death of a baby under one year of age. Because many sudden infant death syndrome (SIDS) babies are found in their cribs, some people call SIDS "crib death," but cribs do not cause SIDS. SIDS is the leading cause of death in babies after one month of age, and most typically among babies between two and four months of age. Race appears to be linked with SIDS, since African-American babies are two times more likely to die of SIDS than white babies.

While experts do not know the exact cause of SIDS, they do know that these deaths tend to happen in colder months and that babies placed to sleep on their stomachs are much more likely to die of SIDS than babies placed on their backs to sleep.

Prevention

There are certain things parents can do to lower the risk for their infant. Parents should always place babies on their backs to sleep, even for naps. This is the safest sleep position for a healthy baby to reduce the risk of SIDS. Babies should always sleep on a firm mattress, such as in a safety-approved crib. Research has shown that placing a baby to sleep on soft mattresses, sofas, sofa cushions, waterbeds, sheepskins, or other soft surfaces can increase the risk of SIDS. Soft, fluffy, and loose bedding, quilts, and stuffed toys and other soft items should be removed from a baby's sleep area.

Parents should make sure the baby's face and head stay uncovered during sleep and should keep blankets and other coverings away from the baby's mouth and nose. Dressing the baby in sleep clothing will avoid having to use any covering over the baby. If parents do use a blanket or covering, they should make sure that the baby's feet are at the bottom of the crib, the blanket is no higher than the baby's chest, and the blanket is tucked in around the bottom of the crib mattress. Parents should not smoke before or after the birth of the baby, and no one should smoke around the baby at any time.

In addition, babies should not get too warm during sleep. The baby's room should be at a temperature that is comfortable for an adult. Too many layers of clothing or blankets can overheat a baby.

There is no risk of choking when babies sleep on their backs, because babies automatically swallow or cough up fluids. Doctors have found no increase in choking or other problems in babies sleeping on their backs. Back sleeping is also safer than side sleeping, because babies who sleep on their sides can roll onto their stomachs. While there are some products that have been designed to keep a baby in one position, these have not been tested for safety and are not recommended.

Babies can be placed on their stomachs for "tummy time," as long as they are awake and someone is watching. When the baby is awake, time spent on the tummy is good because it helps strengthen baby's neck and shoulder muscles.

While it is true that babies who sleep on their backs may develop flat spots on the back of the head, these flat areas will go away a few months after the baby learns to sit up. Tummy time during awake periods is one way to reduce flat spots. Another way is to change the direction a baby sleeps; doing this means the baby is not always sleeping on the same side of the head.

Other ways to prevent SIDS include:

- eating the right foods during pregnancy
- avoiding smoking, taking drugs, or drinking alcohol while pregnant
- getting frequent prenatal checkups
- breast-feeding

- taking the baby for scheduled well-baby checkups
- making sure the baby gets shots on time.

Possible Causes

Many researchers favor a theory that brain-stem birth defects somehow affect arousal reflexes, so that babies do not wake up when problems arise with breathing, heart rate, blood pressure, or temperature. However, some experts believe that such brain abnormalities may not be enough to cause death on their own.

Another serious possibility is that an overwhelming infection leads to SIDS. Recent research suggests that infection with the common bacterium *E. coli* may be linked to SIDS, since a shock-producing by-product of *E. coli* was found in the blood of all SIDS babies tested, but in none of the infants used as a comparison.

Autopsies tend to show wet, heavy lungs with small hemorrhages on the heart and lungs, and the blood of SIDS babies is unclotted, which is something never seen in suffocation cases. Furthermore, SIDS deaths captured on medical monitors have shown that these babies died of a shock-like process. In addition, the blood from babies who have died of SIDS is toxic to chick embryos and mice, which indicates the presence of a toxin. Sometimes, *E. coli* bacteria produce a protein called curlin, which scientists suspect may help the bacteria compete for a foothold in the competitive germ environment in the intestines. The bacteria itself was found in the intestines of all the SIDS babies, but only in 80 percent of the healthy babies. However, curlin was detected in the bloodstream of all SIDS babies and none of the others. This indicated that curlin could be responsible for SIDS deaths, given the fact that curlin causes shock in laboratory mice.

Other scientists believe the deaths might be triggered by infection, or might be due to a combination of genetic factors, such as a brain stem defect or an impaired immune system, and environmental factors, such as the baby sleeping on its stomach or breathing in cigarette fumes.

The basic theory that some serious, overwhelming acutely acquired infection is the cause of SIDS is a legitimate hypothesis. Many experts believe that SIDS may have a variety of different causes in individual infants.

suicide Suicide is the third leading cause of death for 15- to 24-year-olds (approximately 5,000 young Americans) and the sixth leading cause of death for five- to 14-year-olds. The rate of suicide for these age groups has nearly tripled since 1960, making it the leading cause of death in adolescents and the second leading cause of death among college age youth.

Children and Suicide

Most people do not realize that children under age 12 are capable of killing themselves. Over the last few decades, the suicide rate among young children has risen dramatically. Between 1980 and 1996 the suicide rate among children 10 to 15 has skyrocketed by 100 percent.

Most suicides among children between ages five and 14 are among the older children; it is fairly rare (although not unheard of) for children under age 10 to take their own lives. The reason why suicide is rare before puberty is not known, but it is universally true for all cultures. It may be that critical risk factors such as DEPRESSION or exposure to drugs and alcohol are rare in very young children.

Experts believe that many suicides among children are unreported or misreported as accidents in young children, and that the actual number of youth suicides may be two to three times higher than official statistics indicate.

In the United States youth suicide rates are highest among the western states and Alaska, and lowest in the southern, north-central, and northeastern states. Overall, the U.S. suicide rate for children under age 15 is twice the rate for all other countries combined. For suicides involving firearms, the suicide rate for children in the United States is almost 11 times higher than the rate for *all* other countries combined.

Teenagers and Suicide

Over the last several decades, the suicide rate in adolescents has increased dramatically until by 1997 suicide was the third leading cause of death in 15- to 24-year-olds (11.4 of every 100,000 persons) following unintentional injuries and homicide. Suicide also was the third leading cause of death in 10- to 14-year-olds, with 303 deaths among 19,097,000 children in this age group. In 1998 among youth ages 10 to 19, there were 2,054 suicides. For those aged 15 to 19, there were 1,802 suicide deaths among 19,146,000 teens.

Although the overall suicide rate has declined over the past 20 years from 12.1 per 100,000 in 1979 to 11.3 per 100,000 in 1998, the suicide rate for teens 15 to 19 years old has increased by 6 percent. For adolescents 10 to 14 years old, the suicide rate increased by more than 100 percent over that time period. And while youth suicide rates did decrease significantly between 1993 and 1998, suicide was still the third leading cause of death for young people 10 to 19 years old in 1998. More teenagers died from suicide than from cancer, heart disease, AIDS, birth defects, stroke, pneumonia and influenza, and chronic lung disease combined.

Gender Issues

Teenage boys are about four times more likely to kill themselves than are teenage girls. Among young people 20 to 24 years of age, there were 2,384 suicide deaths among 17,488,000 people in this age group, and the gender ratio in this age range was about six boys to every one girl.

While more boys die from suicide, more girls attempt suicide and report higher rates of depression. Experts believe the gender difference in suicide completion is most likely due to the differences in suicide methods, since boys are more likely to use firearms, which are more likely to lead to a fatal outcome.

Culture Issues

In 1998 white boys accounted for 61 percent of all suicides among youth aged 10 to 19, and white boys and girls together accounted for more than 84 percent of all youth suicides. However, the suicide rate among Native American teenage boys is exceedingly high in comparison with the overall rate for boys 10 to 19 (19.3 per 100,000 vs. 8.5 per 100,000).

The suicide rate has been increasing most rapidly among African-American boys aged 10 to 19—more than doubling from 2.9 per 100,000 to 6.1 per 100,000 from 1981 to 1998. On the other hand, a 1999 national survey of high school students found that Hispanic boys and girls were significantly more likely than white students to have reported a suicide attempt (12.8 percent vs. 6.7 percent). Among Hispanic students, girls (18.9 per-

cent) were almost three times more likely than boys (6.6 percent) to have reported a suicide attempt. The most likely explanation for ethnic rate differences is the variations in cultural factors that promote or inhibit suicide.

Homosexuality

It has been widely reported in the media that gay and lesbian youth are at higher risk to complete suicide than other youth and that a significant percent of all attempted or completed youth suicides are related to issues of sexual identity. However, there are no national statistics for suicide completion rates among gay, lesbian, or bisexual persons, and in the few studies examining risk factors for suicide completion where an attempt was made to assess sexual orientation, the risk for gay or lesbian persons did not appear any greater than among heterosexuals, once mental and substance abuse disorders were taken into account.

Several state and national studies have reported that high school students who report homosexual or bisexual activity have higher rates of suicide thoughts and attempts compared to youth with heterosexual experience. Experts do not agree about the best way to measure reports of adolescent suicide attempts or sexual orientation, however, so the data are subject to question.

Suicide Attempts

Many more youths attempt suicide each year than complete it. Suicide attempts are difficult to count, because many may not be treated in a hospital or may not be recorded as self-inflicted injury. Survey data from 1999 indicate that 19.3 percent of high school students had seriously considered attempting suicide, 14.5 percent had made plans to attempt suicide, and 8.3 percent had made a suicide attempt during the year preceding the survey. All suicide attempts should be taken seriously.

Warning Signs

The challenge for family and friends of teens is to be able to tell the difference between normal teen moodiness and actual despair. Luckily, many experts agree that there are recognizable warning signs. Ninety percent of suicidal teens are depressed, and depression tends to cause certain types of behavioral changes—a cluster of changes in behavior and mood, in sleep and eating patterns, and energy level. Other warning signs include dramatic changes in behavior or appearance, in weight, or in performance in school. Any talk about wanting to die or commit suicide should be seen as a real risk factor. Another strong signal is continuing alcohol or drug use, because one of the first things troubled teens try to do is to medicate themselves by drinking or taking drugs instead of seeking psychological help.

Risk Factors

Suicide is a complex behavior that is usually caused by a combination of factors. Researchers have identified a number of risk factors associated with a higher risk for suicide, and factors that may reduce the likelihood of suicidal behavior. It is important to note, however, that the importance of risk and protective factors can vary by age, gender, and ethnicity.

Previous attempts If a teen has attempted suicide in the past, there is a higher chance of recurrence in the future. If a teenage boy has attempted suicide in the past, he is more than 30 times more likely to complete suicide, while a female with a past attempt has about three times the risk. About a third of teenage suicide victims have made a previous suicide attempt.

Mental disorders or substance abuse Research shows that more than 90 percent of teenagers who complete suicide have a mental or substance abuse disorder or both, and that most are depressed. In a 10- to 15-year study of 73 adolescents diagnosed with major depression, 7 percent of the adolescents had completed suicide sometime later. The depressed adolescents were five times more likely to have attempted suicide as well, compared with a control group of age peers without depression.

Almost half of teenagers who complete suicide have been seen by a mental health professional. In addition, aggressive, disruptive, and impulsive behavior is common in youth of both sexes who complete suicide.

Family history A high proportion of suicides and attempters have had a close family member who attempted or completed suicide, which may be either linked to imitation or genetics. Many of the mental illnesses which contribute to suicide risk appear to have a genetic component.

Stressful life event or loss Stressful life events often precede a suicide or suicide attempt, such as trouble at school or with the police, fighting, or breaking up with a friend. Rarely a sufficient cause of suicide, these events may act as precipitating factors in young people.

Gun access There is a direct link between the accessibility and availability of firearms in the home and the risk for youth suicide. The more guns there are and the easier they are to retrieve, the higher the risk.

Exposure to suicidal behavior Whether a real or fictional account of suicide, research suggests this can trigger suicide in vulnerable teens. In addition, local epidemics of suicide have a contagious influence. Suicide clusters nearly always involve previously disturbed young people who knew about the others' deaths but rarely knew the other victims personally.

Incarceration Data suggest a high prevalence of suicidal behavior in juvenile correctional facilities. One study found that suicide in juvenile detention and correctional facilities was more than four times greater than youth suicide overall. According to another recent study, more than 11,000 juveniles engage in more than 17,000 incidents of suicidal behavior in juvenile facilities each year.

Other risks Other identified risk factors include a family history of mental or substance abuse disorders, a history of physical and/or sexual abuse, low levels of communication with parents, the possession of certain cultural and religious beliefs about suicide (for instance, the belief that suicide is a noble resolution of a personal dilemma), and lack of access or an unwillingness to seek mental health treatment.

The impact of some risk factors can be reduced by interventions (such as providing effective treatments for depressive illness). Those risk factors that cannot be changed (such as a previous suicide attempt) can alert others to the heightened risk of suicide during periods of the recurrence of a mental or substance abuse disorder, or following a significant stressful life event.

Protective Factors

Factors that protect against suicide include a teen's genetic or neurobiological makeup, attitude and behavior characteristics, and environment. Problem solving skills, impulse control, conflict resolution, and nonviolent handling of disputes all help reduce risk, together with family and community support, access to effective mental health care and support, restricted access to guns, and cultural and religious beliefs that discourage suicide and support self-preservation instincts.

Measures that enhance resilience or protective factors are as essential as risk reduction in preventing suicide. Positive resistance to suicide is not permanent, so programs that support and maintain protection against suicide should be ongoing.

Methods

Firearms are the most common method of suicide by both boys and girls, and younger and older teens for all races. More than 60 percent of youth suicides between the ages of 10 and 19 in 1998 were firearm-related. The rate of youth suicides involving a firearm increased 38 percent between 1981 and 1994, and although firearm-involved suicides declined more than 20 percent from 1994 to 1998, these numbers are still high.

Prevention

Despite this very real threat during the teen years, many families feel uncomfortable about discussing the topic with their children, fearing that if they bring up the subject it will plant a suggestion where none before existed. In fact, talking with a teenager about their negative feelings can help ease the sense of hopelessness the child may have.

Parents who worry that their child might be suicidal should seek help from a mental health professional (either a psychologist, psychiatrist, psychiatric nurse, school counselor, religious counselor, or social worker). Pediatricians and family doctors also can help, although they may have less training in suicidal crises. In case of a suicide emergency, parents can call 911 or take the child to a hospital emergency room.

Although it is not possible to prevent every case of suicide, parents who closely watch their teenagers and work hard at maintaining communication have the best chance of saving their child's life.

sulfonamides (sulfa drugs) A large group of synthetic drugs used to treat bacterial infections derived from a red dye (sulfanilamide). Drugs in this class prevent the growth of bacteria (bacteriostatic); they do not *kill* bacteria (bactericidal).

Given by mouth, these drugs are effective against a wide variety of infections such as URINARY TRACT INFECTION. Most (including sulfamethoxazole and sulfaphenazole) are quickly absorbed from the stomach and small intestine and should be taken at regular intervals. Others are long-acting (such as sulfadoxine, used to treat leprosy and MALARIA) and only need to be taken once a day.

Side effects may include anemia or jaundice, especially if taken for longer than 10 days. More severe side effects include blood disorders, skin rashes, and fever. These drugs are not given during the last trimester of pregnancy or to young babies because of the risk of MENTAL RETARDATION. The drugs are prescribed with caution to patients with kidney or liver problems. In general, patients using these drugs should avoid exposure to direct sunlight.

sunblock See SUNSCREENS.

sunburn Inflammation of the skin as a result of overexposure to the sun that occurs when the sun's ultraviolet rays destroy skin cells in the outer layer of the skin, damaging tiny blood vessels underneath. Sunburn is a particular problem in light-skinned children whose skin does not produce much melanin (the protective pigment that can protect against damage from the sun).

Symptoms

Sun-exposed skin turns red, becomes very painful, and may develop blisters; if the burn is severe, the child also may experience symptoms of sunstroke, including vomiting, fever, and collapse. Several days after the skin has burned, it may shed its dead cells by peeling. Repeated exposure to sunlight over the years may result in prematurely aged skin and skin cancer; even one blistering sunburn before age 20 increases the risk of melanoma.

Treatment

The best idea is to avoid getting sunburned in the first place. While there are many so-called sunburn remedies, none are highly effective. Sunburn should be treated as a medical emergency in a baby under one year of age. If the child is over age one, a doctor should be consulted if there are severe pain, blistering, lethargy, or fever over 101°F.

If a child gets sunburned, she should drink water or juice to replace fluids. Acetaminophen should be given for fever over 101°F. The skin should be soaked in tepid, clear water, followed by application of a light moisturizing lotion. If touching the skin is painful, lotion should not be applied. Dabbing plain calamine (without antihistamine) lotion may help. Compresses may help the pain, using a variety of ingredients such as skim milk and water, aluminum acetate baths (as contained in Buro-Sol antiseptic powder or Domeboro's powder), oatmeal, or witch hazel. Soap or bubble baths should not be used on sunburned skin because these products can irritate tender flesh. Alternatively, a cornstarch paste, raw cucumber or potato slices, yogurt, or tea bags soaked in cool water may ease the sting. Aloe (the oil from the aloe plant) may be applied directly to the skin for sunburn relief for children who are not allergic to aloe.

Alcohol should not be applied, because it may cool the skin too much. Likewise, no medicated cream (such as hydrocortisone or benzocaine) should be used unless the baby's doctor prescribes it. The child should be kept completely out of the sun until the burn is healed.

Prevention

Limit exposure to strong sunlight 15 minutes on the first day, especially in children with fair skin, increasing exposure slowly each day. Until the skin has tanned, it should be protected with a high-protection SUNSCREEN of at least 15 sun protection factor (SPF). Fair children and those who are sensitive to the sun should use a sunscreen with an SPF of 30 or higher. Children should avoid going out into the sun between the hours of 10 A.M. and 3 P.M.

Aspirin and nonsteroidal anti-inflammatory drugs (NSAIDs) can prevent sunburn only if taken before exposure to the sun; once the skin is burned, they are not effective. New types of protective clothing are now available which are equivalent to an SPF of 30; typical clothing is only about as effective as SPF 6.

sun poisoning A temporary condition of red, itchy bumps that occurs in about 10 percent of children after excessive exposure to the sun. The bumps should disappear within a week as long as the child remains out of the sun. Patients should see a doctor if weeping, oozing blisters develop, since this may indicate a possible infection. Cool compresses and over-the-counter hydrocortisone cream or oral antihistamines. (See also SOLAR WARNING INDEX; SUNBURN; SUNSCREENS.)

sun protection factor (SPF) A rating system for SUNSCREEN products that measures how effectively the sunscreen works. The higher the sun protection factor (SPF) rating, the greater the amount of protection from the sun. For example, an SPF of 15 means that a child using the sunscreen could spend up to 15 times longer in the sun without burning than if he was not wearing it. However, the SPF applies only to ultraviolet-B (UVB); no rating for ultraviolet-A (UVA) currently exists.

Experts suggest that sunscreen should have a minimum SPF of 15 to avoid the burning, drying, and wrinkling that result from overexposure to the harmful rays, which are the single most damaging element to the skin. On the other hand, experts at the Food and Drug Administration (FDA) criticize sunscreens with SPFs up to 50, charging that consumers may have a false sense of security by using products with very high SPF values.

An SPF of 50 implies that a person can tolerate 50 times the amount of sun that it would normally take to burn, which is not necessarily true. Even a sunscreen with an SPF of 50 lets *some* UVB rays through, so using it does not allow a person to bake for hours in the sun without any risk of cancer or wrinkling, according to some dermatologists.

In addition, the higher the SPF number, the faster the proportional increase in protection diminishes. For example, the difference between an SPF of 45 and one of 30 is only a few percentage points. As a result of these concerns, the FDA recently proposed legislation that would limit SPF labeling to 30.

There are still some physicians and sunscreen manufacturers who believe that higher SPFs should be available for those who choose to use them. Rather than cut off protection at 30, these physicians suggest that the FDA ask manufacturers to explain the percentage of ultraviolet rays blocked by each of the different SPF numbers.

For overseas travelers, it is important to realize that not all SPFs are the same. In Europe the SPF is called DIN (Deutsches Institut für Normung, the company that developed the system). The DIN uses lower numbers than the American SPF system for equivalent sun protection. For example, an SPF 12 is equal to DIN 9; SPF 19 is DIN 15.

sunscreens Products that protect the skin from the harmful effects of sunlight's radiation; all sunscreen products protect against ultraviolet-B (UVB); some products protect against both ultraviolet-A (UVA) and UVB. Sunscreens are used primarily to avoid SUNBURN, although they can also be used to prevent the rash caused by SUN SENSITIVITY.

While some skin exposure to sunlight is necessary for the body to produce VITAMIN D, overexposure can have a range of harmful effects, especially in fair-skinned children. The danger is significant, since even one blistering sunburn during childhood can result in skin cancer many years later.

Most sunscreens, including those preparations containing para-aminobenzoic acid (PABA), work by absorbing ultraviolet rays of the sun. Products containing other substances (such as titanium dioxide, an uncolored relative of zinc oxide) *reflect* the sun's rays.

However, researchers have found that while sunscreen protects against sunburn, it may impair the ability of immune cells to fight melanoma. In one study, despite wearing sunscreen, mice exposed to ultraviolet light had a higher incidence of melanoma than did mice who were not exposed to the UV light.

Sunscreens are designed to protect against UVB light, the type of radiation that causes sunburn. Most common sunscreens are not designed to protect against UVA, another kind of ultraviolet light produced by the sun that used to be considered less dangerous because it did not directly damage skin. However, more recent research suggests that UVA can cause malignant melanoma simply because sunlight contains so much of it, and it also contributes to aging. (Think UVA-*aging*, UVB-*burn*).

Only a few sunscreens offer protection from UVA rays; those that do list the ingredient "Parsol 1789" (avobenzone), the only ingredient approved by the Food and Drug Administration (FDA) specifically for blocking the UVA rays.

Many more products that contain certain other ingredients are also allowed to claim UVA protection, but none can say how much. Since each of these chemicals block only part of the UVA spectrum, it is a good idea to choose a product with more than one of them. Check the label for some of these names: dioxybenzone, oxybenzone, sulisobenzone, methyl anthranilate, octocrylene, and octyl methoxycinnamate (also called ethylhexyl p-methoxycinnamate).

The best sunscreens offer a broad spectrum of protection and include such ingredients as oxybenzone, titanium dioxide, zinc oxide, or Parsol 1789.

While sunscreens are not perfect, they can prevent a burn, which is important since studies show burns are likely to develop into skin cancer. Sunscreen can also protect against *some* future freckling and brown spots, and they can lower the risk of developing actinic keratoses (precancerous lesions) and skin cancer. However, the only way to completely protect yourself against skin cancer is to avoid the sun.

Sun Protection Factor (SPF)

Sunscreen products are labeled with a sun protection factor (SPF), which is a measure of how effectively the sunscreen works; the higher the number, the more the protection (up to about SPF 30; after that, there is not much additional protection). Sunscreen should have a minimum SPF of 15; an SPF of 15 means that children using the sunscreen could spend up to 15 times longer in the sun without burning than if they were not wearing it. However, the SPF applies only to UVB; no rating for UVA currently exists.

An SPF 15 blocks 94 percent of UVB rays, an SPF 30 blocks 98 percent, and an SPF 50 also blocks 98 percent of the UVB rays. So even if you do not burn, you will still be exposed to some UVB rays. And since some people skimp when applying sunscreen, or apply it unevenly, experts rationalize that if you skimp when applying SF 15 you might end up with the equivalent of an SP 6, whereas if you skimp using an SPF of 50, you'll still get adequate protection.

However, the FDA established guidelines for safety of sunscreens in 1978; they are currently revising sunscreen labeling to include a maximum

SPF 30 on all sunscreens, the use of the terms "water-resistant" and "very water-resistant" instead of "waterproof," charts to match skin types with the appropriate SPF numbers, and stricter guidelines on antiaging claims.

Sunscreen and Infants

Infants under age six months should not be given sunscreen and should be kept out of the sun entirely by using carriage hoods, canopies, and tightly woven umbrellas, along with a lightweight but tightly woven hat. Time in the sun should be limited to short trips, with the baby kept in the shade as much as possible. Since sand, concrete, snow, and water reflect ultraviolet radiation, it is better to park the carriage on grass instead of a patio. When at the beach, the baby should stay away from the water. Even on overcast days, as much as 80 percent of the sun's harmful radiation can still penetrate the clouds.

How to Apply

Parents should look for a sunscreen with an SPF of 15 or higher, and for an SPF 15 lip balm for face and hands; the waxy form stays on and does not sting or taste bad. Toddlers can apply it themselves. Do a patch test by applying a small amount of sunscreen on the inside of a child's wrist the day before it is going to be used all over. If irritation or rash develops, ask a physician to recommend a nonirritating alternative.

Sunscreens should not be used on infants under six months of age. After a baby reaches six months of age, experts agree on the importance of using sunscreen especially made for children. Most of these do not contain PABA, which can be irritating to the skin. Unscented sunscreens are a better choice because they do not attract insects. The SPF should be at least 15, manufactured by a major drug company and purchased at a store with a large turnover. Look for an expiration date (lack of one probably indicates there are no ingredients that will deteriorate).

Sunscreen should be applied in all exposed areas and under thin clothing, 15 to 30 minutes before exposure (it takes that long for the ingredients to penetrate the skin). When applying sunscreen, the child's skin should be well coated, including hands, ears, nose, lips, and areas around the eyes. The eyes or eyelids should be avoided. It may help to apply sunscreen to your hands first, and then rub it on a young child.

Sunscreen should be applied before going into the sun, and every two hours thereafter (more often if the child plays in water or sweats a lot).

Zinc oxide on the nose and lips may give more protection. However, parents should never put baby oil on the child before going outdoors; it makes the skin translucent, letting the sun's rays pass through more easily.

Sunscreen should be applied before going outside even in cloudy weather, since 80 percent of the sun's rays break through the clouds, and then reapplied every two hours and again after swimming. Waterproof or water-resistant sunscreens can be applied less often, but experts recommend an extra application after swimming if there is any uncertainty about the need for more.

Sunscreen Allergies

Some people are allergic to the chemicals contained in sunscreens and can develop a skin rash (especially when using those products containing PABA). But people may also be allergic to other ingredients, such as benzophenone and cinnamate. Children who break out when wearing a sunscreen should consult a dermatologist, who will do a patch test to determine what ingredient is to blame for the rash. Children, in particular, are extremely sensitive to PABA and should use special sunscreens designed for their sensitive skin.

Fortunately, new chemical-free sunscreens are now being developed which contain physical sunblocks (such as titanium dioxide and talc) broken down into tiny particles that can be formulated into clear, invisible lotions instead of the white zinc-oxide creams. The nonchemical sunscreens block both UVA and UVB rays far better than most chemical sunscreens.

Other Protective Factors

A more controversial approach to sunscreen developments is the addition of other protective factors, such as vitamins E and C (antioxidants that neutralize free radicals, which are unstable oxygen molecules that damage skin). The goal is to prevent or delay damage to skin cells by screening out some of the premature-aging effects of sunlight while allowing the triggering of vitamin D, but many dermatologists are skeptical. Because the wavelength of light that triggers vitamin D production is UVB, experts believe it is best to block all the UVB light. Since it takes only 15 minutes two or three times a week to spur vitamin D synthesis in the skin, very few people have to worry about not getting enough sun exposure.

Rating Sunscreens

The Skin Cancer Foundation rates many sunscreens; consumers should look for their seal of approval on all sunscreen products. Sunscreens that have the foundation's seal on the label have met stringent criteria that exceed those of the FDA; in order to rate the foundation's approval, the product must prove that it helps prevent sun-induced damage to the skin. The product must have an SPF of 15 or higher and include substantiation for any claims that a sunscreen is waterproof, water- or sweat-resistant. The seal is also granted to self-tanning products that include a sunscreen; this sunscreen must meet the same requirements as regular sunscreen. Clothing is still considered to be the best protection against sun-induced skin cancer of all types. (See also SUN POISONING; SOLAR WARNING INDEX.)

SAFE EXPOSURE TIMES USING SUNSCREENS

Skin Type	SPF 4	SPF 8	SPF 15
	Safe Exposure Time		
Fair	10 minutes	40–80 minutes	1.5–2 hours
Medium	50–80 minutes	2–2.5 hours	5–5.5 hours
Dark	1.5–2 hours	3.5–4 hours	all day
Black	4 hours	all day	all day

sun sensitivity A toxic skin reaction to the sun that can be caused by a variety of substances, such as some prescription medications and consumer products, as well as some physical disorders. It often occurs because a substance (called a "photosensitizer") has been ingested or applied to the skin; examples of these photosensitizers include certain drugs, dyes, chemicals in perfumes and soaps, and plants such as buttercups, parsnips, and

mustard, and fruits such as limes and lemons. Any abnormal reaction to the sun causing exaggerated sunburn, painful swelling, hives, or blistering should be considered to be a sign of photosensitivity. A photosensitive reaction can occur in less than half an hour or it can take from 48 to 72 hours after exposure.

Drugs are the primary cause of photosensitivity, including tetracyclines, griseofulvin, sulfonamides, and nalidixic acid; phenothiazine, piroxicam and naproxen, tretinoin (RETIN-A), diphendramine, and birth control pills. Other medications that may cause a problem include anticancer and photochemotherapy drugs, ANTIDEPRESSANTS and ANTIPSYCHOTICS, ANTIHISTAMINES, antiparasitic drugs, diuretics, and hypoglycemics.

Sun sensitivity can also be triggered by the coal tars in some medicated soaps and shampoos, or the oil of bergamot in certain perfumes, toilet soaps, lemons, and limes. Topical photosensitizers can be found in cosmetics, face creams, perfumes, and aftershave lotions. In addition, plants such as celery, wild carrots, limes, and meadow grass contain photosensitizing compounds. Industrial contaminants and air pollutants such as tars and polycyclic aromatic hydrocarbons are also potent photosensitizers.

Photosensitivity can also be caused by some disorders, including LUPUS erythematosus and the porphyria group of blood disorders.

Fortunately, relatively few people ever become photosensitive; the risk is higher for those who only have intermittent exposure to the sun, who have light skin, and who tend to burn instead of tan.

About 10 percent of individuals have an adverse reaction to sunlight in the absence of photosensitizing medications. These individuals suffer from polymorphic (or polymorphous) light eruption, an itchy eruption which is characterized by red papules 24 to 72 hours after sun exposure and lasting several days after the person avoids the sun. Frequently known as "sun poisoning," this reaction often develops on the first sunny outing in the spring or during a winter holiday to a sunny destination. It is usually mild, but the itch, swelling, and rash can be so severe that it can ruin a holiday. It can be prevented by getting small amounts of sun before going on holiday, or with pretreatment (PUVA or PUVB).

COMMON PHOTOSENSITIZING DRUGS

Antibiotics
aureomycin (Chlortetracycline)
griseofulvin (Fulvicin)
minocycline (Minocin, Dynacin)
quinolone (Aprofloxacin, naladoxic acid)
sulfa drugs
tetracycline (Tetracycline)

Antiarrythmics
quinidine (Cin-Quin, Duraquin, etc.)

Antidepressants
amitriptyline (Elavil)
desipramine (Norpramin)

Tranquilizers
chlordiazepoxide (Librium)
chlorpromazine (Thorazine)

Diuretics
hydrochlorothiazide (Esidrix)
chlorothiazide (Diuril)
chlorathalidone (Hygroton)
furosemide (Lasix)
triamterene (Dyrenium)

Treatment

Prevention is the best option; a child using a known photosensitizer should avoid exposure to sunlight. Treatment of lesions depends on the type, extent, and severity of response. Cool tap water compresses can be applied continually or intermittently; topical application of corticosteroid cream or lotion can reduce inflammation. Systemic antihistamines may lessen the itch. If the process is severe and extensive, systemic corticosteroids (such as those used in extensive poison ivy cases) may be needed.

sunstroke   Also called heatstroke, this condition involves a very high body temperature and lack of sweating followed by loss of consciousness due to excess exposure to heat and the sun. Very young children are particularly vulnerable to sunstroke. This condition is potentially fatal unless treated quickly. It is a particular problem for young athletes training during hot and humid temperatures.

Even a rise of a few degrees from the body's normal temperature can have profound effects on the way the metabolism works.

Symptoms

Very often, a child exposed to very hot temperatures will first experience "heat exhaustion," which is characterized by dizziness, fatigue, headache, rapid pulse, rapid breathing, and muscle cramps. The warning signs that this is becoming a potentially fatal sunstroke are:

- hot, flushed skin
- no sweating
- a high body temperature
- confusion
- nausea and vomiting
- loss of consciousness

Cause

Exposure to extreme heat can cause a breakdown in the body's ability to lower its own temperature through sweating, and body temperature can soar to 107°F or higher. If the body is dehydrated and cannot cool the skin through sweat evaporation, this can cause the failure of many of the body's vital systems, such as the heart, lungs, kidney, and brain. The sufferer can fall into shock and unconsciousness.

Treatment

Quick cooling is the most important aspect of treatment for sunstroke, and the quicker treatment is given, the more likely a child can make a full recovery. An ice bag or crushed ice should be applied immediately; alternatively, a sheet should be hosed down with cold water and wrapped around the patient until emergency medical help arrives.

suntan   The result of the body's attempt at protecting itself from the damage of the sun's ultraviolet rays. During exposure to the sun, the skin begins to produce more of the dark pigment called melanin to absorb the damaging rays. The result is a darkened skin tone. While a suntan is widely considered to be desirable, it is in fact a sign that the skin has been damaged. Melanin does provide some protection from skin damage; that is the reason dark, thick, oily skin gets fewer wrinkles than badly sun-damaged fair skin.

Even with frequent applications of SUNSCREEN, sunbathers may be at risk for developing melanoma (the most serious form of skin cancer). In fact, skin cells can undergo changes not just by exposure to the sun's ultraviolet-B (UV-B) light (rays between 280 and 320 nanometers) but also light with longer wavelengths, including ultraviolet-A (UV-A) light.

In the past scientists had linked melanoma to damaged DNA because those who inherit a defect in their ability to repair DNA are more than 1,000 times more likely than others to get this type of cancer. Because DNA absorbs only UV-B energy, many researchers believed that only this type of light caused the damage. Others *suspected* UV-A light but lacked hard evidence of a link between the light and cancer.

While studying light exposure with fish susceptible to the development of melanoma, scientists at Brookhaven National Laboratory in Upton, New York, found that exposure to a wavelength of 365 nanometers (UV-A used in black lights) resulted in tumors in 38 of 85 fish tested. Of the 61 fish treated with violet light (405 nanometers), 18 developed melanoma; only one of 20 control fish kept in subdued yellow light got cancer. It is believed that melanin absorbs light, setting off a chemical reaction that produces compounds damaging to DNA. (See also SUNBLOCK; SUNBURN; SUN PROTECTION FACTOR.)

surgery and children   See HOSPITALIZATION.

swimmer's ear   A painful infection in the delicate skin of the outer ear canal caused by frequent exposure to water that moistens the canal skin and provides an ideal environment for bacteria and fungi to grow. The resulting irritation may first cause itching, followed by swelling of the skin of the ear canal, and drainage. This may be accompanied by severe pain that is worsened when the ear lobe or other outside part of the ear is touched.

Treatment

The child's doctor will probably prescribe ear drops containing antibiotics and/or corticosteroids to help fight the infection and reduce the swelling in the ear canal. The drops are usually given several times a day for up to 10 days. Over-the-counter pain relievers also may help until the antibiotics begin to work.

If the ear swelling is severe, the doctor may place a cotton wick into the ear canal to help the medication get carried into the ear. For even more severe infections, oral antibiotics may be prescribed, and a sample of ear discharge may be sent to a laboratory to determine exactly which germ is causing the infection.

In addition to the medication, the child must not go swimming, take showers, or shampoo the hair until the infection clears (generally 10 to 14 days).

Prevention

Swimmer's ear can be prevented. Acid alcohol drops (available over-the-counter) are an effective way to prevent the problem. After swimming, three or four drops should be put into the ear canal while the child is lying down on her side. The area in front of the ear canal should be gently massaged to allow the drops to penetrate the ear. The child should remain in that position for a full minute before having drops in the other ear.

For a child with normal ears, earplugs are not as effective as drops in preventing swimmer's ear. For a child with a hole in the eardrum or ear tubes, however, earplugs are useful. Earplugs work best for surface swimming only; the effectiveness of an earplug cannot be guaranteed underwater.

swimmer's itch   An itchy skin inflammation caused by schistosome bites, which cause a distinctive rash after swimming in water populated by ducks and snails. On the saltwater tributaries of Long Island Sound it is known as "clamdigger's itch." This type of dermatitis is a potential risk whenever people use an aquatic area with animals and mollusks who harbor the schistosomes. In the United States, the worst outbreaks occur in the lake regions of Michigan, Wisconsin, and Minnesota, although it may also occur in saltwater areas.

Symptoms

After exposure to water affected by the schistosomes, a prickling or itchy feeling begins that can last up to an hour while the flukes enter the skin. Small red macules form, but there may be swelling or wheals among sensitive children. As these lesions begin to disappear, they are replaced after 10 or 15 hours by discrete, very itchy papules surrounded by a red area. Vesicles and pustules form one or two days later; the lesions fade away within a week, leaving small pigmented spots. Different symptoms depend on how sensitive the patient is to the schistosome; each reexposure causes a more severe reaction.

Prevention

The best way to alleviate the problem is to destroy the snails by treating the water with copper sulfate and carbonate, or with sodium pentachlorophenate. A thick coating of grease or tightly woven clothes can protect against infestation; bathing with a hexachlorophene soap before swimming may help to some degree. Briskly rubbing the skin with a towel after swimming may help remove some organisms.

Treatment

Calamine lotion or oral antihistamines may help control the itch until the lesions begin to disappear on their own.

swimming and disease Recreational water illnesses have been associated with swimming at ocean beaches. Some common germs can live for long periods of time in salt water, and lakes and rivers can become contaminated with germs from sewage, animal waste, water runoff, as well as direct human contamination from fecal accidents and germs rinsed off the bottoms of swimmers.

Children should avoid swimming in areas that have been identified as unsafe by state/local health departments that release information about germ-testing results for local recreational water. Some germs that live in freshwater normally do not infect humans. (See also POOLS AND PARASITES.)

swimming pool safety See POOLS AND PARASITES.

syphilis A sexually transmitted disease (STD) that causes a skin sore and rash and may be transmitted from an infected mother to her unborn child during delivery. Syphilis was first recorded as a major epidemic in Europe during the 15th century, after Columbus returned from his trip to America. Today the infection is transmitted almost exclusively by sexual contact. Between 1999 and 2000 the national rate of congenital syphilis decreased by 7.6 percent, from 14.5 to 13.4 cases per 100,000 live births.

Cause

Syphilis is caused by a spirochete that enters broken skin or mucous membranes during sex, by kissing, or by intimate body contact with an open syphilitic sore. The rate of infection during a single contact with an infected person is about 30 percent.

Symptoms

During the first (primary) stage, a sore appears between three to four weeks after contact; the sore has a hard, wet, painless base that heals in about a month. In males, the sore appears on the shaft of the penis; in girls it can be found on the labia, although it is often hidden so well that the diagnosis is missed.

Six to 12 weeks after infection, the patient enters the secondary stage, which features a skin rash that may last for months. The rash has crops of pink or pale red round spots. The latent stage may last for a few years or until the end of a person's life. During this time the person appears normal; about 30 percent of these patients will develop end-stage syphilis, which usually begins about 10 years after the initial infection. At this point a person's tissues begin to deteriorate, involving the bones, palate, nasal septum, tongue, skin, or any organ of the body. The most serious complications in this stage include heart problems, brain damage leading to insanity, and paralysis.

Treatment

Penicillin is the drug of choice for all forms of the disease; early syphilis can often be cured by a single large injection. Later forms of the disease require multiple doses of penicillin over time.

Incidence

The 5,979 cases of syphilis reported in 2000 were the fewest cases ever reported in the United States, most of which occur in a few counties in the south.

Indeed, half of all syphilis cases were reported from only 21 counties in the United States. Cook County, Illinois, has the most cases, followed by Marion County, Indiana, Wayne County, Michigan, and Shelby County, Tennessee. However, the highest rate per 100,000 was Robeson County, North Carolina, where 49 of every 100,000 people are infected with syphilis. Between 1999 and 2000 the national rate of congenital syphilis decreased by 7.6 percent, from 14.5 to 13.4 cases per 100,000 live births.

Although there are big differences in the reported rates among racial and ethnic groups, these differences have been declining over the past five years. For example, the syphilis rate reported for 2000 among African Americans was 21 times the rate reported among whites, reflecting a substantial decline from 1996, when the rate among African Americans was 50 times greater than that among whites.

syrup of ipecac   See IPECAC, SYRUP OF.

systemic lupus erythematosus (SLE)   The more serious and potentially fatal form of the chronic autoimmune disease lupus erythematosus that affects many systems of the body. The milder form is discoid lupus erythematosus (DLE). Systemic lupus erythematosus (SLE) is probably not one but several conditions; while many systems of the body may be affected, it is also possible that the disease may affect just the skin. Although typically a disease of girls and young women, it can affect either sex and all age groups without regard to race. The disease commonly waxes and wanes, and its etiology is affected by heredity, autoimmunity, certain drugs, sex hormones, ultraviolet light, and viruses.

SLE accounts for about 70 percent of all lupus patients as well as a higher percentage of pediatric patients. Although SLE typically develops during the 20s, 30s, or 40s, about 15 to 17 percent of patients with systemic lupus first notice symptoms during childhood or adolescence. Most of these symptoms are seen in children 10 years or older; it is extremely rare to see symptoms in children younger than five. (Although there are no definitive data, it has been estimated that between 5,000 and 10,000 children in the United States have SLE.)

The relationship between DLE and SLE is controversial. Between 2 and 20 percent of patients who are first diagnosed with DLE go on to develop SLE. It is not uncommon for typical SLE to go into remission, leaving lesions of chronic DLE. On the other hand, DLE may spontaneously subside, remain constant, worsen, or progress to active SLE after some stress.

The prognosis for patients with SLE depends on which organs are involved; kidney or central nervous system involvement implies a poor prognosis. In most patients the disease is chronic; more than 90 percent of patients survive for at least 10 years.

Symptoms

Typically there is a red scaly rash on the face, affecting the nose and cheeks, arthritis, and progressive kidney damage; the heart, lungs, and brain may also be affected by progressive attacks of inflammation followed by the formation of scar tissue. In the milder form (DLE) only the skin is affected. Patients with lupus often have fever, weakness, fatigue, or weight loss. They may experience muscle aches, loss of appetite, swollen glands, hair loss, or abdominal pain, which can be accompanied by nausea, diarrhea, and vomiting. Sometimes the person's fingers, toes, nose, or ears will be particularly sensitive to cold and will turn white in cold temperatures, a condition known as Raynaud's phenomenon.

Diagnosis

SLE can be difficult to diagnose, because no two patients have the same symptoms, which also can be mistaken for those of other diseases. SLE may be serious and life-threatening or very mild. To make diagnosing SLE easier, the American College of Rheumatology has published a list of 11 symptoms that are typically seen in SLE; a patient who has at least four of these symptoms probably has SLE:

- rash across the cheeks and the bridge of the nose
- circular, red raised patches of skin that often occur on the face, neck, or chest
- sensitivity to ultraviolet light
- painless ulcers in the nose or mouth

- arthritis that does not destroy the bones around the joints
- inflammation of the lining around the heart, abdomen, or lungs
- kidney problems, either mild (with no early symptoms) or severe
- neurological disorders, such as seizures or psychosis
- blood problems, such as a low red blood cell count (anemia), a low white blood cell count (leukopenia), or a low platelet count (thrombocytopenia)
- problems with the immune system
- positive test for antinuclear antibodies (ANA), specific proteins that are a hallmark of rheumatic or autoimmune disease

Treatment

Local corticosteroid creams and ointments, or a therapeutic trial of salicylate are used to treat SLE. Immunosuppressive agents are sometimes used, especially among those who have experienced side effects from corticosteroids.

Tay-Sachs disease (TSD)   A fatal genetic disorder in children that causes progressive destruction of the central nervous system, bringing blindness, dementia, paralysis, seizures, and deafness. It is usually fatal within the first few years of life. Most babies with Tay-Sachs disease (TSD) are of eastern European Jewish origin.

The disease was named for Warren Tay, a British ophthalmologist who in 1881 described a patient with a cherry-red spot on the retina of the eye, and for Bernard Sachs, a New York neurologist whose work several years later provided the first description of the cellular changes in Tay-Sachs disease.

Cause

Tay-Sachs is a genetic disease that occurs most often among Jews of central or eastern European descent. When two parents are carriers, a child has a one in four chance of having the disease, which is caused by the absence of a vital enzyme called hexosaminidase A (Hex-A). Without Hex-A, a fatty substance builds up abnormally in cells of the brain, gradually damaging the cells. The disease begins during early pregnancy, although the disease is not clinically apparent until the child is several months old.

Every human has genes in pairs along 23 pairs of chromosomes. Tay-Sachs is controlled by a pair of genes on chromosome 15 (these are the genes that code for the enzyme Hex-A). If either or both Hex-A genes are active, the body produces enough of the enzyme to prevent the development of Tay-Sachs. Carriers of TSD (people with one copy of the inactive gene along with one copy of the active gene) do not have Tay-Sachs disease, but they could possibly pass the inactive gene to their children. A carrier has a 50 percent chance of passing the inactive gene on; any child who inherits one inactive gene is a Tay-Sachs carrier like the parent.

If both parents are carriers and their child inherits the inactive TSD gene from each of them, the child will have Tay-Sachs disease, since he or she has inherited two inactive recessive genes and therefore cannot produce any functional Hex-A. When both parents are carriers of the inactive Tay-Sachs gene, they have a one in four chance (25 percent) with each pregnancy that their child will have Tay-Sachs disease, and a three in four chance (75 percent) that their child will be healthy. Of their unaffected children, there is a two in three chance that each child will be a carrier, like the parents. This pattern of inheritance is called autosomal recessive.

Symptoms

A baby with Tay-Sachs disease appears normal at birth and seems to develop normally until about six months of age. The first signs of TSD appear at different ages in affected children. First development slows down and the child begins to lose peripheral vision, developing an abnormal startle response. By about age two, most children with the condition have recurrent seizures and diminishing mental function. Skills are slowly lost, one by one, until the child is unable to crawl, turn over, sit, or reach.

Other symptoms include increasing loss of coordination, progressive inability to swallow, and breathing difficulties. Eventually, the child becomes blind, mentally retarded, paralyzed, and unresponsive.

By the time a child with TSD is three or four years old, the nervous system is so badly affected that the child will die. Even with the best of care, all children with classical TSD die early in childhood, usually by the age of five.

Diagnosis/Treatment

Although there is not any treatment for this disease, there is a test to help parents determine if they are carriers of the gene.

TB   See TUBERCULOSIS.

teething   The eruption of an infant's first teeth typically starts between four and seven months, although it is perfectly normal to begin earlier or later than this. The first teeth to erupt are usually the two bottom front teeth (the central incisors) followed four to eight weeks later by the four front upper teeth (central and lateral incisors). About a month later will come the two teeth flanking the bottom front teeth (lower lateral incisors). These are followed by the first molars (the back teeth used for grinding food), and then the pointed eye-teeth in the upper jaw.

Most children have all 20 of their primary teeth by their third birthday. Rarely, children will be born with one or two teeth or will have a tooth emerge within the first few weeks of life. Unless the teeth interfere with feeding or are loose enough to pose a risk of choking, this should not be a problem.

Teething is usually accompanied by increased drooling and the desire to gnaw on things. Most babies do not have much pain, but some may experience brief periods of irritability, and some may be cranky for weeks. While some discomfort is normal, extreme irritability should be reported to the pediatrician. Although tender and swollen gums could cause a slight rise in temperature, teething normally does not cause a high fever or diarrhea.

What Parents Can Do

There are some things parents can do to make their teething infants feel more comfortable, including:

- wiping the baby's face often to remove the drool and prevent rash
- giving the baby something to chew on, such as a cold wet washcloth or a rubber teething ring
- rubbing the baby's gums with a clean finger.

Tooth Care

Even though the first set of teeth will fall out, it is important to take care of these baby teeth, because tooth decay can make teeth fall out early and interfere with the spacing of the permanent teeth.

Daily dental care should begin before the baby's first tooth emerges. Parents should wipe the baby's gums daily with a clean, damp washcloth or gauze, or brush them gently with a soft, infant-sized toothbrush and water without toothpaste. As soon as the first tooth appears, it should be brushed with water. Toothpaste may be used once the child is old enough to know how to spit it out and not swallow it (usually about age three).

By the time all the baby teeth are in, parents should be brushing the child's teeth at least twice a day (after breakfast and before bed), and flossing as well. Flossing can be started as soon as the first two teeth start to touch.

Finally, babies should never fall asleep with a bottle, because the milk or juice can pool in the mouth and cause tooth decay. The American Dental Association and the American Academy of Pediatric Dentists recommend that children see a dentist by age one or when six to eight teeth appear in order to spot any potential problems and advise parents about preventive care.

television and children   While television can be a wonderful educational tool, too much TV—or the wrong type of shows—can be harmful to children. According to the American Academy of Pediatrics (AAP), children who watch a great deal of television on a regular basis may be at risk for obesity and aggressive behavior. In fact, research suggests that the more time preschool children spend watching TV, the more likely they are to be overweight. Placing a television set in a child's room also seems to further increase the likelihood that a child will become overweight.

Other studies suggest that excessive TV watching may be associated with more problems with school, social skills, and attentiveness.

For this reason, experts recommend that children younger than age two avoid TV altogether, and that those over two watch less than two hours of TV each day. Parents can help influence their children's TV habits by reducing their own TV viewing. Rather than simply expecting children to turn off the TV, parents should also limit their own viewing. Instead of automatically turning on the TV, experts suggest that parents sit down and plan what shows the family will watch together. When those shows are over, the TV should then be turned off.

Some families ban TV on school nights and tape weekday shows they want to watch for viewing on the weekends.

tendonitis Inflammation of a tendon that usually occurs after excessive exercise but is sometimes caused by a bacterial infection or generalized rheumatic infection. Treatment involves rest or splinting the nearby joint, together with corticosteroid injections into the sore area around the tendon.

tension headaches See HEADACHE.

testicles, undescended The common name for "cryptorchidism," in which one or both testicles fail to descend from the abdomen into the scrotum by age one. Undescended testicles is a common childhood problem that affects about a third of premature babies and 3 percent of full-term infants.

Incomplete testicle descent is not just a physical abnormality; it also can lead to infertility and testicular cancer later in life. Normally, the testicle will descend by the time a child is born, or by the end of the first year of life. However, if the testes remain in the abdomen, sperm production (and fertility) is usually impaired. If not repaired by age six, the condition can cause permanent infertility.

If only one testicle has descended, the boy will have a low sperm count, whereas if both remain in the abdomen, there is usually no sperm in the semen. Researchers believe that this is because the higher temperature in the abdomen destroys the enzymes and proteins needed for normal sperm production. There are several types of cryptorchidism.

In true undescended testes, the testicles are positioned within the normal route of descent, but they cannot be manually lowered into the scrotum. "Retractile testes" usually occurs between age three and six and is caused by hyperactivity of the abdominal muscles that raises the testes. Ectopic (displaced) testes are found outside the normal route of descent in areas such as the upper groin, floor of the pelvis, penile shaft, or thigh. Many researchers believe there is less chance of cancer in ectopic testes than in true undescended testes.

Cause

Most cases of undescended testicles have no known cause.

Symptoms

Undescended testicles should be suspected if the testis cannot be felt in the scrotum, or if the testis is very soft and small.

Treatment

Doctors disagree about whether to treat this condition surgically or with hormonal therapy, although most experts recommend some form of treatment between a child's first and second birthday. In the United States most doctors prefer to treat one undescended testicle with surgery, placing the testis in the normal position before the second birthday, so that it has a chance of developing normally and producing sperm cells.

If both testicles are undescended, many specialists prefer a combination of surgery and hormone therapy with human chorionic gonadotropin (hCG) or gonadotropin-releasing hormone (GnRH) or both. European doctors usually rely on hormone therapy alone as the primary treatment for all patients with undescended testicles.

Unfortunately, if the testes have been injured by their failure to descend, this usually cannot be corrected. Men with undescended testicles are more likely to have hormone problems or abnormal testicular ducts. Some doctors report improvements in sperm quality among men who receive medical therapy with clomiphene citrate (an antiestrogen drug) and hCG.

tests There are a wide variety of medical tests that can help diagnose diseases and conditions in children. These include scans (CT, MRI, nuclear), echocardiography, ultrasounds, X ray, and scans of bone, kidney, lung, thyroid, and urinary bladder.

CT Scan (Computed Tomography, or CAT scan)

CT scans provide many cross-sectional images of the body by using special X rays and computer enhancement to create an image that is much more sensitive than a simple X ray. After x-raying the body from many angles, the X rays are then analyzed by a computer to provide a picture of the body that can be viewed on a monitor or printed out as a photograph. The images show a composite slice of the body (usually the head, chest, or abdomen).

In this procedure, a child lies flat on a movable table that moves into the center of the CT scanner.

As the child remains still, X rays are beamed into the body. If the child cannot remain still, sedatives are administered. Sometimes a dye or other contrast material is injected to better reveal blood vessels. Results are interpreted by radiologists and then reported to the child's doctor, who will analyze and interpret them for the parents.

Echocardiography

This procedure uses a special device to detect the sound that is reflected from a beating heart. Sometimes called "diagnostic cardiac ultrasound," this test uses reflected sound waves to show if a child has congenital heart defects, fluid around the heart, valve disorders, or weakened heart muscles. It is possible to actually see the heart move as the images are projected on a monitor. The direction of blood flow into and out of the heart can be seen in different colors on the monitor.

In this procedure, a child lies on his back, tilted slightly to the side. A special jelly is applied to the skin on the area of the heart, and the transducer is positioned over the heart. As sound waves are reflected back to the transducer, an image becomes visible on a monitor that can be turned into printouts from the screen. This test produces no radiation and the child experiences no discomfort. Although images are produced immediately, they must be interpreted by a cardiologist and sent to the child's doctor, who will interpret them for the parents.

MRI (Magnetic Resonance Imaging)

Another way to take pictures of the inside of the body involves the use of magnetism and radio waves to produce much more detailed images than an X ray because of its ability to separate different types of soft tissues. As radio waves are sent to a specific part of the body, the atoms emit their own radio waves that are translated into images by a computer. MRI can be used to look at any area of the body and is especially useful in diagnosing disease of the soft tissues of the head, spinal cord, kidneys, urinary tract, pancreas, and liver. MRIs are also the procedure of choice to detect sports injuries involving tendon and ligament damage.

After removing any metal objects, a child lies on a table that slides into a tube so that radio waves can be directed at the body, triggering the body's atoms to create radio waves that are picked up by the MRI scanner. The information is then used to create a composite slice that can be viewed on a monitor and printed for further study. Although the process is painless, it can frighten some children because they are confined in the tube during the procedure. For this reason, sedatives may be given. Because it tends to be very noisy inside the tube, earplugs are usually given to help eliminate the noise; alternatively, earphones are usually available for children who would like to listen to tapes. The scan takes 30 to 60 minutes.

Some hospitals offer an open MRI, which does not require confining a child to the tunnel; this procedure is faster and less noisy, making it ideal for children. MRI results are interpreted by a radiologist and sent to the child's doctor, who will present them to the parents.

Radioisotope (Nuclear) Scan

A number of tests use very small quantities of radioactive materials (radioisotopes) to reveal parts of the body. The radioisotope is attached to another substance that is injected, inhaled, or swallowed, so that special devices can sense their position and produce an image of them as they appear in a child's internal organs. Although it may seem dangerous to swallow a radioactive substance, the quantity and duration of radioactivity in these tests have been designed to be safe in humans, and should not cause any harmful effects.

Bone Scan

A bone scan can detect changes in bone growth and identify cancer, infections, or the reason for unexplained bone pain, such as a break that did not show up on an X ray. This test evaluates how a radioactive isotope collects in the bone. The radioactive isotope is injected into a vein and is absorbed by the bones; as the tracer isotope emits radiation, it is detected by a scanner. It takes about two to four hours after the injection before enough of the radiation has collected in the bones for the scan to be done.

During the test, a child lies flat on a table while a special camera records the distribution of the tracer isotope. An abnormal distribution of the isotope indicates a problem. The bone scan is interpreted by a radiologist and sent to the child's doctor, who will present the findings to the parents.

Kidney Scan

The kidney scan uses radioisotopes to identify problems with the structure and function of the kidney. These scans are used after kidney transplants and to diagnose kidney failure, disorders, and infections.

In this test, the child lies on a table and a substance with a small amount of a radioisotope is injected into a vein. Then the kidneys are scanned, and images are sent to a computer. Results will be read by a radiologist and sent to the child's doctor, who will present them to the parents.

Liver or Gallbladder Scan

The liver or gallbladder scan uses radioactive isotopes to look for liver or gallbladder damage: hepatitis, cirrhosis, abscess, infection, cancer, or injury. After a radioisotope is injected into a vein, it is absorbed by the liver or gallbladder. During the test, the child lies on a table under a scanner; the radioactive material is then picked up by a scanner, which transmits images to a computer. The radiologist interprets the findings and sends them to the child's doctor, who will present them to the parents.

Lung Scan

A nuclear lung scan helps to determine the presence of a blood or abnormal formation of the lung. In this test, radioactive gas lung tracers are given by inhalation or injection so that the chest can be scanned. These scans can also be used to study malformations of the lung. The results will be read by a radiologist and sent to the child's doctor, who will present them to the parents.

Thyroid Scan

Thyroid scans are not often performed in children because there is not much risk of thyroid disease in children. The thyroid scan uses radioisotopes to discover problems with the structure or function of the gland. These tests can help determine if a patient has thyroid problems, including hyperthyroidism and cancer or other growths.

In this test, a radioisotope is injected into a vein so that the neck can be scanned with a camera to display an image of the thyroid gland in several views. The thyroid scan will be read by a radiologist and sent to the child's doctor, who will present the results to the parents.

Urinary Bladder Scan

This test is also called a radionuclide voiding cystogram, and it is used to detect whether urine is flowing backward from the bladder to the kidney, which can be associated with an infection. In this test, a small amount of radioisotope is added to a fluid, which is inserted into the bladder by a catheter. After the bladder is filled, the child urinates and images are obtained throughout the test to detect reflux.

Ultrasound

Ultrasound can examine many parts of a child's body by using high-frequency sound waves to bounce off internal organs and create pictures. Some of the organs that can be examined by painless ultrasound include the kidneys, liver, spleen, brain, female pelvis, and the hips. A special jelly is applied to the skin on the area that is tested; as the transducer is positioned over the area, sound waves are reflected back to the transducer, and the image appears on a monitor. Printouts are then made from the screen. Although the images are created immediately, they must be interpreted by a radiologist; results will be reported to a doctor, who will interpret them for parents.

X Ray

X rays consist of electromagnetic radiation (like light), but with a shorter wavelength, that penetrates the body and forms an image on film. Any part of the body can be x-rayed, and the procedure is particularly useful in diagnosing injuries or changes in bones. Chest X rays can detect pneumonia or other lung diseases, and determining heart size. Some tests use dyes or other materials (such as barium) that show up on X rays to outline structures within the body.

In an "upper GI," for example, the child swallows a contrast material, and an X ray examines the progress of the material through the stomach and upper small intestine. The contrast material gives the radiologist a better look at the shape of the gastrointestinal tract.

A myelogram is an X-ray test of the spine in which dye is injected into the spinal fluid to outline the spinal cord.

An arthrogram is an X ray of a knee or hip joint in which a dye is injected to make the picture clearer and to enable detection of a tear in the cartilage or other joint abnormalities.

In fluoroscopy, a moving picture of the body is seen as the test is performed and is recorded on videotape or as still images. This technique can be used to evaluate the gastrointestinal tract, the respiratory system, and the bladder, among other things. Fluoroscopy and other specialized tests are performed by a radiologist with the assistance of a technologist.

An intravenous pyelogram (IVP) uses a contrast dye to outline the kidneys, ureters (the tubes that carry urine from the kidney to the bladder), and bladder on an X ray. The dye, which is given through a vein, helps the radiologist evaluate kidney function as well determine any abnormalities in the structure of the urinary system.

In an X-ray test, the child is positioned so that the machine can take a picture of the area being investigated. The painless test is usually performed by a technologist in the radiology department of the hospital, and results are interpreted by a radiologist.

tetanus   An acute, often-fatal infectious disease commonly known as "lockjaw" because the condition causes the jaw muscles to lock. In the United States, four out of every 10 people who get tetanus will die. The disease is not passed from one person to the next, because the illness is caused by toxins produced by bacteria. The tetanus vaccine has been available since the 1940s.

Cause

Tetanus is caused by a bacterium belonging to the *Clostridium* genus, which thrives in the absence of oxygen. It is found almost everywhere in the environment—most often in soil, dust, manure, and in the digestive tract of humans and animals. The bacteria form spores, which are hard to kill and highly resistant to heat and many antiseptics.

Tetanus bacteria enter the body through a wound (even one as small as a pinprick). More typically, the wound that leads to tetanus is a deep puncture caused by a nail or knife; because these wounds are hard to clean, bacteria remains deep within the wound. In the presence of dead tissue, tetanus spores can grow and produce the deadly exotoxin that causes symptoms. While tetanus bacteria are found almost everywhere, natural immunity is rare, which is why immunization is so important.

It is also possible to contract tetanus from animal scratches and bites, in wounds where the flesh is torn or burned, in crushing wounds, and in frostbite. It may even follow minor wounds such as splinters, and it can develop after surgery.

tetracycline   Any of a group of broad-spectrum antibiotics derived from cultures of *Streptomyces* bacteria that are used to treat many bacterial and rickettsial infections. Because tetracycline may cause permanent discoloration of the teeth, it is not used during the last half of pregnancy or during a child's first eight years of life. Children with significant liver or kidney problems should not use this drug.

theophylline   A bronchodilator used in the treatment of ASTHMA and to prevent attacks of APNEA (cessation of breathing) in premature infants. The drug is also used to treat heart failure, since it stimulates heart rate. Brands such as Theo-Dur, Slo-Phyllin, and Theobid are less commonly used today.

thermometers   Devices to record body temperature at one time all contained mercury, which has now been deemed unsafe. Mercury is a toxic substance that can harm both humans and wildlife. Many different products, including thermometers, contain mercury.

If mercury thermometers are thrown away in the regular garbage and that garbage is burned in an incinerator, mercury vapors will be released into the air. Mercury in garbage sent to a landfill can seep into the groundwater or can be released into the air as a toxic vapor. Airborne mercury eventually falls to the earth, often into rivers and lakes.

There are several types of alternative thermometers are available commercially. These include:

- digital thermometers
- glass gallium-indium-tin (galinstan) thermometers

- flexible forehead thermometers
- ear canal thermometers

All of these are acceptable alternatives to the older mercury-filled instruments. Mercury is a high priority toxic substance targeted for elimination by the U.S. Environmental Protection Association (EPA). Many communities across the country have sponsored "Thermometer Exchanges," in which citizens could bring in their mercury thermometers to local pharmacies for exchange with alternative devices.

thimerosal A common preservative found in vaccines that, as it metabolizes, can produce ethyl mercury, an organic derivative of mercury. Since the 1930s thimerosal has been added to some vaccines and other products because it is effective in killing bacteria and in preventing bacterial contamination, particularly in multidose containers. Not much is known about the effects of thimerosal exposure on humans and how this compares to methyl mercury exposure.

Mercury is a naturally occurring chemical element found throughout the environment as a pure metal (as in thermometers), as inorganic salts, and as an organic derivative. Humans and wildlife are exposed to all three forms. Most mercury in the environment is either metallic or inorganic. Because mercury is everywhere, it is not possible to prevent all exposure to it. High levels of mercury are toxic.

Methyl mercury, the most common organic derivative of mercury, is produced by microorganisms in water and soil and is of particular concern because it can accumulate in certain edible freshwater and saltwater fish, to levels that are much higher than in the surrounding water. Methyl mercury can also accumulate in humans who eat these fish. Exposure to high levels of methyl mercury is toxic and can cause MENTAL RETARDATION, CEREBRAL PALSY, and seizures. A fetus is especially sensitive to methyl mercury exposure, and may suffer brain damage or even death if exposed to high levels. This is why pregnant women are advised to limit their consumption of certain fish.

The only known side effects of receiving low doses of thimerosal in vaccines have been minor reactions such as redness and swelling at the injec-

tion site. However, in July 1999 the Public Health Service (PHS) agencies, the American Academy of Pediatrics (AAP), and vaccine manufacturers agreed that thimerosal should be reduced or eliminated in vaccines as a precautionary measure and to reduce exposure to mercury from all sources. Today all routinely recommended licensed pediatric vaccines that are currently being manufactured for the U.S. market are either thimerosal-free or contain markedly reduced amounts of thimerosal. However, thimerosal remains in some vaccines given to adults and adolescents, as well as some pediatric vaccines not on the Recommended Childhood Immunization Schedule.

The decision to reduce or eliminate thimerosal in vaccines was based on the various federal guidelines for methyl mercury exposure and the assumption that the health risks from methyl mercury and ethyl mercury were the same. Methyl mercury exposure is primarily through fish consumption. People who regularly eat mercury-contaminated fish can accumulate methyl mercury in their body over time. Some of this methyl mercury may be passed from the mother to the fetus before birth and to infants through breast milk. The fetus is most sensitive to damage by this exposure. During vaccination, infants are exposed to ethyl mercury by intramuscular injection, not by fetal exposure or by ingestion. Furthermore, infants receive limited quantities of ethyl mercury from vaccines that are administered days or months apart, while methyl mercury guidelines assess a child's risk based on a continuing daily mercury exposure. More research is needed to determine if the guidelines for methyl mercury exposure are also appropriate guidelines for thimerosal.

throat culture A test to determine the type of organism causing disease in the throat (especially STREP THROAT). For this test, a health-care worker obtains a specimen from deep in the throat with a long-handled sterile swab. The specimen is placed on a culture plate and read at 24 and 48 hours.

Rapid strep tests are now widely used; these tests react with certain proteins in the bacteria, giving results in just three minutes. They are about 90 percent accurate, compared to throat cultures. Many health-care workers do both the rapid test and a backup throat culture to make sure all cases of strep throat are diagnosed.

throat, sore   See SORE THROAT.

thrush   A yeast infection of the mouth, found often in infants and young children and in those with an impaired immune system.

Cause
A yeast infection is a fungal infection, but not all fungi are yeasts. In the case of thrush, the yeast that causes the infection is *Candida albicans*. While there are many different kinds of *Candida* species, *albicans* causes most human infections and almost all cases of thrush.

An infant may be infected during delivery if the mother has a vaginal yeast infection at birth; infants also may contract thrush from infections on a caregiver's hands or from bottle nipples. Babies born to diabetic mothers are more susceptible to thrush, as are those born with birth defects of the palate or lip. A child is infectious as long as there are lesions in the mouth.

Symptoms
Pain in the mouth area, together with raised patches in the mouth that look like milk curds on cheek and tongue and roof of the mouth.

Diagnosis
Tests are not needed; the disease can be identified by inspecting the mouth. The patches may be swabbed and examined for yeast cells under a microscope; alternatively, the fungus can be cultured.

Treatment
The mouth can be painted with nystatin suspension. Rinsing the mouth often can discourage the spread of thrush.

Prevention
Mothers with the symptoms of yeast infections should be treated in the last three months of pregnancy. No one should put fingers in a new baby's mouth. If the infant is bottle-fed, nipples and bottles should be boiled and hands washed before feeding. Children with impaired immune systems (including those with AIDS or those taking corticosteroid drugs or chemotherapy) should be careful to brush the mouth and tongue regularly and rinse the mouth often.

tics   Repeated involuntary movements that may vary in complexity from a twitch to a well-coordinated action. Tics may be either vocal, motor, or mental. See also TOURETTE'S SYNDROME.

ticks and disease   The tiny blood-sucking pests that plague American dogs and cats also can transmit disease to children. These tick-borne conditions include BABESIOSIS, CAT-SCRATCH DISEASE *(Bartonella)*, EHRLICHIOSIS, Colorado tick fever, LYME DISEASE, ROCKY MOUNTAIN SPOTTED FEVER, tick paralysis, and tularemia.

Depending on its species, a tick may take less than a year or up to several years to travel through its entire four-stage life cycle. Ticks need a blood meal at each stage after hatching; some species can survive years without eating anything.

When walking in the woods, hikers should stay on trails and avoid brushing up against low bushes or tall grass. Ticks do not hop, jump, fly, or descend from trees, although they may blow in a strong breeze. To prevent bites, hikers should wear protective clothing, light-colored, long-sleeve shirts, and light-colored pants tucked into boots or socks, so that ticks can be more easily spotted.

An insect repellent preferably containing no more than 30 percent DEET may be used on bare skin and clothing. All insect repellent should be used with caution on children and should not be applied to the hands or face.

Ticks and their hosts (chipmunks, voles, mice, and other small mammals) need moisture and a place hidden from direct sun to hide. Therefore, the clearer the area around a house, the less chance there will be of getting a tick bite. All leaf litter and brush should be removed as far as possible away from the house. Low-lying bushes should be pruned to let in more sun. Leaves should be raked every fall, since ticks prefer to overwinter in fallen leaves. Woodpiles are favorite hiding places for mammals carrying ticks; woodpiles should be neat, off the ground, in a sunny place, and under cover.

Gardens should be cleaned up every fall; foliage left on the ground over the winter provides shelter for mammals that may harbor ticks. Stone walls on the property increase the potential for ticks.

Shady lawns may support ticks in epidemic areas; lawns should be mowed and edged. Entire fields should be mowed in fall, preferably with a rotary mower.

Bird feeders attract birds that carry infected ticks, so feeders should not be placed close to the house. The ground under the feeder should be cleaned regularly. Bird feeding should be stopped during late spring and summer, when infected ticks are most active. Building eight-foot fences to keep out deer may significantly reduce the abundance of ticks on large land parcels. Pets allowed outside on a daily basis should be examined regularly; tick and flea medications can prevent infestations.

TICK TESTING/IDENTIFICATION

Any tick can be accurately identified and tested for the presence of the bacteria that causes Lyme disease *(Borrelia burgdorferi)* at the Tick Research Lab. Tick identification takes only a few minutes. Testing ticks for the presence of Lyme disease spirochetes can also be done with any tick, alive or dead, at any stage of development. Cost for identification and evaluation of the tick is $45. Tick identification alone is $15.

For more information contact Tick Research Lab, Biological Sciences Dept., University of Rhode Island, 100 Flagg Rd., Kingston, RI 02881 or contact the lab's email address at: ticklab@uriacc.uri.edu

---

tinea The medical term for ringworm, a group of common fungus infections of the skin, hair, or nails caused by various species of the fungi *Microsporum, Trichophyton,* and *Epidermophyton;* it also affects animals. Ringworm is highly contagious and can be spread by direct contact or via infected material; infections may be picked up from other people, animals, soil, or an object (such as a shower stall). The term "tinea" is often followed by the Latin term for the part of the body affected by the fungus, such as "tinea pedis," or ATHLETE'S FOOT.

Symptoms

Symptoms vary according to the part of the body affected by the infection; the most common area is the foot, causing athlete's foot, with cracking, itchy skin between the toes. Tinea cruris, or JOCK ITCH, is more common in males, and produces a red, itchy area from the genitals outward over the inside of the thighs; tinea corporis (ringworm of the body) is characterized by itchy circular skin patches with a raised edge. Tinea capitis (ringworm of the scalp) causes round, itchy circles of hair loss found most commonly in children in large cities or overcrowded conditions. Tinea unguium (ringworm of the nails) is characterized by scaling of soles or palms with thick, white, or yellow nails.

Treatment

Antifungal drugs (creams, lotions, or ointments) can successfully treat most types of tinea. For widespread infection (or those affecting hair or nails), the drug is given as a tablet (usually griseofulvin). Treatment should continue after symptoms have faded to ensure that the fungi have been destroyed. Mild infections on the surface of the skin may be treated for four to six weeks; toenail infections may require treatment for up to two years.

tinea capitis The medical term for RINGWORM of the scalp. (See also TINEA.)

tinea corporis The medical term for RINGWORM of the body. (See also TINEA.)

tinea cruris The medical term for JOCK ITCH. (See also TINEA.)

tinea manuum This RINGWORM infection is most often caused by *Tinea rubrum,* usually found together with a foot infection. The condition is characterized by thickened outer skin of palms and fingers, especially in the creases of the skin.

Treatment

Topical antifungal preparations such as Whitfield's ointment may help, although newer topical imidazole antifungals are preferred. However, topical agents alone do not usually cure this problem; an oral antifungal drug, such as griseofulvin or ketoconazole, is usually required for between two to three months. (See also TINEA.)

tinea pedis   The medical term for ATHLETE'S FOOT. (See also TINEA.)

toeing in/out   This is a common gait problem in young children. Some babies are born with the condition, but others develop it as they begin walking. Toeing in often occurs with bow legs and can cause problems if it makes a child trip while walking. Toeing out (also called "duck walking") is more rare. Many children have a slight outward turn of the feet of about 10 degrees while walking, but toeing out at an angle of more than 30 degrees is considered abnormal.

Causes

Congenital toeing out occurs if the shinbone or the hip bone is twisted outward as a result of an abnormal position in the womb.

Toeing in is much more common than toeing out in childhood and is eventually outgrown. It is often caused by the baby's position before birth. Most hooked feet get better without treatment during the baby's first year, although sometimes a cast may be necessary.

If a child does not start toeing in until after beginning to walk, this may be caused by a twisting of the shinbone that can occur if the child regularly sleeps or sits with knees flexed and feet turned inward. Abnormal twisting also can occur in the hip joint, rotating the entire leg inward, and the feet whip out to the sides when running.

Treatment

In most cases, no treatment is required. Many babies toe in or out when learning to stand and walk. They may toe in when shifting the body weight to the middle of the foot to compensate for knock-knees, which usually develop during the third year of life and disappear by age seven. Some parents fear that toeing in and toeing out will permanently harm a child's feet and ankles, but these fears are largely unfounded.

A temporary deformity caused by an abnormal position in the womb can often be corrected by stretching the baby's feet gently several times a day. If this does not work, a temporary cast or night splint that holds the feet in a normal position may be necessary. Some doctors recommend reversing the baby's shoes for a while (placing the left shoe on the right foot and vice versa) to correct toeing in.

A twisted shinbone often corrects itself, but corrective splints may be necessary if the deformity is severe and persists after the child has started walking. Hip abnormalities that cause toeing in and out usually require no treatment, except to avoid sleeping and sitting positions that might worsen them.

toe-walking   Walking on the toes is common among toddlers first learning to walk, especially during the second 12 months of life. Generally, the tendency is gone by age two, although in some children the habit persists.

Intermittent toe-walking is not serious; the only time it is a problem is when it is associated with other problems. Children who walk on their toes almost exclusively and continue to do so after age two should be medically evaluated to rule out conditions such as mild CEREBRAL PALSY.

Treatment

Persistent toe-walking, with no other symptoms, occasionally requires treatment. This involves casting the foot and ankle for about six weeks, which usually corrects the problem.

tonsillitis   Infection or inflammation of a tonsil caused by a virus or bacteria. Acute tonsillitis is often caused by a STREPTOCOCCAL INFECTION. If tonsillitis caused by a strep infection is untreated, it may lead to rheumatic fever or kidney disease.

Symptoms

Symptoms include severe sore throat, fever, headache, fatigue, swallowing problems, earache, and enlarged, tender lymph nodes in the neck. Acute cases may also be accompanied by SCARLET FEVER.

Treatment

Tonsillitis can be treated with systemic antibiotics and painkillers, together with warm liquids and soft foods. While a tonsillectomy is still sometimes performed for recurrent cases, this surgical procedure is done much less often today than in earlier decades.

tonsils   A mass of lymphoid tissue on either side of the back of the mouth that is one of the body's ways of dealing with invading infections. The tonsils make up part of the lymphatic system, which is an important part of the body's defense system against infection. Along with the adenoids at the base of the tongue, the tonsils protect against upper respiratory tract infections. They gradually get bigger after birth, reaching full size at about age seven; after that, they shrink substantially.

An infection of the tonsils is called TONSILLITIS, a common infectious disease of childhood. Although the removal of tonsils during childhood to treat infection was once a common treatment, it is rarely performed today.

Tourette's syndrome A neurological disorder characterized by tics, or rapid, sudden movements that occur involuntarily and repeatedly in a consistent fashion. To be diagnosed with Tourette's syndrome, an individual must have multiple motor tics as well as one or more vocal tics over a period of more than one year. These need not all occur simultaneously, but in general the tics may occur many times a day, usually in brief, intense groupings, nearly every day, or intermittently.

Common simple tics include eye blinking, shoulder jerking, picking movements, grunting, sniffing, and barking. Complex tics include facial grimacing, arm flapping, coprolalia (use of obscene words), palilalia (repeating one's own words), and echolalia (repeating another's words or phrases).

For individuals with Tourette's, tics may vary over time in terms of their frequency and severity, as well as in type and location. In some cases, symptoms may disappear for a period of weeks or even months. Although there is an involuntary quality to the tics experienced by individuals with Tourette's, most persons have some control over their symptoms, at least briefly, and even for hours at a time. However, suppressing them tends simply to postpone a more severe outburst, since the impulse to express tics is ultimately irresistible and must be expressed. Tics often will increase in response to stress and become less frequent with relaxation or intense focus on a task.

Many patients with Tourette's syndrome have other conditions at the same time, such as ATTENTION DEFICIT HYPERACTIVITY DISORDER (ADHD), OBSESSIVE-COMPULSIVE DISORDER, or LEARNING DISABILITIES.

Up to 20 percent of children have at least a transient tic disorder at some point. Once believed to be rare, Tourette's syndrome is now known to be a more common disorder that represents the most complex and severe manifestation of the spectrum of tic disorders.

Symptoms

Obsessions, compulsions, impulsive behavior, and mood swings. Tourette's is commonly associated with other syndromes, including attention deficit hyperactivity disorder, anxiety, mood, or panic disorders, obsessive-compulsive disorder, behavior problems, and learning disabilities.

In most children, Tourette's syndrome fluctuates; anxiety, stress, and fatigue often intensify tics, which are usually significantly reduced during sleep or when the child is focused on an activity. Psychoactive drugs (especially cocaine and stimulants) tend to worsen tics.

In most cases, tics peak in severity between ages nine and 11, but between 5 and 10 percent of children continue to have unchanged or worsening symptoms into adolescence and adulthood. There is no reliable way to predict which children will have a poorer prognosis.

Cause

An abnormal metabolism of the neurotransmitters dopamine and serotonin is linked to the disorder, which is genetically transmitted. Parents have a 50 percent chance of passing the gene on to their children. Girls with the gene have a 70 percent chance of displaying symptoms, boys with the gene have a 99 percent chance of displaying symptoms.

Diagnosis

The single most important component of managing the condition is to get an accurate diagnosis. Tics occur suddenly during normal activity, unlike other movement disorders such as:

- *Chorea* A pattern of nonrepetitive irregular movements
- *Stereotypy* Constant, repetitive behaviors performed for no obvious reason
- *Dystonias* A slow, constant repetitive behavior

The doctor will want to rule out any secondary causes of tic disorders. A complete general physical examination is important, with specific attention to the central nervous system. The thyroid-stimulating hormone (TSH) level should be measured in most patients, since tics often occur together with hyperthyroidism. A throat culture should be checked for group A beta-hemolytic streptococcus, especially if symptoms get worse or better with ear or throat infections. The evidence of strep infection with a single occurrence of worsening tics is not enough to make a diagnosis of streptococcus-induced, autoimmune-caused Tourette's syndrome.

An electroencephalogram is useful only in children in whom it is difficult to differentiate tics from manifestations of EPILEPSY. Imaging studies are not likely to be helpful, and the importance of other studies depends on symptoms. For example, a urine drug screen for cocaine and stimulants should be considered in the case of a teenager with sudden onset of tics and inappropriate behavior symptoms. A child with a family history of liver disease associated with a Parkinsonian or hyperkinetic movement disorder should undergo a test for copper in the blood to rule out Wilson's disease.

The basic workup is usually appropriate in a child with a gradual onset of symptoms, a developmental progression of tics, and a family history of tics or obsessive-compulsive disorder.

Treatment

Positive reinforcement programs appear to be most helpful in managing tic disorders. Target behaviors may be categorized into two groups, skill deficiencies (areas that initially require concentration to build social and academic skills) and behavior excesses, in which the goal is to help the patient decrease the frequency of these behaviors. Managing behavior excesses needs to be handled carefully, however, since some children who undergo behavior modification to directly target the Tourette's symptoms experience a worsening of symptoms.

Drug Treatment

The goal in tic control is to use the lowest dosage of medication that will bring the patient's functioning to an acceptable level. Often this will require only modest levels of tic reduction. The most common drug treatments are haloperidol (Haldol), pimozide (Orap), risperidone (Risperdal), and clonidine (Catapres). Guanfacine (Tenex) is not labeled for use in children under 12 years of age. Less often, clonazepam (Klonopin) may be prescribed. For tics of mild to moderate severity, or in patients who are wary of drug side effects, an initial trial of clonidine or guanfacine may be tried. These medications are modestly effective in tic control and have a range of less specific benefits. Many children taking them may be less irritable or less impulsive, and manifestations of ADHD may improve as well.

Side Effects

These include sedation, weight gain, poor school performance, social anxiety with school refusal in children, and unusual body movements, including tardive dyskinesias, a potentially irreversible drug-caused movement disorder that may be difficult to distinguish from tics. When pimozide is used, baseline and follow-up electrocardiograms are recommended.

Most children with Tourette's syndrome require medication for up to one to two years. About 15 percent of patients require long-term medication for tic control. When tics appear to be stable and adequately controlled for a period of four to six months, a slow and gradual reduction in medication should follow. With such a strategy, occasional drug holidays may be possible in some patients as tics lessen. If tics increase, incremental increases in medication may be needed.

Because many children with Tourette's syndrome have other conditions, treatment for these conditions may be necessary. Treatment of ADHD with Tourette's has been controversial because of reports that stimulants hasten the onset or increase the severity of tics in some patients. This observation alone may not be a contraindication for stimulant treatment in patients with significant symptoms of ADHD. Stimulants alone may not substantially worsen the course or severity of the disorder. In some cases, it may be necessary to treat both the ADHD and the Tourette's syndrome with a stimulant in combination with either clonidine or guanfacine, or with a neuroleptic agent. A trial of clonidine or guanfacine alone may be sufficient to adequately treat both conditions. When possible, multiple drugs should not be used, especially in children.

toxic shock syndrome (TSS) An uncommon condition caused by infection with *Staphylococcus* bacteria, characterized by a distinctive skin rash resembling sunburn on the palms and soles of the feet. The condition, first recognized in the 1970s, is associated with the use of certain brands of highly absorbent tampons (now taken off the market). About 70 percent of cases occur in girls and women who were using tampons when symptoms begin. The U.S. Food and Drug Administration estimates that one out of every 100,000 menstruating girls and women develops toxic shock syndrome (TSS) each year.

About three percent of TSS cases are fatal. Since 1984 there have been 69 reports of death related to tampon use; all but three were caused by TSS. However, the risk of death from TSS is higher in cases not related to menstruation.

Symptoms

When related to menstruation, TSS symptoms may not begin until the first few days after a girl's period and tend to appear quickly. In addition to the skin rash, symptoms include sudden high fever, vomiting and diarrhea, headache, muscular aches and pains, dizziness, and disorientation. Blood pressure may drop rapidly and shock may develop. The sunburn-like rash may not develop until the patient is very ill, or it may go completely unnoticed if it appears in a small area. The skin on palms and feet may flake and peel. Once a person has had TSS, she is more likely to get it again.

Death usually occurs as a result of a prolonged drop in blood pressure or lung problems.

Cause

The condition is caused by a toxin produced by *Staphylococcus aureus*. Scientists first described TSS as a distinct disease in 1978; two years later, reports of the problem increased among girls who had become ill during or just after menstruation. Studies showed that the use of the high-absorbency tampons was associated with the problem, but the exact connection remains unclear.

While it is most common in connection with menstruating girls and women using tampons, TSS also occurs in newborns, children, and men, primarily as a result of infection after surgery.

Scientists believe that for TSS to develop, the staphylococcus bacteria must release one or more toxins into the bloodstream. While these bacteria normally live without causing problems in the nose, skin, and vagina, they can sometimes lead to serious infection after a deep wound, surgery, or during extended tampon use.

Treatment

Antibiotic drugs and intravenous infusion (to prevent shock), plus treatment for any complications as they occur. Recurrence is common; girls and women who have had toxic shock syndrome should not use tampons, cervical caps, diaphragms, or vaginal contraceptive sponges.

Prevention

The best way to prevent TSS is not to use any kind of tampon. Because the risk of TSS rises with increased tampon absorbency, it is a good idea to use products with the lowest absorbency and to change tampons very often.

toxocariasis Infection with the larvae of *Toxocara canis* (the common roundworm of dogs and cats). Children between age one and four who eat dirt are at particular risk for this disease. Older children and adults in households with an infected younger child may show evidence of light infection.

Cause

Ingesting the eggs that are often found in soil leads to the spread of tiny larvae throughout the body. In the United States dogs are often infected with worms which are passed to them as pups before birth or while nursing. Adult worms pass eggs in the dogs' feces, which then may find their way into soil or sandboxes. These eggs can remain viable for many weeks and even months. When a child eats soil or sand containing these eggs, the larvae hatch in the child's small intestine, penetrating the intestinal wall and migrating throughout the body. After some time, the larvae in the child will die. It is also possible to be infected by eating unwashed vegetables grown in contaminated soil. However, humans cannot pass the infection from one to another.

Symptoms

Most people have no signs of the infestation, and there is a long incubation period. Children who swallow large numbers of worms may be sick with breathing problems, enlarged liver, fever, anemia, fatigue, skin rash, and eye problems.

Diagnosis

An abnormal blood count with a high number of a certain type of white blood cell and antibodies suggests a diagnosis of toxocariasis.

Complication

If the larvae migrate to the liver, lungs, or abdomen, they can cause an enlarged liver, PNEUMONIA, and stomach pain. They may reach a child's eyes and damage the retina. Symptoms of complications include breathing problems, rash, and fever.

Treatment

There is no specific drug treatment that will cure the infestation. The disease is usually self-limiting even without treatment. In severe cases, two drugs may treat symptoms: thiabendazole or diethylcarbamazine. Steroids have helped some people with heart or nervous system problems.

Prevention

Worming of pets can help prevent the spread of this disease. All pets at age three weeks should be dewormed, followed by a deworming every two weeks until the pet has had three treatments. They should be wormed every six months thereafter.

toxoplasmosis   A disease of mammals and birds, especially the cat, that causes a mild disease in children (and more severe problems in those with impaired immune systems). Cats get the disease by eating infected mice.

At least 50 percent of everyone in the United States has been infected with toxoplasmosis by the age of 50; the vast majority of infections produce no symptoms.

Cause

The parasite *(Toxoplasma gondii)* can be transmitted to children via undercooked meat, contaminated soil, or by direct contact. Most often, a cat may be involved. The parasite excretes eggs into the cat's feces, where it then travels to the child. The eggs of the *T. gondii* migrate to an animal's muscles, where they remain infectious for a long time. Eating undercooked beef, mutton, or lamb from an infected animal can transfer the infection. Children also can get the disease by drinking unpasteurized goat's milk from infected goats, drinking water contaminated with cat feces, or by handling cat feces or infected soil.

Symptoms

If symptoms appear, they are usually mild, with a slight swelling of lymph nodes at various sites in the body together with a low-grade fever, tiredness, sore throat, or slight body rash. The disease is often misdiagnosed as infectious MONONUCLEOSIS. Symptoms usually appear between five and 20 days after exposure. Children are not infectious to each other.

However, in children with impaired immune systems, the infection can be quite severe, involving multiple organs in the body.

Most serious of all is infection during pregnancy. While 90 percent of such infected babies are born without disease, 7 percent have minor abnormalities and 3 percent have severe damage. The highest risk occurs if the mother is infected during the first six months of pregnancy. Infant abnormalities include eye problems, water on the brain, microcephaly, low levels of iron in the blood, jaundice, vomiting, fever, convulsions, or mental retardation. In a newborn the parasite continues to divide, but symptoms may not appear for several years. Postnatal disease may include fever, headache, facial pain, and lymph node swellings. Severe disease includes heart problems (myocarditis), meningoencephalitis, and PNEUMONIA.

Diagnosis

Blood tests can reveal the disease; antibodies will remain for life. If a pregnant women thinks she may have been exposed or her symptoms resemble the disease, blood tests can detect antibodies; some women with an infection during early pregnancy may choose to end the pregnancy. Unfortunately, there is no test that can show whether or not the fetus has been infected by the disease.

Tests taken of newborns can detect those who may have been infected while in the womb; those babies with possible infection can be treated with antibiotics for one year, which can reduce the risk that the baby will have permanent damage. At present, however, this filter paper blood specimen test is not done routinely in all states.

Complications

Complications of infection during pregnancy in the first trimester can include miscarriage, premature birth, and poor growth in the womb. Infants who appear normal at birth may develop eye problems or mental retardation by age 20.

Children with impaired immune systems (such as in AIDS) are at risk for complications, including pneumonia, heart infection, and death. These patients often suffer with infection in the brain, especially if dormant organisms that have remained in muscle tissue for years reactivate. (This does not happen to people with healthy immune systems.)

Treatment

Severe cases are treated with sulfonamides and pyrimethamine. Healthy children do not need treatment. Pregnant women cannot take pyrimethamine, which can damage the fetus. Pregnant women with suspected or proven toxoplasmosis need counseling to understand the risks and options, since no safe and effective drug exists that can be used during pregnancy.

In Europe the drug spiramycin is used in these cases, where it has proven to decrease (but not eliminate) the risk of infection to the fetus. This drug is not approved for use in the United States but it is available here for physicians only as an investigational drug requiring special permission to be dispensed. It is available to an individual researcher for the treatment of pregnant women with toxoplasmosis.

Prevention

Pregnant women and those with impaired immune systems should avoid eating raw or undercooked meat. Pregnant women should not touch or even clean cat litter. Cat boxes should be cleaned daily before the feces dry; the eggs are infectious for the first 24 to 48 hours. Hands should be washed after handling cats (especially before eating). Indoor cats should be kept indoors, away from infected mice. Stray cats should not be allowed in the house; raw meat should not be fed to cats. At-risk individuals should not work in gardens accessible to cats.

traumatic brain injury The common general term for brain injuries that impair thinking as a result of physical trauma severe enough to cause loss of consciousness or damage to the brain structure. Each year, about two million Americans sustain a brain injury—about one every 15 seconds. More than a million of these are sustained by children, 30,000 of whom will have permanent disabilities.

Boys are twice as likely to be injured as girls, especially between the ages of 14 and 24, followed by infants, and then the elderly. Children are more likely to incur traumatic bran injury during the spring and summer. Traffic accidents account for almost half of the injuries; about 34 percent occur at home and the rest in recreation areas.

Traumatic brain injury includes both open and closed head injury, both of which can cause severe learning problems. In an open head injury, the force of impact can cause scalp injuries and skull fractures, together with blood clots and bruising. This type of injury usually affects one place in the brain, producing specific problems.

A closed head injury can cause more widespread damage as the force of impact causes the brain to smash against the opposite side of the skull, tearing nerve fibers and blood vessels. This type of injury may affect the brain stem, causing physical, intellectual, emotional, and social problems. The entire personality of the person may be forever changed.

In young children, abuse is the primary cause of this type of injury; 64 percent of babies under age one who are physically abused have brain injuries, usually caused by shaking. In children under age five, half are related to falls. Cars and biking accidents and suicide attempts are the primary causes of traumatic brain injury in school-age children and adolescents.

Some children may experience coma after a brain injury; the degree of the coma severity is measured by the Glasgow Coma Score, which assigns a number to the degree to which patients can open their eyes, move, or speak. X rays and brain scans may help if a skull fracture is suspected.

Symptoms

The signs following a traumatic brain injury may be elusive, but it is important to understand that head injuries tend to get worse over time. Obvious warning signs include:

- lethargy
- confusion
- irritability
- severe headaches
- changes in speech, vision, or movement
- bleeding
- vomiting
- seizure
- coma

More subtle signs of head injury may also appear, over time, and may include:

- long- and short-term memory problems
- slowed thinking
- distorted perception
- concentration problems
- attention deficits
- communication problems (oral or written)
- poor planning and sequencing
- poor judgment
- changes in mood or personality

Sometimes, certain behavior may appear long after the traumatic brain injury occurs. These behaviors may include overeating or drinking, excessive talking, restlessness, disorientation, or seizure disorders.

Treatment

Rehabilitation should begin as soon as possible after the accident, focusing on the problem areas. Treatment may include physical or occupational therapy, or speech and language therapy.

Prevention

Traumatic brain injury can be prevented by taking appropriate safety precautions, such as insisting that children wear helmets when biking, riding a scooter, or skating, sledding, and skiing. Children should wear seat belts and ride in the back of the car. (See also SCOOTER SAFETY.)

traveler's diarrhea A type of diarrhea that results from eating or drinking water contaminated with feces while traveling in other countries. Up to half of all Americans who visit the tropics pick up traveler's diarrhea (or "Montezuma's revenge") or, in Spanish-speaking countries, "turista." Areas of high risk include the developing countries of Africa, the Middle East, and Latin America.

Traveler's diarrhea is more common in younger people. The risk of infection varies depending on where the child eats, from a low risk (in private homes) to high risk (food from street vendors).

Cause

Most traveler's diarrhea is caused by a special strain of the common intestinal bacteria ESCHERICHIA COLI. Other bacteria responsible for SALMONELLA POISONING and SHIGELLOSIS can also cause diarrhea, as can the parasitic conditions of GIARDIASIS and amebiasis.

Symptoms

Diarrhea, nausea, bloating, urgency, and malaise that usually lasts from between three to seven days. Even if traveler's diarrhea is not treated, it will go away by itself in most cases. Diarrhea that lasts more than four days or is accompanied by severe cramps, bloody stools, dehydration, or foul-smelling gas should be reported to a physician.

Treatment

Drink plenty of fluids to replace water; add oral rehydration packets to fluids to replace lost minerals. Several prescription and over-the-counter drugs will relieve symptoms or kill bacteria. One of the best treatments for early diarrhea is the antibiotic combination trimethoprim/sulfamethoxazole (Bactrim), which is 90 percent effective against the organisms that cause traveler's diarrhea. Bactrim can usually shorten the illness and ease the symptoms.

The most widely used antidiarrheal medication is the over-the-counter drug Pepto-Bismol (bismuth subsalicylate), which treats the symptoms instead of killing the bacteria. Pepto-Bismol appears to be effective in preventing traveler's diarrhea (two ounces four times a day, or two tablets four times a day), but this is not recommended for more than three weeks at a time. Side effects of this preventive treatment include temporary blackening of the tongue and stools, occasional nausea and constipation, and rarely, ringing in the ears. Pepto-Bismol should be avoided by those allergic to aspirin or who have kidney problems, seizures, or gout. Parents should discuss this preventive treatment with a doctor before giving it to children or teens.

Scientists at West Virginia University have discovered that wine is capable of killing bacteria that cause diarrhea much faster than did Pepto-Bismol, tap water, tequila, or pure alcohol. In the case of salmonella, for example, the wines destroyed about 10 million bacteria in just 20 minutes; it took the Pepto-Bismol two hours to reach the same effect.

Prevention

Since most diarrhea-causing organisms are water-borne, they can be passed on in untreated water or on food handled by people who have not properly washed their hands. Before leaving for a trip, a physician can provide a prescription to take along for antidiarrheal medicine. In order to prevent this type of diarrhea while traveling, children and their parents should avoid:

- drinking tap water or using it to brush teeth (even in good hotels)
- ice in sodas or alcoholic drinks
- mixing alcohol with water
- milk or dairy products unless they have been pasteurized

Instead, travelers should:

- boil water for tooth brushing for five minutes, or add water purification tablets
- avoid bottled water unless it is carbonated (the carbonation process inhibits bacterial growth)
- drink carbonated beverages, beer, wine, coffee, or tea
- wipe off bottle or can tops before drinking
- not eat raw vegetables, fruits, meat, or seafood
- avoid cold buffets left in the sun for several hours

- avoid garden or potato salads or food from street vendors
- eat only hot cooked meals, fruit with peels, and packaged foods

trichinellosis   See TRICHINOSIS.

trichinosis   A food-borne disease caused by the microscopic intestinal roundworm *Trichinella spiralis.* Any child who eats undercooked meat of infected animals can develop trichinosis; pork products are most often responsible, although cases have appeared after eating infected bear and walrus. The parasite may be found in a wide variety of animals, including pigs, dogs, cats, rats, and many wild animals (such as fox, wolf, and polar bear).

The disease is found only among those who eat pork, primarily in North America and Europe. Up to 5 percent of Americans have had an infestation, usually without symptoms. It is almost never a problem in countries such as France, where pigs eat root vegetables, not garbage.

Cause

Worm larvae exist as cysts in the muscles of infested animals. Within four to six weeks after a child eats undercooked or raw meat of an infested animal, the larvae are released from the cysts and develop into adults in the child's intestines. The adult worms produce fresh larvae, which travel in the blood to tissues and organs including the heart, tongue, eye, and brain, and to the muscles, where they form cysts. The disease does not spread by person to person contact, but infected animals are infectious for months and the meat from these infected animals remains infectious unless properly cooked.

Symptoms

The incubation period varies depending on the number of parasites in the meat and how much was eaten. Infestation with only a few worms causes no symptoms, whereas a heavy infestation may cause diarrhea and vomiting, PNEUMONIA, heart failure, or respiratory failure.

Usually within 10 to 14 days after infection, symptoms of fever, muscle aches, pain, and swelling around the eyes will begin. Thirst, profuse sweating, chills, weakness, and tiredness may develop. If the parasite becomes imbedded in the diaphragm (thin muscle separating lungs from abdominal organs), chest pain may result. When the larvae attach to the lining of the intestines, the intestines become inflamed, causing abdominal pain, diarrhea, and weakness. As the larvae begin to increase in length and form cysts in the muscles, muscle soreness and pain in muscle fibers will begin. Very rarely, a child becomes seriously ill and dies. Those who survive severe infection maintain a partial immunity.

Diagnosis

A physician may suspect trichinosis from the symptoms; it is confirmed by blood tests which detect antibodies to the larvae, or by a muscle biopsy which reveals the larvae themselves.

Complications

Warning signs include breathing problems, swelling, or shortness of breath. Heart failure may be fatal either in the first two weeks after infection, or between the fourth and eighth week.

Treatment

Painkillers and thiabendazole and corticosteroids may relieve symptoms. Bed rest is recommended to prevent relapse and possible death. After two or three months, the organisms cause no more symptoms. Once the larvae migrate to muscle, mebendazole is the treatment of choice.

Prevention

The best way to prevent the disease is to ensure pork products or wild game are properly cooked to at least 150°F for 35 minutes per pound. Freezing infected meat no higher than −13°F for 10 days will destroy the parasite. Pork or pork products should never be eaten raw, and even smoked or salted meat may still harbor organisms. Pork should not be ground in the same grinder as other meats; the grinder should then be cleaned well after grinding pork. Routine inspection of carcasses for trichinella organisms is not performed in the United States because the disease is on the decline. Irradiation of pork carcasses can also eradicate the larvae.

trichotillomania The habit of pulling out the hair, often associated with mental illness or psychotic illness (such as SCHIZOPHRENIA). Hair-pulling may also take place among disturbed children who are anxious and frustrated. Typically, the patient will pull, twist, or break off chunks of hair, leaving bald spots; children sometimes eat the removed hair, which may cause a hairball in the stomach. Adults may sometimes pull out their pubic hair. The condition is treated with psychotherapy and/or antipsychotic drugs.

triple X syndrome A rare chromosomal abnormality that affects only girls, in which the child will have three X chromosomes instead of two. Normally, everyone has 46 chromosomes; two of these 46 chromosomes are sex chromosomes and define whether a person is a boy or girl. Girls typically have two X chromosomes, and boys have one X chromosome and one Y chromosome.

Triple X syndrome is also called triplo-X, trisomy X, XXX syndrome, and 47 XXX.

Diagnosis

Triple X may be found during prenatal genetic testing, such as amniocentesis, or it may be identified later as part of an evaluation of developmental delay in a child.

Symptoms

Some girls with triple X have no symptoms, but the type of symptoms a girl has may vary a great deal from one patient to the next. Symptoms may include:

- tall stature
- delayed development of certain motor skills and speech and language
- LEARNING DISABILITY such as DYSLEXIA
- delayed puberty
- infertility
- small head
- vertical skin folds that may cover the inner corners of the eyes
- mental retardation (rarely)

Treatment

There is no specific treatment for this condition. The parents of a daughter with triple X syndrome may be referred to a pediatric geneticist for counseling. Other specialists that may help treat the child may include a pediatric endocrinologist for puberty delays, a child psychologist for delays in mental development, and a speech pathologist for a speech delays.

trisomy 21 See DOWN SYNDROME.

tuberculin test A skin test used to determine whether or not a child has been infected with TUBERCULOSIS (TB); the test is used to diagnose suspected cases of tuberculosis, prior to vaccination against the disease.

During the test, the skin is first disinfected and a small dose of tuberculin (a protein extract of the tuberculosis bacilli) is introduced into the skin in one of a variety of ways. In the Mantoux test the extract is injected into the skin with a needle; in the Sterneedle test the extract is dropped on the forearm as a spring-loaded instrument circled with a sharp prong forces the tuberculin into the skin.

After 48 to 72 hours, the skin is inspected at the site; if the skin is unchanged, the reaction is negative, indicating the person has never been exposed to tuberculosis and has no immunity. Skin that becomes red, hard, and raised after the injection indicates that the person has been exposed to tuberculosis, either through vaccination or infection.

tuberculosis (TB) A serious respiratory disease spread from person to person through the air. Children usually contract tuberculosis (TB) from close contact with a diseased adult. Because infants and young children do not have very strong immune systems, they are susceptible to TB, as are those with impaired immune systems.

Once known as "consumption," "scrofula," or "wasting," this disease is less common today in the United States, but it infects half of the rest of the world's people. TB usually affects the lungs, although it can also affect other parts of the body (such as the brain, kidneys, or spine). It was once the leading cause of death in the United States.

Children with TB infection but not the disease have the bacteria that causes the infection within their bodies, but the germs are inactive. They cannot spread the bacteria to others, but they may develop TB later on. Because of this, they are often treated to prevent them from developing the disease.

In 1993 the World Health Organization (WHO) declared a "global TB emergency" because of the massive TB epidemic that was spreading around the world. In its 1996 report on TB, the WHO concluded that worldwide, the disease is the leading killer of women and the leading killer of HIV-positive patients. (Among those with HIV, one in 10 per year will develop active TB.) TB kills more adults than all other infectious diseases combined and leaves more orphaned children than any other infectious disease. In 1995 more people died of TB than in any other year in history. If current trends continue, at least 30 million people will die from TB in the next 10 years. For every person who died in 1995 of the Ebola virus, more than 12,000 people died of TB.

About eight million new cases of TB occur each year; the number of cases reported in the United States has increased each year since 1985. In 1993 there were 215,313 cases reported in this country. Between 10 to 15 million Americans are infected with the TB germ; these people may develop TB sometime in the future. In industrialized countries the steady drop in TB began to level off in the mid-1980s and then began to increase. This may be due in part to immigration from countries with a high rate of TB.

Treatment

Of most concern is the fact that cases of TB resistant to more than one drug have been reported in 17 states in the United States since 1989. Because of this, it is essential to treat TB patients with a recommended four-drug regimen of isoniazid, rifampin, pyrazinamide, and ethambutol, or streptomycin, since it is less likely that bacteria can become quickly resistant to multiple drugs at the same time.

Cause

TB is caused by three species of mycobacteria: *Mycobacterium tuberculosis, M. bovis,* and *M. africanuum.* Once inhaled, the bacteria settle in the lungs and grow; from here, they can travel through the blood to other parts of the body (such as the kidney, spine, or brain). TB in the lungs or throat is mildly infectious, but the bacteria in other parts of the body are not usually contagious.

TB bacteria are sprayed into the air when a child with the disease of the lungs or throat coughs or sneezes. People with active TB are most likely to spread it to those they spend time with every day (such as family members or coworkers). Infectiousness is directly related to the number of bacilli expelled into the air. Patients are more likely to be infectious if they have TB in the lungs or larynx, have a cavity in the lung, and cough a lot. Infectiousness is also related to not covering the mouth when coughing and not receiving adequate treatment.

While TB is infectious, it is not highly infectious and is not nearly as contagious as MEASLES or WHOOPING COUGH. Letting fresh air blow through a room will eradicate most of the infectious germs exhaled by a sick patient every day. The bacteria are also sensitive to ultraviolet rays, which means that infection rarely occurs outside in daylight. Indeed, only half of the people who live with an infected patient will contract the disease themselves.

People with TB are most likely to transmit the disease before it has been diagnosed and treated, and at least 12 weeks must pass before a person who has been exposed to the disease will test positive. Infectiousness seems to decrease quickly once treatment begins; those who have been treated for two to three weeks, whose symptoms have improved, and who have three consecutive negative sputum tests can be considered "noninfectious."

Most people who breathe in the bacteria and become infected are able to fight off the disease; the bacteria become inactive, but they remain alive in the body and can become active later. This is called TB *infection*. People with TB infection have no symptoms, do not feel sick, and cannot spread the disease. However, they usually have a positive skin test for TB and they can develop the disease later in life if they do not receive preventive treatment. Many people who have the infection never develop the disease, however. In these people, the bacteria remain inactive for a lifetime.

Symptoms

The illness does not cause symptoms at first. TB growing in the lungs may cause a bad cough that lasts longer than two weeks and pain in the chest. The patient may cough up blood or phlegm from the lungs. Other symptoms include fatigue or weakness, weight loss, appetite loss, chills, and fever.

Diagnosis

A tuberculin skin test determines if a person has the TB organism, but it cannot identify those with active disease. For this skin test, a small amount of fluid (tuberculin) is injected under the skin in the lower part of the arm. Two or three days later a health-care worker looks for a reaction on the arm.

A positive reaction usually means that the person has been infected with the TB germ, but not necessarily that they have an active infection. Other tests (chest X ray and sample of phlegm) are necessary to identify active disease.

People should be tested for TB if they have spent time with someone with infectious TB, have HIV, come from a country where TB is common (most countries in Latin America, the Caribbean, Africa, and Asia except for Japan). Others at high risk are those who inject drugs or who live in the United States where TB is common (homeless shelters, migrant farm camps, prisons, and some nursing homes).

Because it may take several weeks after infection for the immune system to react to the TB skin test, it may be necessary to be retested 10 to 12 weeks after the last exposure to TB. If the reaction to the second test is negative, there is probably no TB infection present.

The skin test is mandatory in some states and countries for immigrants and students from Africa, Asia, and Latin America, as well as for personnel in schools, hospitals, prisons, food handlers, group homes, child-care centers, and substance abuse centers. At the moment, screening of children entering kindergarten or day-care centers is not required in all school districts, but the government recommends that school children be tested for TB to ensure that all U.S. citizens are tested at least once in their lives.

A new test can now diagnose TB in a clinical lab much more quickly than in the past. The new test can confirm a TB diagnosis in just six hours, as opposed to the current two to six weeks required to confirm TB bacteria in culture. This new test is under consideration for approval by the U.S. Food and Drug Administration. The new test appears to have a low rate of false positives, which has been a problem with other tests in the past.

Treatment

Up to the 1700s it was thought that the touch of a king or queen would cure TB; today, scientists know that TB is cured by taking several drugs for up to nine months. If patients stop taking the drugs too soon, or if they do not take the drugs correctly, the TB organisms may become resistant. TB that is resistant to drugs is harder to treat.

Within a month after treatment begins, the patient should feel well, regain weight, and have no fever. Coughing should have slowed down, and there should be improvements on X ray. If the disease was severe, however, complete end of treatment may not occur for a year.

If there is no improvement within three months, a change in therapy may be needed. Relapses usually occur within six months after treatment ends and are usually due to patients who do not follow correct drug procedures.

When TB becomes active again in a patient who had been treated before, there is a very good chance that these bacteria will be drug-resistant. If the microorganism is resistant to standard drugs, it may be necessary to use more toxic drugs to treat the infection.

Prevention

Some people who have the TB germ but not active disease are more likely than others to develop an active case. These high-risk individuals include those with HIV infection, those who were recently exposed to someone with TB disease, and those with certain medical conditions.

For patients who have TB germs but not the active disease, physicians recommend taking isoniazid for up to 12 months. Infants and children who have spent time with someone who is infected are often given preventive therapy even if their skin test is negative.

There is a vaccine for TB disease that is used in many countries but is not widely used in the United States. Called BCG (Bacillus Calmette-Guérin), this vaccine does not completely prevent people from getting TB. Those who have been vaccinated with BCG can be given a tuberculin skin test; although the vaccine can cause a positive reaction to the test, it is more likely that a positive reaction is caused by TB infection if the reaction is large, the person was vaccinated a long time ago, the person has been around someone with TB disease, or the person is from a country where TB is common.

While there is some question as to how effective the BCG vaccine really is against adults, the World Health Organization recommends its use in newborns in developing countries, because it appears to offer some protection in children.

A relatively new TB vaccine from "naked" DNA might work better with less risk of infection than the current BCG vaccine. The traditional BCG vaccine is made from an altered, weakened form of the disease that infects cows. But in 1996 researchers reported that they had made a new vaccine out of a gene taken from the human version of TB. The use of use one gene (known as "naked DNA") instead of the many genes contained in TB DNA, appears to be as effective as the earlier cow vaccine. However, trials in humans have not yet been done.

Unlike traditional vaccines, which stimulate the human body to produce disease-fighting antibodies, naked DNA vaccines are incorporated by the cells and the immune response begins there. There is also a lower risk of infection with this new vaccine. While this did not occur often with the old vaccine, it did happen in certain rare cases.

Scientists also have recently discovered that it is possible to transmit TB on an airplane. In the spring of 1994, a woman on an eight-and-a-half-hour United Airlines flight from Chicago to Honolulu infected four passengers sitting near her; all tested positive for the disease, but none have yet become ill. A few days later, the woman died from TB. Because this showed transmission is possible on airlines, the Centers for Disease Control and Prevention (CDC) recommended that when airlines learn that a passenger or crew member has traveled with the disease (especially on long flights) they should contact passengers and crew members and inform them. The CDC pointed out that only those passengers sitting near the woman were infected; others sitting farther away breathed air that passed through the plane's filtration system.

tuberous sclerosis (TS)   A disorder that causes benign growths ("tubers") on several different organs within the body, including the brain, eyes, kidneys, heart, skin, and lungs; it occurs in about one in 6,000 births.

Cause

There is a 50 percent chance that a parent with tuberous sclerosis (TS) will have a child with the disease.

Symptoms

The condition is often first recognized in children who experience epileptic seizures or who exhibit developmental delays. The severity of TS varies from mild skin abnormalities to very severe cases that cause MENTAL RETARDATION or kidney failure.

Treatment

Treatment usually includes medication to prevent SEIZURES, treatments to address skin problems, surgery to remove tumors (to reduce the risk of cancer as well as for cosmetic reasons), and the management of high blood pressure caused by kidney disease. As with all of the neurocutaneous syndromes, a child's prognosis depends on the severity of the case.

Tuberous Sclerosis Alliance   A nonprofit organization formerly known as the National Tuberous Sclerosis Foundation, which was founded in 1974 by four mothers to provide fellowship, generate awareness, and provide hope to those who shared the common bond of TUBEROUS SCLEROSIS (TS). The group was reorganized and renamed the Tuberous Sclerosis Alliance in 2000. Today the group serves more than 20,000 constituents, including 11,000 family members and adults personally impacted by TS. The group is currently expanding its research agenda through its Center Without Walls (CWW) research program and offers a range of brochures and books, together with a wide range of events. (For contact information, see Appendix I.)

typhoid fever   A serious bacterial infection of the intestinal tract and sometimes the bloodstream caused by eating food or drinking water contaminated with *Salmonella typhi.* An almost identical disease called PARATYPHOID FEVER is caused by a related bacterium.

Typhoid fever today is an uncommon disease in the United States, but it is still common in Latin America, Africa, and Asia. In 1942 there were 4,000 reported U.S. cases, but since 1964 only about 400 cases have occurred each year, mostly imported from Mexico or India. An estimated 16 million cases of typhoid fever and 600,000 related deaths occur worldwide, and 2.6 cases of typhoid fever were reported to the U.S. Centers for Disease Control and Prevention (CDC) per 1 million U.S. citizens and residents traveling abroad between 1992 through 1994.

Before the advent of antibiotics, 12 percent of victims died. Today fewer than 10 percent of cases are fatal; these occur in malnourished infants and children. About 3 percent of those who recover from a mild illness become chronic carriers. Carriers are infectious for years unless they are treated with antibiotics.

Thomas Willis first described typhoid fever in 1643; typhoid fever was often confused with "typhus" fever until the two were distinguished in 1837, and the name "typhoid" fever—meaning *typhoid-like*—was coined.

Cause

Typhoid fever is caused by the bacterium *Salmonella typhi,* a species of salmonella. While the common salmonella species in the United States live in animals and infect humans via contaminated food (chicken, eggs, etc.), *S. typhi* lives in the intestinal tract of humans. Once ingested, the bacteria lodge in the lower small intestine, where it multiplies and invades the bloodstream.

The disease is contracted from food or water that has been contaminated by the feces of patients or carriers, or from intimate contact with an infected person. It occurs in developing countries from eating shellfish taken from contaminated beds, eating raw fruits, or drinking tainted water supplies. It can also be contracted from food left outdoors accessible to flies. Anyone can get typhoid fever, but today the greatest risk is to children visiting countries where the disease is common.

Children are infectious as long as the bacteria are being shed in feces (usually three to four weeks), but some may remain infectious up to three months. To be considered uninfectious, a child must have stool cultures every week until there are three negative cultures in a row.

The most important modern source of the typhoid bacillus (found throughout the world) is the typhoid carrier; these carriers at times contaminate water, milk, or food and set off typhoid epidemics.

Symptoms

Between eight and 14 days after ingesting bacteria, symptoms of fever, headache, joint pains, sore throat, and constipation begin. There may be appetite loss and abdominal pain. Most children have a mild illness and recover without antibiotics. Untreated, the fever will continue to rise for two or three days, remain high for up to two weeks (103° to 104°F) and then fall. Nosebleed and bronchitis are often present. At the height of the fever, the child appears extremely ill and can be delirious.

Even when symptoms pass, the child may still carry *S. typhi*. Relapses occur in 10 percent of untreated patients and 20 percent of treated patients about two weeks after the fever abates. If the fever returns, antibiotics must be restarted. Some patients notice rose spots on chests and abdomens during the second week. Infection confers some immunity, but not enough to protect a patient if there are large numbers of bacteria ingested a second time.

Diagnosis

The diagnosis is confirmed by obtaining a culture of typhoid bacteria from a sample of blood during the first week; feces and urine tests reveal the bacillus during the second. A blood test reveals the presence of antibodies against typhoid bacteria.

Complications

Children with serious cases can go on to experience frothy, bloody diarrhea in later stages and become apathetic. Typhoid fever can inflame the intestines, and in severe cases intestinal ulcers can perforate, causing severe infections. This can also lead to severe intestinal bleeding, which kills 25 percent of untreated patients.

Treatment

Antibiotics can shorten the disease and reduce chances of complications and death. Otherwise, it can take months to recover. Doctors may prescribe chloramphenicol, ciprofloxacin, ceftriaxone, or cefoperazone. In addition, patients need bed rest and good nutrition. Aspirin, enemas, or laxatives should not be given.

Gloves should be worn when nursing a typhoid patient, and rigorous hand washing is critical. Because the germ is passed in the feces of infected patients, only those with active diarrhea who cannot toilet themselves (infants and some handicapped people) should be isolated.

With early diagnosis and proper treatment, the outlook is usually excellent. Permanent immunity usually follows an attack of typhoid, although relapses are common if the disease is not fully eradicated by thorough antibiotic treatment.

Most infected children may return to school when they have recovered, as long as they wash hands after toilet visits. Children in day care must obtain the approval of the local or state health department before returning to school.

Prevention

Typhoid fever is a reportable disease. Typhoid vaccination is not required for international travel, but it is recommended for travel to high-risk areas, including the Indian subcontinent and other developing countries in Asia, Africa, and Central and South America. Vaccination is particularly recommended for those who will be traveling in smaller cities, villages, and rural areas. However, typhoid vaccination is not completely effective and is not a substitute for careful selection of food and drink.

An oral vaccine (Ty21a) was licensed in 1990 that provides fewer side effects than the older vaccine. This new version provides between 70 and 90 percent protection and is recommended for any child over age six who is traveling off tourist routes (or for a long time) in Latin America, Asia, or Africa.

The oral vaccine includes four capsules taken every other day for seven days. All four must be taken to provide maximum protection. The capsules should be kept refrigerated until they are taken with a cool liquid a half hour before a meal. Antibiotics or the antimalarial drug mefloquine should not be taken at the same time. The entire four-dose series should be repeated every five years for those who need protection. There are few side effects with this drug, although some people notice nausea, vomiting, cramps, and skin rash. The older injected vaccine caused fever, headache, and local pain and swelling in about one-third of patients. This oral vaccine is approved for children over age 6.

The alternative is an injected vaccine called Typhim Vi is available in Canada and the United States and is equally effective with few side effects. It is approved for children over age two and should be taken two weeks before travel to allow immunity to develop.

Further preventive measures for travelers include drinking only pasteurized milk products, boiled or bottled water, or carbonated beverages; eating only cooked food or fruit with that is peeled by the diner; eating shellfish boiled or steamed at least 10 minutes; and controlling flies with screens and sprays.

ulcerative colitis See INFLAMMATORY BOWEL DISEASE.

ulcers See HELICOBACTER PYLORI.

underweight See ANOREXIA NERVOSA; EATING DISORDERS.

upper respiratory infections Any infection of the upper respiratory system, which can include the common COLD, LARYNGITIS, SORE THROAT, SINUSITIS, or TONSILLITIS.

urethritis Inflammation of the urethra usually caused by one of a variety of infectious organisms, the best known of which is the bacteria that causes GONORRHEA.

Cause

Nonspecific urethritis may be caused by one of a number of different types of microorganisms, including bacteria, yeasts, or chlamydia. Bacteria may spread to the urethra from the skin or rectum.

Symptoms

A burning sensation and pain when urinating that can be severe are the symptoms of urethritis. The urine may be stained with blood; if gonorrhea is the underlying cause, there may be yellow pus-filled discharge. The infection may be followed by scarring that narrows the urethra, which can make urinating more difficult.

Treatment

Treating the underlying infection will cure the urethritis. Gonorrhea is usually cured by penicillin or another antibiotic. Treatment of nonspecific urethritis depends on what organism is causing the infection. If the urethra is scarred, a physician may try to stretch and widen the tube while the patient is under anesthesia.

urinary tract infection (UTI) An infection that occurs when microorganisms (usually bacteria from the digestive tract) cling to the opening of the urethra and begin to multiply.

Cause

Most infections are caused by one type of bacteria (*Escherichia coli*) that normally live in the colon. In most cases, bacteria first begin growing in the urethra and then move on to the bladder, causing a bladder infection (cystitis). If the infection is not treated right away, bacteria may move up the ureters to infect the kidneys.

Chlamydia and mycoplasma also may cause UTIs, but these infections tend to remain limited to the urethra and reproductive system. Unlike *E. coli*, chlamydia and mycoplasma may be sexually transmitted, and infection requires treatment of both partners.

Any abnormality of the urinary tract that obstructs the flow of urine sets the stage for an infection. Catheters are a common source of infection (bacteria on the catheter can infect the bladder, so hospital staff must take special care to keep the catheter sterile and to remove it as soon as possible). Children with diabetes have a higher risk of getting UTIs because of changes in the immune system—in fact, any disorder that suppresses the immune system raises the risk of a UTI.

UTIs are more common in girls and women because their urethra is relatively short, allowing bacteria quicker access to the bladder. Further, a woman's urethral opening is located near sources of bacteria from the anus and vagina. Some girls and women suffer from frequent UTIs; nearly 20 percent who have one UTI will have another, and 30 percent of those will have yet another.

Symptoms

Symptoms of a urinary tract infection include:

- frequent urge to urinate
- painful, burning feeling in the area of the bladder or urethra during urination
- fatigue
- weakness
- uncomfortable pressure above the pubic bone
- little urine passed despite constant urge to urinate
- milky, cloudy, or reddish tint to urine

If the infection reaches the kidneys, symptoms may include:

- fever
- pain in the back or side below the ribs
- nausea
- vomiting

Diagnosis

To diagnose a UTI, a doctor will test a urine sample for pus and bacteria. Although the doctor may begin treatment before the lab report comes back, the lab cultures will confirm the diagnosis and may mean a change in antibiotic. If treatment fails to clear up an infection, the doctor may order a test that makes an image of the urinary tract to identify whether there are structural problems contributing to the infection or interfering with treatment.

Prevention

To help avoid UTIs, some doctors suggest drinking cranberry juice, which in large amounts inhibits the growth of some bacteria by acidifying the urine. Vitamin C (ascorbic acid) supplements also acidify the urine. Drink plenty of water every day. It is important to encourage children to urinate when they feel the need. Girls should be taught to wipe from front to back after toileting to prevent bacteria from the anal area from entering the vagina or urethra. Girls should avoid using feminine hygiene sprays and scented douches, which may irritate the urethra.

urticaria pigmentosa An uncommon rash that usually affects the neck, arms, legs, and trunk of children and young adults. The rash consists of reddish-brown spots that turn into hives when they are rubbed hard or scratched. Sometimes the spots will blister.

Cause

The spots in urticaria pigmentosa contain a large number of mast cells (infection-fighting cells that live in the skin). Mast cells make a substance called histamine, which causes hives, itching, and flushing. Experts do not know why people with urticaria pigmentosa have abnormal collections of mast cells in the skin.

Most children who develop urticaria pigmentosa before the age of five will grow out of the condition by adolescence or early adulthood. When urticaria pigmentosa starts after the age of five, the abnormal collections of mast cells will sometimes involve the internal organs and the disease does not always go away. These patients need blood tests and other studies.

Treatment

There is no satisfactory treatment for urticaria pigmentosa, although antihistamines such as Benadryl can help control itching, hives, and flushing. Patients should avoid aspirin, codeine, opiates, procaine, alcohol, polymyxin B, hot baths, and vigorous rubbing after bathing and showering, since these can release histamine, which can cause itching, flushing, and hives.

vaccination See IMMUNIZATION.

Vaccine Adverse Events Reporting System (VAERS)
A cooperative reporting program for vaccine safety that tracks any unusual event that occurs after a vaccination was given. Vaccine Adverse Events Reporting System (VAERS) is a post-marketing safety surveillance program, collecting information about side effects that occur after the administration of U.S. licensed vaccines. Reports to the VAERS program are welcome from all patients, parents, health-care providers, pharmacists, and vaccine manufacturers. The Center for Biologics Evaluation and Research and the Centers for Disease Control and Prevention (CDC) jointly manage the Vaccine Adverse Event Reporting System.

In order to collect all information that may be of value, there is no restriction on the time lapse between the vaccination and the start of the event, or between the event and the time the report is made. The toll-free VAERS information line is (800) 822-7967. Consumers are encouraged to get help from their family doctors in reporting the event.

In addition to any reports by consumers, the NATIONAL CHILDHOOD VACCINE INJURY ACT OF 1986 requires health-care providers to report specific adverse events after the administration of those vaccines outlined in the Act.

vaginal infections Any infection of the vagina caused by bacteria or yeast. Together with a physical exam and history, lab tests are needed to examine vaginal fluid microscopically. Some vaginal infections cause VAGINITIS, an inflammation of the vagina that may include discharge, irritation, and itching. Some of the most common vaginal infections are bacterial vaginosis, trichomoniasis, and vaginal yeast infection. A girl may contract a vaginal infection by improper toileting habits.

vaginal warts See WARTS.

vaginitis Any mild infection or inflammation of the vagina, which also may be called bacterial vaginosis or nonspecific vaginitis.

Cause
The bacterium *Gardnerella vaginalis* has been associated with vaginosis, although recent studies suggest a mixture of bacteria may be associated with the illness. Most of these bacteria are normally found in the vagina, but in vaginitis the numbers are much higher than normal.

It is not clear how girls get vaginitis, although those teens who are sexually active and those who have more than one partner have higher rates of disease and more infections than older women. While vaginitis may be related to sexual activity, it cannot be passed directly from one person to another.

Symptoms
Gray or frothy vaginal discharge with a foul or fish-smelling odor is the hallmark of this disorder. It rarely causes itch, burning, or irritation.

Diagnosis
Inspection of the vaginal discharge can diagnose the disease.

Treatment
Vaginitis is easily treated with the antibiotic metronidazole (Flagyl), which is also used to treat trichomoniasis. Sexual intercourse and douching are not recommended during treatment. Patients

should bathe or shower daily with plain soap and water; bubble baths and bath salts or oils should be avoided until the infection clears.

vaginosis   See VAGINITIS.

valacyclovir (Valtrex)   A new antiviral drug used to treat herpes infections. Easily absorbed and converted in the body to ACYCLOVIR, it is available for use by the body in concentrations three to five times greater than that of acyclovir. In the body the drug interferes with viral reproduction. Several large studies have shown that it is safe and well tolerated.

In SHINGLES, Valtrex reduces the fever and lesions and shortens the duration of the infection. It is able to shorten the pain that occurs after shingles. Although valacyclovir will not cure shingles or genital HERPES, it does help relieve the pain and discomfort and helps the sores heal faster. Valacyclovir works best if it is used within 48 hours after the first symptoms of shingles or genital herpes (for example, pain, burning, or blisters) begin to appear. For recurrent outbreaks of genital herpes, valacyclovir works best if it is used within 24 hours after the symptoms begin to appear.

Side Effects
Valacyclovir can cause nausea and headache and may be involved in kidney damage. Because of the potential kidney problems, children with existing kidney damage should be careful using valacyclovir.

vancomycin-resistant enterococci (VRE)   Bacteria infecting children in hospital intensive-care units that resist vancomycin, the most powerful antibiotic available. Vancomycin-resistant enterococci (VRE) infection represents an increasing public health concern.

Enterococci normally live in the stomach and intestines and on the skin; generally they do not cause disease, but they can cause infections (especially in children weakened by another illness). What makes these particular bacteria so dangerous is that many strains are able to resist antibiotics, including penicillins, cephalosporins, and aminoglycosides. As a result, for many years doctors relied on vancomycin to treat serious enterococcal infections.

In the late 1980s, however, strains of enterococci began to appear that resisted even this drug of last resort. They now cause 10 percent of all hospital-acquired infections. VRE were first documented in Europe in the 1980s and are now emerging as a new threat to patients in the United States.

In 1993 infection with enterococci bacteria occurred in about three or four cases per 10,000; of these, about 14 percent were resistant to vancomycin. As many as 73 percent of patients who contract VRE die.

Recent information suggests that in the United States, VRE are most commonly found in teaching hospitals and hospitals with more than 500 beds. Reports also suggest that it is rare for a patient who has not been in a hospital to have VRE. However, in Europe VRE can be found in waste waters and in the feces of both nonhospitalized patients and healthy volunteers.

In one recent study reported in the British medical journal *Lancet,* researchers found that of 38 patients admitted to intensive care, nine brought the infection with them, 12 became infected on the unit, and one person who had one strain of the bacteria on admission developed a second different variety while hospitalized. Of these 13, 11 were infected by a strain that had spread from another patient.

There is no proven treatment for VRE; the infection is transmitted by hand contamination. Chlorhexidine (but not regular soap) kills the bacteria.

Because VRE can live on telephones, walls, and patient charts, hospitals are trying to improve housekeeping and make sure all health-care workers wash their hands often. Moreover, doctors should not prescribe antibiotics for viral illnesses (such as colds) or in low doses or for just a few days. Weak prescriptions simply slow down the germs and help create superbugs.

vaporizer   See HUMIDIFIERS.

varicella   See CHICKEN POX.

varicella vaccine   Vaccine against CHICKEN POX that is recommended at any visit at or after age 12 months for any child who has never had the disease. Susceptible people aged older than 13 years should receive two doses, given at least four weeks apart. The vaccine is prepared from weakened, live varicella-zoster virus. See also IMMUNIZATION.

varicella-zoster virus A member of the family of herpes viruses, which causes the diseases varicella (CHICKEN POX) and herpes zoster (SHINGLES). When the virus enters the upper respiratory tract of a nonimmune host, it produces the skin lesions of chicken pox. The virus then passes from skin to sensory ganglia, where it establishes a latent infection. When the patient's immunity to HSV fades away, the virus replicates within the ganglia and results in shingles (herpes zoster).

The virus is highly contagious and may be spread by direct contact or droplets. However, dried crusts of the skin lesions do not contain the virus.

variola Another name for SMALLPOX.

vegetarian diets With careful attention to nutrition, dietary experts agree that a vegetarian diet can be a healthy lifestyle choice for teenagers, as long as the diet includes a variety of food that supplies enough calories and nutrients for normal body growth and function.

Typical types of vegetarian diets include vegan, lacto-vegetarian, and lacto-ovo-vegetarian, depending on whether the teenager prefers to avoid all or only some animal products. A strict vegan diet includes vegetables, fruits, grains, legumes (beans and peas), seeds, and nuts, but no animal products of any type—no meat, no eggs, no dairy products. A lacto-vegetarian diet is identical to a vegan diet, except it also includes dairy foods. A lacto-ovo-vegetarian diet is the same as a vegan diet, except it includes dairy foods and eggs.

Some teens consider themselves vegetarian, but they are technically semi-vegetarians because they also eat fish and chicken.

Teens who are interested in following a vegetarian diet should be careful to eat a balanced diet, making sure to get enough calories, protein, and iron.

Calories

Fruits, vegetables, and grains are relatively high in fiber and low in calories and fat compared with meat, eggs, and dairy products. Teens should make sure to get enough calories, including at least 20 percent from fat.

Protein

Protein supplies amino acids necessary for the growth, repair, and maintenance of body tissues. Teens will get sufficient amino acids by eating a variety of grains, legumes, seeds, nuts, and vegetables. One of the best sources is soy, which is considered to be nutritionally equivalent to the protein found in meat.

Iron

Foods high in iron include dried beans, tofu, green leafy vegetables, whole grains, iron-fortified cereals, and breads. Absorption of iron is improved by eating iron-rich foods along with foods high in vitamin C.

Calcium

Dairy products are high in calcium. Teens who want to avoid eating dairy products can get calcium in calcium-fortified orange juice, green leafy vegetables, tofu, calcium-enriched soymilk, and sardines.

Vitamin B_{12}

This important vitamin is found only in animal foods, including eggs and dairy products. Vegans can get the vitamin B_{12} they need in foods fortified with vitamin B_{12}, such as soymilk or cereal. Teens also should take a multivitamin that includes vitamin B_{12}.

Vitamin D

Vitamin D is added to milk and most soy beverages. The body also makes vitamin D when the sun shines on the skin.

Zinc

The body needs this mineral to fight infections and keep the skin healthy. Good vegetarian sources include whole-grain cereals, nuts, and legumes.

venereal disease See SEXUALLY TRANSMITTED DISEASES.

venereal warts See WARTS, GENITAL.

viral infections One of the most important types of infectious diseases, caused by viruses—the smallest known kind of infectious agent. Much smaller than the smallest bacteria, viruses also have a much simpler structure and method of multiplication. Scientists still debate whether viruses are really living organisms, or just collections of large molecules capable of self-replication under favorable conditions. Viruses take over cells of other organisms, where they make copies of themselves. Outside living cells, viruses are inert and not capable of metabolism, or other activities typically found in living organisms.

Experts believe that there are more viruses than any other types of organism, and they parasitize recognized life forms (even bacteria). More than 200 types of viruses have been identified that cause human disease, including the adenovirus, arenavirus, coronavirus, enterovirus, herpesvirus, poxvirus, picornavirus, rhinovirus, and retrovirus.

Viral infections may be mild (such as the common COLD or WARTS), or they can be extremely serious, such as RABIES, AIDS, SMALLPOX, POLIO, and probably some types of cancer.

There are no specific cures for viral diseases, although some of the newest antiviral drugs can treat symptoms and lessen the seriousness of viral infections. However, it is possible to prevent some of the viral diseases through vaccination, including smallpox, MEASLES, and polio.

visual perception disabilities Students with visual perception disabilities have trouble making sense out of what they see, not because they have poor eyesight but because their brains process visual information differently.

Children with this problem have trouble organizing, recognizing, interpreting, or remembering visual images. This means that they will have trouble understanding the written and picture symbols they need in school—letters, words, numbers, math symbols, diagrams, maps, charts, and graphs.

Because this type of visual problem is subtle, it is not often caught until the child starts having trouble in school. Visual perception skills include the ability to recognize images we have seen before and attach meaning to them, to discriminate among similar images or the words, and to separate signif-

icant figures from background details, and to recognize the same symbol in different forms. For example, children should understand that the letter D is the letter D whether it is upper or lower case, in different colors or fonts. Sequences are another important visual perception skill; a child with a visual sequencing problem may not understand the difference between the words *saw* and *was*.

Students with visual perception problems are usually slow to learn letters and numbers and often make mistakes, omissions, and reversals. They often have trouble with visual memory and visualization and may be extremely slow readers.

vitamins A proper balance of vitamins is vital to healthy childhood development. While most doctors believe that a vitamin supplement is not critical for children who eat a variety of foods, a multivitamin may be appropriate for a very picky child.

Vitamin A
This vitamin is necessary for healthy skin, and is contained in many foods. Especially good sources include liver, fish-liver oils, egg yolk, milk and other diary products, margarine and a wide range of fruits and vegetables.

Deficiency of this vitamin is rare in the United States; a serious lack or too much vitamin A can both cause dry, rough skin, among other problems. Contrary to popular belief, getting too much carotene by eating huge amounts of carrots does not cause excess levels of vitamin A; however, it can produce carotenemia (high blood levels of carotene), which colors the skin deep yellow.

Synthetic vitamin A-like compounds called "retinoids" applied directly to the skin have been used to treat skin wrinkling and mottled pigmentation caused by chronic sun exposure.

Vitamin B$_2$ (Riboflavin)
While a balanced diet usually provides adequate amounts of riboflavin, some children are susceptible to a deficiency, which may cause chapped lips and sore tongue and mouth corners. Children taking phenothiazine antipsychotic drugs, tricyclic antidepressants, oral contraceptives, or those with malabsorption disorders may develop a deficiency. It also may result from serious illness or injury, or surgery.

Vitamin B₆ (Pyridoxine)

This vitamin plays a vital role in the activities of various enzymes and hormones involved in keeping skin healthy. Good dietary sources of vitamin B_6 are found in liver, chicken, pork, fish, whole grains, wheat germ, bananas, potatoes, and dried beans. A balanced diet will provide sufficient amounts of this vitamin, which is also produced in small amounts by intestinal bacteria.

Deficiency of this vitamin causes a variety of skin conditions, inflammation of mouth and tongue, and cracked lips. Children at risk for developing a vitamin B_6 deficiency include breast-fed infants, those with poor diets, those with malabsorption disorders, and those taking certain drugs, including penicillamine, hydralazine, or birth control pills.

Vitamin C

Also known by its chemical name, ascorbic acid, this vitamin plays an important role in healing wounds in the skin, boosting the immune system, and preventing scurvy. The primary dietary sources of this vitamin are fresh fruits and vegetables, especially citrus fruits, tomatoes, green leafy vegetables, potatoes, green peppers, strawberries, and cantaloupe.

A balanced diet usually provides enough vitamin C, but slight deficiencies may occur after surgery, fever, constant inhalation of carbon monoxide in tobacco smoke and traffic fumes, serious injury, or use of oral contraceptives.

Vitamin D

A naturally occurring substance produced by the interaction of sunlight with chemicals in the skin that helps the body absorb calcium from the intestinal tract and provide for the healthy development and growth of bones. About 15 minutes outdoors a day meets the body's requirements for the vitamin, although it is also found in many foods. A deficiency of vitamin D, either through a poor diet or lack of sunlight, can lead to rickets; it has been added to milk since the 1930s as a way to reduce the incidence of rickets.

Many foods (especially milk) are fortified with vitamin D, and supplements are also available. However, because sunlight's interaction with the skin provides vitamin D, unless children drink no milk their chance of a vitamin D deficiency is very low.

Other good dietary sources of vitamin D include oily fish, liver, dairy products, and egg yolks.

Vitamin D is considered to be an antioxidant and anticarcinogen and may play a role in skin pigmentation. It can be absorbed by the skin, and thereby applying this vitamin topically can have an effect on the skin's health.

Vitamin D is toxic in very large amounts, however (between 5,000 and 10,000 International Units (IU) daily for several months for D_3 or D_4), and megadoses should be avoided. Sunbathing, however, will not create an overdose.

Vitamin E (Tocopherol)

This vitamin has a long history of use with skin problems, but research has not found it to be effective when used topically as anything other than a moisturizer. Some people rub contents of vitamin-E capsules or creams and lotions on the skin to treat rashes, acne, wounds, or scars. Except for an occasional allergic reaction, this causes no harm, although it is not likely to be effective since vitamin E cannot penetrate the outer skin's layers. Some studies have found that this vitamin can actually irritate the skin of the face, especially when it is used with an acne product that has a peeling effect. When spray-on vitamin E is forced through the layers of the skin, it can lead to severe allergic reactions.

Overdosing on oral vitamin E can block the absorption of other fat-soluble vitamins such as A and D. Vitamin E is an antioxidant, however, which means that it helps prevent free radical damage.

Vitamin E is found naturally in vegetable oils, including wheat germ oil; most people get an adequate supply by eating a typical American diet.

vitiligo A common disease in which the skin loses pigment due to the destruction of pigment cells so that the skin becomes white, especially in areas such as the groin or armpits, around body openings, and on exposed areas like the face or hands. The unpigmented areas are extremely sensitive to ultraviolet radiation and are especially obvious in dark-skinned people. Most children who have vitiligo are in good health and suffer no symptoms other than areas of pigment loss.

Vitiligo may spread to other areas, but there is no way of predicting whether or where it will spread. In many cases, initial pigment loss will occur; then after several months, the number and size of the light areas become stable and may remain so for a long time. Episodes of pigment loss may appear again later on. Many vitiligo patients report that initial or later episodes of pigment loss followed by periods of physical or emotional stress, seem to trigger further depigmentation in those who are predisposed. Sometimes depigmented areas may spontaneously repigment.

About half of the people who develop this skin disorder experience some pigment loss before the age of 20, and about one-third of all vitiligo patients say that other family members also have this condition.

When vitiligo begins and how severe the pigment loss will be differs with each patient, but illness and stress can result in more pigment loss. Light-skinned people usually notice the pigment loss during the summer as the contrast between the vitiliginous skin and the suntanned skin becomes distinct. People with dark skin may observe the onset of vitiligo at any time.

In severe cases, the pigment loss extends over the entire body surface. The degree of pigment loss can also vary within each vitiligo patch, and a border of abnormally dark skin may encircle a patch of depigmented skin.

Vitiligo often starts with a rapid loss of pigment, which may be followed by a lengthy period when the skin color does not change. Later, the pigment loss may resume, especially if the patient has suffered physical trauma or stress. The loss of color may continue until for unknown reasons it suddenly stops. Cycles of pigment loss, followed by periods of stability, may continue indefinitely. However, it is rare for a patient with vitiligo to regain skin color. Most patients who say that they no longer have vitiligo may actually have become totally depigmented and are no longer bothered by contrasting skin color. While such patients appear to be "cured," they really are not. People who have vitiligo all over their bodies do not look like albinos because the color of their hair and eyes may not change.

Cause

Medical researchers are not sure what causes vitiligo. Some researchers think the body may develop an allergy to its pigment cells; others believe that the cells may destroy themselves during the process of pigment production. Melanin is the substance that normally determines the color of skin, hair, and eyes. This pigment is produced in cells called melanocytes. If melanocytes cannot form melanin or if their number decreases, skin color will become lighter or completely white as in vitiligo.

A combination of genetic and immunologic factors is of major importance in most cases. In more than half the cases, there is a family history of vitiligo or early graying of hair. Many patients do not realize that anyone in the family has had vitiligo, either because they do not know that premature gray hair is a sign of vitiligo or because the affected area is hidden by clothing. In many cases of vitiligo, there is no family history of the disorder, and many vitiligo patients do not have either children or grandchildren with symptoms of pigment loss.

Many people report pigment loss shortly after a severe sunburn. Others relate the onset of vitiligo to emotional trauma associated with an accident, death in the family, or divorce. Patients with vitiligo appear to have normal pigment cells. An increase in something such as nitric oxide may be toxic for pigment cells or there may be a lack of growth factors that are required for normal pigment cells to be viable.

Treatment

There is no cure for this disease, but the symptoms can be treated, although treatment may not be completely satisfactory. There are two basic methods: to try to restore the normal pigment (repigment), or to try to destroy the remaining pigment cells (depigment).

The most common method of repigmenting is a combination of a drug called psoralen (applied to the skin or taken orally) and regulated doses of sunlight. Some clinics use psoralen and indoor ultraviolet light treatments. When psoralen drugs are activated by UVA, they stimulate repigmentation by increasing the availability of color-producing cells at the skin's surface. The response varies among patients and body sites. The psoralen treatment is not always successful, but many patients find that it can help restore some degree of pigmentation to areas of the skin. About 75 percent of the patients who undergo psoralen and UVA light therapy respond to some extent, but complete repigmentation rarely occurs.

The psoralen drugs used for repigmentation therapy are trimethylpsoralen and 8-methyoxypsoralen. A patient takes the prescribed dose by mouth two hours before lying in the sun or under artificial ultraviolet (UVA) light. The ideal time for natural sunlight is between 11 A.M. and 1 P.M. when the sun is highest. Treatment every other day is recommended. Too much ultraviolet light can be harmful. Treatment schedules can be adjusted for each patient. If the day is cloudy or if sun exposure is not possible on a scheduled treatment day, then the patient does not take any medication because the drug does not work without appropriate sunlight.

In the northern United States, patients usually begin therapy in May and continue until September. Moderate repigmentation should take place during this time. Treatment is usually discontinued during the winter. Although artificial sources of UVA light can be used throughout the year, patients should consult a dermatologist to determine whether such treatments are desirable. UVA light systems for home use are expensive and treatment can be time-consuming. Ordinary sunlamps are not effective with the psoralen medications, since only UVA light produces the desired interaction.

After the initial two to three weeks of exposure to sunlight, patients will look worse since the contrast between light and tanned skin increases. With time, however, repigmentation will begin, and the appearance of the skin improves. If patients stop the therapy in winter, most will retain at least half of the color they achieved during the summer months.

A dermatologist's supervision is required during all aspects of repigmentation therapy. Patients with vitiligo should always protect their skin against excessive sun exposure by wearing protective clothing, staying out of the sun at peak periods except during treatment time, and applying sunscreen lotions and creams. Patients with vitiligo should use a sunscreen with a sun protection factor (SPF) of 15 or higher, except during the hours of treatment. During treatment, an SPF of eight to 10 protects against sunburn but does not block the UVA needed for treatment. Sunscreens should be reapplied after swimming or perspiring. To prevent potential damage to the eyes, special sunglasses with protective lenses should be worn during sunlight exposure and for the remainder of the day on which the psoralen drug is taken.

Another method of psoralen treatment, used occasionally for patients with small, scattered vitiligo patches, involves the application of a solution of the drug directly to the affected skin, which is then exposed to sunlight. However, such topical treatment makes a person very susceptible to severe burn and blisters with too much sun exposure.

Hydrocortisone-type compounds applied to the skin slow the process of depigmentation and sometimes even enhance repigmentation. However, the cortisones that are sold without a prescription (such as 0.5 percent hyrocortisone) are too weak to help. On the other hand, very potent cortisones when used daily for a long time produce side effects, such as thinning of the skin. Under the care of a dermatologist it is usually possible to adjust the treatment with topical hydrocortisones so that side effects are at a minimum.

Not everyone is a good candidate for repigmentation. The ideal person should have lost pigment no more than five years earlier. In general, children and young adults respond better than older people, but patients should be at least 10 years old. While treatment is safe for younger children, the method is tedious, and better results are achieved when the child is interested in treatment. In addition, patients should be healthy, and no one with a sensitivity or allergy to sunlight can be treated.

Depigmentation

Children with vitiligo over more than half of the exposed areas of the body are not candidates for repigmentation. Instead, they may want to try removing the pigmentation of the remaining skin so the patient is an even color. However, total depigmentation is tried only in very severe cases of vitiligo.

The drug for depigmentation is monobenzylether of hydroquinone. Many patients with vitiligo are at first apprehensive about the idea of depigmentation and reluctant to go ahead, but those who achieve complete depigmentation are usually satisfied with the end results. Unfortunately, some people become allergic to the medication and must discontinue therapy.

Cosmetics

Most patients, even if they are responding well to treatment, would like to make the vitiligo less obvious. Many find that a combination of cosmetics can de-emphasize the skin disorder. Cosmetics are not just for girls, nor are they only for the face. Anyone can wear them anywhere on their body. Over-the-counter cosmetics exist in a wide range of skin tones; many are waterproof and don't rub off. There are also special dermatological cosmetics that patients even with severe vitiligo find useful. Patients who are interested in dyes and stains should consult a dermatologist for the names of suitable commercial products.

In the Future

Research on pigment cells and vitiligo has increased since the 1990s. Some studies are trying to stop vitiligo by the use of hydrocortisone compounds applied to the skin. Others are studying the possibility of melanocyte transplants, in which pigment cells from an unexposed normally pigmented patch of skin are grown in culture and returned into a white patch.

vomiting Vomiting is very common during infancy and childhood and is usually caused by an illness or stomach upset. In infants it is important to distinguish between vomiting and "spitting up," which is very typical in babies. Babies spit up if they are fed too fast or too much, and this is not considered to be a problem.

Mild vomiting in children likewise is not serious, but severe vomiting can strain the stomach and esophagus and may cause internal bleeding. Continual vomiting also can lead to dehydration, shock, or metabolic problems; if the vomited material is inhaled into the lungs it can cause PNEUMONIA.

Intentional vomiting in teenagers (BULIMIA) can lead to tooth problems and electrolyte disturbances that can affect the heart's function, and it can be fatal.

Causes

In infancy, spitting up can be caused by improper formula preparation, feeding too much or too fast, too much swallowed air, or improper handling after feeding. Infants who persistently vomit may have an infection, a physical problem, or an inborn error of metabolism. Vomiting during the second through the ninth week may indicate a narrowing of the passage between the stomach and the small intestine (pyloric stenosis).

Vomiting is a very common symptom in a range of infections, such as INFLUENZA, pneumonia, URINARY TRACT INFECTION, and MENINGITIS. It also may be caused by central nervous system disorders, accidents, ulcers, or food poisoning.

Persistent vomiting without any apparent physical cause may be linked to excess stress or an emotional problem. It may be triggered by certain smells, sights, or sounds. Many medications also cause vomiting, including many antibiotics.

When to Call the Doctor

While an occasional vomiting bout is probably not serious, a parent should call the doctor if a child who is vomiting is under age six months, has vomited frequently within 24 hours, or has vomiting plus:

- abdominal pain
- diarrhea
- fever
- sleepiness
- blood in the vomit

Treatment

One of the biggest concerns with vomiting in children is the risk of dehydration, especially when it is accompanied by fever. For this reason, a child who is vomiting needs to restore the fluid levels in the body. Parents should give a vomiting child very small amounts of clear liquids (about half an ounce an hour). Small, frequent liquids are better than one big glass. Frozen or very cold liquids are often tolerated better than room-temperature fluids. Parents may offer ice chips, Popsicles, tea, gelatin, chicken broth or chicken noodle soup, or flat ginger ale or cola. As the vomiting subsides, children may gradually be given solid foods. While vomiting, they should not be given fatty or fried foods.

Vomiting children should not be given antinausea medication, which may cause severe side effects.

Von Hippel–Lindau disease A genetic disorder involving the abnormal growth of blood vessels that usually occurs in certain areas of the body, such as the brain and other parts of the central nervous system, the retina of the eye, the adrenal glands, the kidneys, or the pancreas. The prevalence of the disease is unknown, but a parent who carries the gene that causes Von Hippel–Lindau (VHL) disease has a 50 percent chance of having a child with the disorder.

Blood vessels usually grow like branches on a tree, but in children with VHL they form small tumors called angiomas. Doctors carefully monitor angiomas because in certain areas they can cause other medical problems. For example, angiomas on the retina of the eye may lead to permanent vision loss.

Diagnosis

VHL is diagnosed using a special type of X ray called magnetic resonance imaging (MRI) or a computerized tomography (CT) scan. A thorough physical examination and blood tests are also performed.

Symptoms

There are many symptoms of VHL, and they depend on the size and location of the angiomas. Symptoms include headaches, balance problems, dizziness, weakness, vision problems, and high blood pressure. Fluid-filled cysts or tumors (benign or cancerous) may develop around the angiomas, worsening these symptoms. Children with this disorder have a higher risk of developing cancer, especially kidney cancer.

Treatment

VHL is treated depending on the size and location of the angiomas. The goal of treatment is to treat the tumors while they are small and before they put pressure on any of the major organs, such as the brain and the spine. Surgery may be required to remove the tumors before they create severe problems.

Prognosis

The prognosis for VHL patients depends on both the location and the complications caused by the tumors. If untreated, VHL may result in blindness or permanent brain damage. Fortunately, early detection and treatment can improve a child's treatment outcome.

vulvaginitis Inflammation of the vulva and vagina, usually caused by bacteria, yeast, viruses, parasites, SEXUALLY TRANSMITTED DISEASES, or chemicals (such as bubble bath). It is characterized by profuse vaginal discharge, irritation, itching, odor, and discomfort. Antifungal or antibiotic drugs, cortisone creams, or antihistamines are all used to treat the infection.

warts Generally harmless small, hard, round, raised bumps with a rough surface that usually appear on hands and fingers or around the knees caused by one of more than 58 varieties of PAPILLOMA VIRUS.

Common warts are firm, well-defined growths up to a quarter inch wide, often with a rough surface. They usually appear in areas that are frequently injured, such as the hands, knees, scalp, and face, especially in young children. They often appear in crops and can disappear spontaneously. Sometimes a few of these bumps run together, but they usually appear separately. Tiny black specks in the wart are caused by tiny clots of blood.

Flat (plane) warts are small (about 1/16 inch) tan, flat, round, and grouped together on the face, backs of hands, and shins.

Digitate warts are dark-colored growths with finger-like projections.

Plantar warts are flat, rough warts that appear on the soles of the feet, flattened by the pressure of the body on the bottom of the foot that forces them to grow inward. They appear alone or in groups. Children aged 12 to 16 are most likely to get plantar warts; younger school-age children are more likely to get common and plane warts.

Genital warts are transmitted through sexual contact and are characterized by pink, cauliflower-like groups of growths on the genitals. This type of wart needs prompt treatment, since there is some evidence that these warts infecting the cervix may cause cervical cancer.

Cause

Warts are caused by one of the more than 58 types of human papilloma virus (HPV); the three kinds that affect children are the common, flat, and plan-

tar wart caused by HPV types 1, 2, 3, and 4. Several other types of HPV can cause genital warts.

A child gets a wart by touching someone else's wart, touching something a wart-infected person has touched, or by self-inoculation. Children who bite on their own warts can spread them to other areas of their own bodies.

The incubation period averages between two to three months, but it may be as long as 20 months, and the child is infectious as long as the wart appears.

Diagnosis

Most warts are diagnosed by appearance; rarely, a doctor may biopsy a piece of wart to make a diagnosis.

Treatment

More than 65 percent of warts disappear on their own within two years. There is no cure that will remove all traces of the virus from the body. Instead, treatment aims at removing or shrinking the warts, whether by freezing, using a topical solution or a laser, or surgery. Common, flat, and plantar warts may be removed with liquid nitrogen or a blister-producing agent, corroding acids, or plasters. Surgical removal with a scalpel, electric needle, or laser may also be used. Unfortunately, warts often reappear after treatment. In the doctor's office, liquid nitrogen freezes the wart, forming a blister that lifts off the wart.

Recent research at Children's Memorial Hospital in Chicago and New York University found that the ulcer drug cimetidine may be an effective treatment of multiple warts in children. Multiple warts can be troublesome because they often resist treatment, such as topical medications, freezing, burning, or laser surgery, or they reappear after successful treatment. In the study, young patients whose warts had not responded to other treatment showed signs of improvement after three daily doses of cimetidine. Within six to seven weeks, many of the warts had become flatter and less visible; two months into the study, warts in almost 80 percent of the children had disappeared. Researchers report that cimetidine is safe for children, and does not appear to cause any side effects.

Over-the-counter removal preparations include topical medications containing SALICYLIC ACID and lactic acid that peels off the affected skin (the virus is killed as well, since it is inside the tissue). The skin should be softened first before applying the medicine; a few times a week, the dead skin should be removed with an emery board.

If the warts do not disappear with this treatment, a dermatologist may apply liquid nitrogen to freeze the wart, forming a blister that lifts off the wart. This takes four to six weeks. Sometimes a blister-producing liquid (cantharidin) or a corroding acid liquid or plaster may be used. Some doctors may use heated electrical needles.

Since wart treatment can be painful and cause scars, many doctors prefer to wait for the warts to disappear on their own. (See also WARTS, GENITAL.)

warts, genital   Genital WARTS are the most common viral SEXUALLY TRANSMITTED DISEASE in the United States, outranking even genital HERPES; almost two million Americans are treated for genital warts each year. Most cases are diagnosed in teenage girls; older women may have the virus, but their immune systems control the outbreaks. Those who are most at risk are people with more than one sex partner and those who do not use condoms.

Cause

Eight different types of human PAPILLOMAVIRUS (HPV) are associated with genital warts; a few (types 16 and 18) cause cervical cancer. These types of warts are not usually visible. The different types of warts can only be distinguished in a research lab.

The wart virus is transmitted during unprotected sex with an infected partner. A person is infectious when visible warts are present in the genital area; however, even if the warts have disappeared, the virus may still be present in the body.

Symptoms

Genital warts are pink to gray, soft, raised or flat, and may cause itching, burning, or bleeding around the genital area. They may appear alone or in clusters, ranging in size from pinpoint to a small mass. Boys and men usually notice the warts on the penis, although they can also appear in the anus or the urethra and are often completely missed. Girls and women may find warts on the vulva, vagina, or anus; occasionally they may occur on the cervix. Incubation period is unknown. The warts are not painful, but they can grow and block the openings of the vagina, anus, urethra, or throat.

Diagnosis

A doctor can diagnose the condition from the wart's appearance; a magnifying glass may be needed to find small warts. Odd-looking warts may require biopsy.

Treatment

There is no cure that will remove all traces of the virus from the body. Instead, treatment aims at removing or shrinking the warts, whether by freezing, using a topical solution or a laser, or surgery. Unfortunately, warts often reappear after treatment.

Infected partners should avoid sex when the warts are large, bleeding, or painful. A doctor should be consulted if warts block rectal openings or if there is trouble urinating.

Podophyllin topical solution is applied by a doctor to external genital warts only (it should not be used in the cervix, rectum, or during pregnancy). The solution must not touch the surrounding skin, as it can be irritating. If there are no results after four weeks, another treatment method should be used. Podofilox 0.05 percent is a prescription topical solution that can be applied by the woman for external warts. It works by killing wart tissue.

Cryotherapy freezes the wart off; it is sometimes used for cervical or rectal warts. Laser therapy is performed in a doctor's office and is sometimes used for cervical warts. *Electrosurgery* is also performed in a doctor's office for rectal warts. As a last resort, a doctor may turn to surgical removal if the warts are very large or causing problems. Still, 20 percent of the time warts grow back after this treatment.

Prevention

All women with anogenital warts need a Pap test every six to 12 months to detect early signs of cervical cancer. Young girls with cervical HPV should have regular Pap tests to discover any changes in the cervix. Most cervical problems take care of themselves, but those with a positive Pap test should seek medical help regularly to monitor the changes.

Anyone who has genital warts or who has been diagnosed in the past should always use a condom during sexual intercourse.

Complications

Some strains of the HPV virus are associated with a higher risk of cervical cancer, especially among women with persistent warts and many sex partners. However, most girls and women who have genital warts are not considered to be at increased risk for developing cervical cancer. The association between this type of cancer and HPV is not well understood.

Occasionally, babies exposed to warts in the birth canal develop warts in the throat, and a few develop warts on the genitals or eyes. Warts may also multiply and grow larger among those with weakened immune systems or diabetes.

weight problems   See OBESITY; EATING DISORDERS.

well-baby care   Pediatricians usually like to schedule an infant for well-baby visits to make sure the child is growing and healthy. The American Academy of Pediatrics recommends well-baby checkups at one month, at two, four, six, nine, 12, 15, 18, and 24 months, and yearly after that. (However, not all doctors follow this schedule, so parents should ask the pediatrician for the well-baby checkup schedule.)

During these visits, the doctor will weigh and measure the child and check general development and health, including hearing and vision. Vaccines are also an important part of well-baby visits, which will continue though age two. At that point, a yearly "well child" visit is often recommended.

Parents should bring along written questions to the well-baby visit, and jot down specific instructions regarding special baby care during the visit. At this time, the doctor will update the infant's permanent medical record, tracking growth and any problems.

These well-baby checkups are an important way to assess growth, feeding and sleeping habits, and allow the doctor to monitor any areas of concern that may have appeared during the last checkup. The checkups will probably include most of these things:

- weight, length, and head circumference measurements
- vaccinations
- physical exam with special attention to any previous problems
- physical/emotional development (how well can baby hold up the head or interact with parents)
- advice about feeding and vitamins
- what to expect during the coming months

Vaccinations

At one to two months of age the baby will probably receive the second dose of the hepatitis B vaccine (the first was probably given just after birth.) At two months (and again at four months), the baby will be given several vaccines:

- diphtheria, tetanus, and acellular pertussis (DTaP) vaccine
- *Haemophilus influenzae* type B vaccine
- polio vaccine

Some of these safeguards against serious childhood illnesses can cause reactions (usually mild), such as fever or irritability. Parents should discuss side effects with the doctor and obtain guidelines for what to do if there are any reactions.

Four to Seven Months

From four to seven months is a time of incredibly rapid growth. In addition to continuing concerns about eating and sleeping, parents may begin to wonder whether the child is growing and developing properly. During this stage, the doctor will monitor the baby's progress and answer any questions.

The doctor will probably want to see the baby at four months and at six months, although this may differ from one doctor to the next. Of course, if there has been any problem in the past, the doctor may want to schedule extra visits. Well-baby visits vary from doctor to doctor, but may include:

- length, weight, and head circumference measurements (baby's growth will be plotted on his own growth chart)
- physical exam
- check of the baby's soft spots (the fontanelles) at the top and back of the head
- examination of the baby's mouth for signs of teething

The doctor also will likely review the baby's physical and emotional development (Is the baby holding up her head or rolling over? Is there any stranger anxiety?) and will probably ask if parents are using an appropriate car seat. If the baby can pull himself up, the doctor may ask if parents have removed mobiles and bumpers from the crib. The doctor will discuss baby's eating habits and will probably mention the start of solid foods, which may be introduced soon.

The doctor also may want to check the baby for anemia (low levels of iron in the blood). A simple finger prick provides enough blood for testing; other than that, most babies do not need any routine lab tests at this age.

At the fourth-month visit, vaccines include:

- DTaP vaccine (second dose)
- *Haemophilus influenzae* type B (HIB) vaccine (second dose)
- polio vaccine (second dose)

At the six-month visit, the baby may receive the following:

- DTaP vaccine (third dose)
- hepatitis B vaccine (third dose, if first two doses have been given earlier; otherwise, some time before the checkup at 18 months)
- *Haemophilus influenzae* type B (HIB) vaccine (third dose)

Eight to 12 Months

Most pediatricians generally see babies twice during this stage, once at nine months and again at 12

months. The well-baby visits at nine and 12 months are much the same as earlier exams, although parents may spend more time talking about behavior as the baby becomes more active and independent. The pediatrician may want to know if parents have baby-proofed the home and if the baby rides in an appropriate safety seat in the car.

Nutrition is another important area the doctor will discuss, asking about whether the child is eating more finger foods from the high chair tray, using a cup, or if he is weaned. Most doctors advise a switch from bottle to cup by the first birthday so that the bottle does not interfere with normal tooth development (and to avoid fighting with a toddler later on). By one year most babies can be given cow's milk, citrus fruits, and eggs.

Typically the doctor will check:

- baby's length, weight, and head circumference
- normal function of the limbs, hands and feet, reflexes, eyes, ears, heart, and so on
- baby's soft spots (the fontanel at the back of the head will probably be closed; the one on top may be closed or much smaller)
- baby's mouth for signs of new teeth

If the baby missed shots at previous visits because of illness or scheduling problems, she will probably be brought up to date now. At a baby's 12-month visit, she will receive:

- the first of two measles, mumps, and rubella (MMR) vaccines
- fourth *Haemophilus influenzae* type B (HIB) vaccine (the last of the series)
- tuberculin skin test
- Between 12 and 18 months, babies usually receive a polio vaccine and may receive a varicella (chicken pox) vaccine.

Fifteen Months to Two Years

Barring problems, most pediatricians will want to see a child this age three times, typically at 15, 18, and 24 months of age. These well-baby visits during the child's second year are much the same as earlier ones, although as the child grows more time will be spent discussing behavior and habits. At the 15-month visit most doctors will:

- measure length, weight, and head circumference
- check body, reflexes, eyes, ears, abdomen, heart
- examine the mouth for new teeth

At this well-baby visit, the doctor will ask about the child's physical and emotional development. By 18 months the toddler will probably be able to say about 15 words and walk with a regular heel-toe walking pattern. By age two, a toddler should be able to:

- put two words together to form a sentence
- follow simple directions
- imitate actions
- push and pull a toy

If the child is not doing all these things by these ages, the parents may want to mention this to the child's doctor. However, not all babies perform all of these tasks "on time." Typical safety questions the doctor will ask at this well-baby visit include whether she uses a car seat and whether she wears a safety helmet while on riding toys. Nutrition is also important, and the doctor may discuss the child's eating habits, weaning, and cup use.

If the child missed immunizations at earlier visits because of illness or scheduling problems, he will be brought up-to-date now. Since he is becoming more and more mobile and is coming in contact with other children more often, parents should make sure his immunizations are given close to the recommended times. The doctor will discuss possible vaccine reactions and offer advice on when to call with unusual problems. Vaccines at this age may include:

- *Haemophilus influenzae* type B (HIB) vaccine
- Measles, mumps, rubella (MMR) vaccine may be given at 15 months if your toddler did not receive them at his 12-month visit.
- Varicella (chicken pox) vaccine may be recommended if your child did not receive it at his 12-month visit or has not yet had chicken pox.
- diphtheria, tetanus, pertussis (DTaP or DTP) vaccine; fourth dose should be given before 18 months
- polio vaccine (possibly)

West Nile virus   A virus that can cause a fatal ENCEPHALITIS, commonly found in humans and birds in Africa, Eastern Europe, West Asia, and the Middle East. Until 1999 the virus had not been documented in the Western Hemisphere. In 1999, 62 cases of severe disease, including seven deaths, occurred in the New York area, followed by 21 more cases the next year, including two deaths. In 2003, 9,858 people caught the virus and 262 died. The United States also suffered the biggest reported outbreak of West Nile encephalitis in the world in 2002.

Symptoms

West Nile virus rarely kills, but about one in 150 people who get it will develop its potentially deadly encephalitis or MENINGITIS. Most people who are infected with the virus will not get sick; about a fifth of those will develop a fever, headache, body aches, and sometimes a rash and swollen lymph glands. Symptoms for West Nile encephalitis or meningitis include headache, high fever, neck stiffness, disorientation, and sometimes paralysis.

Cause

The virus is transmitted to humans via the bite of infected mosquitoes, which become infected when they feed on infected birds. The virus is located in the mosquito's salivary glands. During feeding, the virus may be injected, multiplying in a person's blood and crossing the blood-brain barrier to reach the brain, where it inflames brain tissue and interferes with central nervous system function. Among those with severe illness due to West Nile virus, the fatality rates range from 3 percent to 15 percent.

However, even in areas where mosquitoes do carry the virus, very few mosquitoes (less than 1 percent) are infected. If the mosquito is infected, less than 1 percent of people who get bitten and become infected will be severely ill. The chances that any one person will become severely ill from a single mosquito bite are extremely small.

The virus is not spread by touching or kissing a person who has the disease, or from a health-care worker who has treated someone with the disease. Although ticks infected with West Nile virus have been found in Asia and Africa, their role in the transmitting the virus is uncertain. There is no information to suggest that ticks played any role in the cases identified in the United States.

While experts do not know where the U.S. virus originated, it is most closely related genetically to strains found in the Middle East. West Nile virus was first isolated from a feverish woman in the West Nile district of Uganda in 1937. The virus became recognized as a cause of severe inflammation of the spinal cord and brain in elderly patients during an outbreak in Israel in 1957. Equine disease was first noted in Egypt and France in the early 1960s. It first appeared in North America in 1999, with encephalitis reported in humans and horses.

West Nile virus has been described in Africa, Europe, the Middle East, west and central Asia, and most recently, North America. Recent outbreaks of West Nile virus encephalitis in humans have occurred in the Democratic Republic of the Congo in 1998, Russia in 1999, the United States in 1999–2001, and Israel in 2000.

Although the vast majority of infections have been identified in birds, the virus can infect horses, cats, bats, chipmunks, skunks, squirrels, and domestic rabbits. While there is no evidence that a person can get the virus from handling live or dead infected birds, people should avoid bare-handed contact when handling any dead animals and use gloves or double plastic bags to place the carcass in a garbage can. Normal veterinary infection control precautions should be followed when caring for a horse suspected to have this or any viral infection.

Prevention

To prevent being bitten by infected mosquitoes, people should:

- stay indoors at dawn, dusk, and in the early evening
- wear long-sleeved shirts and long pants outdoors
- spray clothing with repellents containing permethrin or DEET
- apply insect repellent sparingly to exposed skin. An effective repellent contains 35 percent DEET (higher concentrations provide no additional protection).

West Nile virus encephalitis   Normally seen in the Middle East and some parts of Europe and Asia, the WEST NILE VIRUS can cause ENCEPHALITIS in some people. The first outbreak of West Nile Virus encephalitis occurred in 1999 in the Western hemisphere. There were a total of 62 cases of human encephalitis or MENINGITIS and seven fatalities in New York City and adjacent Long Island and Westchester County. In addition, mosquitoes and more than 20 bird species were found to be infected with West Nile virus in New Jersey, Connecticut, New York state, and Maryland. In the hardest hit section of Queens, 2.5 percent of humans tested were found to have been infected with West Nile virus. Fatal infection was also seen in horses on Long Island.

The future impact of West Nile virus is uncertain. States on the eastern bird flyway have received federal funding to conduct monitoring activities and perform diagnostic assays. This effort will be expanded nationwide. While all residents of areas where virus activity has been identified are at risk of getting West Nile encephalitis, people over age 50 are at highest risk of severe disease.

Cause

The virus, which normally circulates in birds and mosquitoes, crosses to humans who are bitten by an infected mosquito. The virus then multiplies in the person's blood and eventually crosses the blood-brain barrier to reach the brain. At this point, the virus interferes with normal central nervous system functioning and inflames brain tissue.

Symptoms

Most human illness from West Nile infection is mild, but severe disease is more common in the very young and very old, or those people with a weakened immune system. From three to 15 days after infection, symptoms may appear including fever, headache, and body aches, occasionally with skin rash and swollen lymph glands. More severe infection may be marked by headache, high fever, neck stiffness, stupor, disorientation, coma, tremors, convulsions, muscle weakness, paralysis, and, rarely, death.

Less than 1 percent of those infected with West Nile virus will develop severe illness; of those who do, between 3 percent and 15 percent will die.

Diagnosis

Patients who are at high risk and who have symptoms of West Nile encephalitis will have a sample of their blood sent to a lab to confirm the diagnosis.

Treatment

Treatment is supportive for the encephalitis or meningitis associated with the infection. Severely ill patients may be hospitalized and given intravenous fluids, airway management, a ventilator, and perhaps antibiotics to prevent secondary infection.

whipworms Parasitic roundworms of the species *Trichuris trichiura* that infect a child's intestinal tract. About two million Americans are affected, primarily children. The eggs of these worms are remarkably hardy and may resist freezing.

Cause

Whipworm infestation occurs when a child comes in contact with or ingests whipworm eggs in fecal-contaminated soil. Whipworms are small worms about one or two inches long that can live in the intestines for up to 20 years. Once the eggs hatch, the whipworm embeds itself into the mucous membrane. While the worms live in the large intestine and the appendix, they may infest the colon as well.

Symptoms

Light infestation causes few symptoms, but a heavier worm load may cause bloody diarrhea that appears to contain mucus.

Diagnosis

Examination of the stool can reveal the presence of whipworm eggs.

Treatment

Mebendazole can kill the worms, although a serious case may require more than one treatment. Recovery is complete.

Complications

In very severe cases, dehydration and anemia as a result of the bloody diarrhea can occur.

whooping cough The common name for pertussis, an acute infection of the upper respiratory tract featuring violent, loud bouts of coughing that end in a whoop. Vomiting usually occurs at the end of the coughing spell. Most serious in young children, whooping cough is highly contagious and will infect virtually all susceptible children who come in contact with the bacterium. It can lead to seizures, PNEUMONIA, brain damage, and death.

Before the vaccine was available in the 1940s about 200,000 children got sick each year and about 8,000 died. Because the disease can be deadly in infants, babies should be isolated from anyone with whooping cough.

While the number of cases has declined since the introduction of the vaccine, it is far from eradicated. In the year 2000 there were nearly 1,900 cases of whooping cough, including 16 deaths in infants under six months of age.

Whooping cough is most serious in infants, who may often develop pneumonia; babies younger than three months of age get the worst cases. Seventy percent of deaths occur in young babies; about one in 200 infected babies will die. The most infectious time is right at the beginning of the illness.

Doctors must report any suspected or confirmed cases of whooping cough to the health department. If the child attends school or child care, the parent must notify the principal so staff and other children can be given preventive medicine.

Cause

The disease is caused by a rod-shaped bacterium called *Bordetella pertussis,* which produces a toxin that invades the lining of the throat, windpipe, and bronchial tubes. The tissue damage produces a very thick, irritating mucus leading to severe coughing spells as the child tries to expel it. The thick mucus often leads to pneumonia. A similar but less common bacterium called *iB. parapertussis* may cause a milder form of the disease.

The disease is spread during coughing, which spews the bacteria outward for several feet. These bacteria can survive on tissue or bed covers for a short time; the disease also can be passed on when another person touches these items. Whooping cough is infectious enough that it will be spread to everyone in the household from one infected patient.

Symptoms

Whooping cough occurs in three stages in children: the first stage starts slowly with cold-like symptoms (sneezing, red or sore eyes, and a low-grade fever). This occurs with an irritating dry cough for one or two weeks (during which the child is most infectious).

These first symptoms are followed by intense, violent spasms of repeated coughing with no time to breathe between spasms. There is a repetitive series of eight or 10 rapid coughs on one breath that often end in gagging or vomiting. The coughs may end in a characteristic "whoop" as the patient tries to take a breath. Babies under six months of age will choke but will not make the whooping sound; these youngest patients can become very sick. The infected child may appear blue, with bulging eyes and a dazed, apathetic expression. Infants may temporarily stop breathing after a coughing spasm. The periods between coughing are comfortable; there is little fever. This stage may last about two weeks.

The final stage dwindles down into a chronic cough for three to four weeks; some children experience a cough of more than two months.

Complications

A child with the disease may have an ear infection or pneumonia. About one in 500 children younger than six months may develop seizures, coma, or brain damage. The chronic cough may cause nosebleeds and bleeding from blood vessels on the surface of the eyes; recurrent vomiting can cause dehydration and malnourishment.

Diagnosis

The disease is diagnosed by identifying the bacterium in a culture grown from a nasal swab taken in the early stages of the illness. There are two tests, neither of which is 100 percent accurate, and there are many false negatives. The rapid test gives results in a few minutes; a blood test done in mid-disease may identify the bacterium or detect antibodies.

Treatment

If the illness is recognized early enough, antibiotics such as erythromycin or clarithyromycin are often given; they may shorten the duration of illness and the period of contagiousness, although they are not particularly helpful once the severe coughing stage of the illness has begun.

Patients should be kept warm, given frequent small meals and plenty to drink, and protected from things that produce coughing, such as smoke. An infant or child who becomes blue or keeps vomiting after coughing needs to be admitted to the hospital.

window safety Falls from windows are the leading cause of nonfatal injury for children under 15 and are responsible for the deaths of 140 children each year in the United States. Another three million are injured, mostly during the summer months when windows are kept open and children are more likely to be playing on fire escapes, roofs, and balconies. Children at greatest risk are those living in urban areas, especially youngsters living in deteriorating, low-income apartment buildings.

However, urban children are not the only ones at risk—falls from the first- and second-floor windows of private homes can also be dangerous, depending on how the child falls and what he lands on. The most common injuries are fractures and head trauma.

Parents should never leave a child unattended around an open window, and a window open only five inches can pose a serious danger to a young child, especially a curious toddler or preschooler. In addition, all furniture should be moved away from open windows, because children as young as one year may be able to use it to climb up to the window.

According to the American Academy of Pediatrics (AAP), parents should install window guards on second-story and higher windows (and require landlords to do the same). For example, after the New York health code was changed to require protective window guards on all multiple-family dwellings, the number of children who fell from windows each year plummeted by about 90 percent. The best window guards are those that are designed to keep children in, but that allow an older child or adult to open the window in case of emergency. Parents should never rely on window screens to protect a child from a possible fall, because the screens are easily lifted, torn, or pushed out. If a landlord has installed window guards in a building, renters should never remove them, even if they obstruct the view.

The AAP also recommends that parents:

- discourage children from playing in high areas, such as balconies, rooftops, fire escapes, and porches

- ensure that building codes require railings to have vertical openings of four inches or less
- plant grass or shrubbery at the base of tall buildings to act as a cushion in case of a fall

wound healing   Cuts and scrapes heal best with a broad-spectrum antibacterial ointment and the right kind of bandage. However, some children may be allergic to some compounds in these ointments, especially those that contain neomycin or preservatives. It is best to keep cuts and scrapes moist and not exposed to the air, which forms scabs that cut down on cell growth. Bandages that keep the wound moist (such as those impregnated with petroleum jelly) enable cells to regenerate rapidly.

written expression, disorders of   Problems in producing writing that do not seem to be linked to a child's overall intelligence. Individuals with writing disorders typically have problems in several areas of writing, such as sentence structure, punctuation, spelling, or generating ideas and language in written form. Their ability to express concepts in writing may generally be far more limited than their ability to do so in spoken language, or it may be consistent with their oral-language functioning. In some cases the quality of the writing produced may be the primary difficulty; this might include problems with syntax, word meanings, spelling, grammar, or structure and organization.

In other cases, some children have problems with the ability to produce written text fluently and continuously in response to prompts; in this case, the child may be able to produce good writing sometimes, while at other times be unable to respond effectively at all.

Sometimes both the quality and production of writing may be impaired. Handwriting may also be a problem area. However, problems in only one area, such as spelling or handwriting, excludes this diagnosis.

Disorders of written expression may have a significant impact on an individual's school or job functioning and may have a particularly severe impact on success in high school and college.

Diagnosis

As with other learning disorders, the assessment of a writing disorder is based on problems that are not related to intelligence, age, education, or other disorders. Disorders of written expression are generally diagnosed together with reading and mathematics disabilities, and they are more often discussed and studied under the general category of LEARNING DISABILITY than in isolation.

Significant problems with written fluency and production may also be linked to a more general learning disability but are often associated with a diagnosis of ATTENTION DEFICIT HYPERACTIVITY DISORDER. Written-output difficulties linked to deficits in attention and executive function are often diagnosed as dysgraphia.

Because "disorders of written expression" is a general diagnostic term, determining effective educational practices depends on a closer analysis of the individual's pattern of deficits and strengths.

For those whose disorder of written expression appears along with a general expressive-language disorder or a reading disability, the development of effective writing skills begins with developing more basic language abilities. These may include intensive study and practice of oral language syntax and vocabulary in order to provide a foundation for the development of written-language skills.

In those individuals who also have a reading disorder, the development of decoding skills through practice in awareness of word sounds, discrimination, and phonics may be an essential starting point. Reading and language enrichment activities on a whole language model may boost comprehension and critical reasoning skills.

Until these skills are developed, direct remediation of written-language deficits will not be effective and may in fact lead to frustration and resistance. At the same time, it is important that some work in the area of writing development begin simultaneously with instruction in oral communication and reading development, in order to reinforce and extend the skills acquired in those areas. Such work should focus primarily on the generation of expressive writing, drawing linkages between oral language abilities and their manifestation in writing.

The concept of writing as a process, and the gradual introduction of various strategies for generating, planning, and organizing text, should all play a central role in instruction. In addition, simple elements such as sentence and paragraph concepts should be introduced. Examples of the mechanics of language, such as punctuation or sentence structure, also may be introduced.

As much as possible, work in spelling should be linked to work in the area of reading development, and spelling should generally be de-emphasized within the context of writing instruction, except as reinforcement and a reminder to apply newly learned skills.

For individuals whose written expression disorder may be associated with a reading and/or spelling disability, but not with an expressive language disorder, instruction should focus first on the introduction of the concept of writing as a recursive process, and on continuing practice with various strategies for planning, generating, and organizing writing. In most cases, engaging generating strategies that draw on oral-communication strengths, such as talking out ideas before writing, will play an effective part in writing development. Students with this pattern of abilities will also benefit from direct instruction in written language structures, rules, and conventions, and from continual reinforcement and practice of this knowledge in writing assignments. Instruction in written-language structures and rules, if embedded appropriately into a process-based classroom, may actually have a facilitative and generating power, rather than serving as a constraint on imagination and the free flow of ideas.

Individuals whose disorder of written expression is linked primarily to problems with written output are often also diagnosed with ADHD and may often possess very strong oral communication and reading skills, as well as the ability to demonstrate excellent basic writing abilities in some contexts. The difficulties such individuals experience with writing may primarily stem from deficits in attention, executive function, and active working memory that severely constrain the process of writing and result in impaired writing production, particularly on complex and unfamiliar tasks. While some direct instruction in written-language structures may be appropriate for such individuals, writing instruction in general should use a coaching model.

yeast infections Skin infections caused by types of fungi, the most important of which is *Candida albicans.* This type of yeast can normally be found in a child's mouth, vagina, and large intestine, but for unknown reasons it can sometimes turn against its host, most commonly in those who take antibiotics, oral steroids, and birth control pills, and in diabetics and the overweight.

This type of yeast causes THRUSH (white patches on the inside of the cheeks), cheesy vaginal discharge, damp red eruptions under the breasts, the foreskin, and under body folds in the obese; and redness and swelling around the nails.

Candidal infections usually respond to topical broad-spectrum antibiotics or specific preparations designed to fight yeasts (nystatin).

yellow fever A short-acting infectious viral disease that gets its name from its symptom of yellowed skin caused by jaundice. The three varieties of yellow fever include urban, jungle, and sylvan and can range from mild to fatal. In general, the disease is a risk only for families who travel to sub-Saharan Africa or tropical South America. Eradication of the mosquito from populated areas has greatly reduced the incidence of the disease; it is fatal only about 5 percent of the time.

Still, epidemics of yellow fever can occur when large numbers of susceptible humans and infected mosquitoes coexist. The disease has been known since the time of the first explorations of Africa; every few years since, many thousands of Africans have gotten yellow fever, and as many as half of those infected will die. Nigerian epidemics between 1986 and 1988 killed 10,000 people.

Epidemics of yellow fever end when the dry season comes and the mosquitoes who carry the virus become less abundant. Epidemics have also ended when the surviving human population becomes immune, either through infection or mass vaccination.

Cause

The yellow fever virus was identified in 1927 and is included in a group of viruses called "flavivirus" (from the Latin word *flavus* meaning "yellow"). This is the same group of viruses that contains St. Louis and Japanese ENCEPHALITIS. There is no difference in the way the three types of yellow fever (urban, jungle, and sylvan) affect victims; the three types differ only in their natural cycles.

Yellow fever virus mostly infects monkeys and mosquitoes, although it sometimes is transmitted via mosquitoes who bite monkeys, who pass it on to humans. In cities ("urban yellow fever") the disease is transmitted between humans by *Aedes aegypti* mosquitoes. This mosquito is found in the southeastern United States, but no disease has been reported since 1905 in New Orleans. However, the potential for the disease to spread in this country remains.

Most yellow fever is of the "jungle" type, which is transmitted between monkeys in Africa by forest mosquitoes.

Sylvan yellow fever is transmitted between forest monkeys in South America by treetop-living species of mosquitoes (not *Aedes*) that only bite humans when they cut down a giant tree, bringing the mosquitoes down to ground level.

While people cannot directly transmit the disease to other humans, they will be infectious to mosquitoes from just before fever appears to about five days into the illness. The infected mosquitoes will remain infectious for their entire lifespan. For these reasons, patient isolation and standard blood and body fluid precautions should be taken by caregivers.

Major epidemics can reappear in towns and cities that do not control the mosquitoes. In the forests the virus cycles in monkeys are carried by forest mosquitoes. When monkey populations increase, there are more nonimmune monkeys and the virus spreads among them. In addition, as the monkey populations increase, more of them venture into farmers' fields, where other mosquitoes become infected and in turn infect the farmers.

Symptoms

Many people have no symptoms, some have a mild illness, and a few (about 10 percent of those infected) become very sick and die. In those who have symptoms, between three and six days after infection there is a sudden fever, headache, and backache, with nausea and vomiting. Characteristic signs are pulse slowing as temperature rises and albumen in the urine; in those with serious disease, those signs progress to nosebleeds, bleeding from the mouth, coffee-ground colored or black vomit due to blood in the stomach, black stool due to digested blood.

In most children, symptoms pass in about three days; others experience neck, back, and leg pain, fever, chills, weakness, restless, irritability. Most recover because their immune systems are able to fight off the disease and develop antibodies that destroy the virus. Recovery in these cases is slow but complete, without permanent damage. One attack of yellow fever in humans provides lifetime immunity.

Diagnosis

Urine tests will show high level of albumin; blood tests reveal low levels of white blood cells. Antibodies to the virus in blood samples will be conclusive.

Complications

Some children begin to feel better but after three to nine days progress to the second stage of yellow fever, including liver and kidney damage, jaundice and kidney failure, and agitation. The gums bleed, vomit contains blood, and stools turn black, and skin and eyes become yellow-tinged. Fatal cases proceed to delirium, coma, and death.

Treatment

No drug is effective against the yellow fever virus, so treatment is aimed at lowering fever, maintaining blood volume via transfusion of fluids, and avoiding liver damage. In mild or moderate cases the prognosis is excellent; 50 to 95 percent of patients will survive.

Prevention

Vaccination confers long-lasting immunity and should always be obtained before traveling through affected areas. Although the vaccination is protective for life, international regulations require revaccinations every 10 years. The vaccine is effective beginning 10 days after the first dose. The yellow fever vaccine must be approved by the World Health Organization and is given only at approved yellow fever vaccination centers.

Reactions to the vaccine are usually mild. Between 2 and 5 percent of vaccinated children have mild headaches, low-grade fevers, or other minor symptoms between five and 10 days later. Immediate hypersensitivity reactions (including rash, hives, or asthma) are extremely uncommon (less than one in a million). They occur primarily in those with egg allergies.

A yellow fever vaccination certificate is required for entry to many countries. If travel plans include a trip to any country in Africa or South America, travelers should get a yellow fever vaccination and certificate before leaving the United States for these locations. In addition, countries where yellow fever is reported are listed every two weeks in the Summary of Health Information for International Travel ("the blue sheet"). This is available 24 hours a day from the CDC Fax Information Service for International Travelers or by calling the CDC international travelers' hotline at (404) 332-4559. The blue sheet is also available from state or local health departments. In Canada information can be found at the Tropical Health and Quarantine Division at the Laboratory Center for Disease Control at (613) 957-8739 or fax (613) 998-6413.

All those who cannot be vaccinated for medical reasons must obtain a medical waiver instead of the yellow fever certificate. This will include a doctor's letter stating the reasons against the vaccine;

the waiver is obtained from the consular or embassy officials of the country to be visited before leaving the United States. A single injection of the vaccine gives protection for up to 10 years, but children under age one should not be vaccinated.

The World Health Organization must be notified within 24 hours about new cases of yellow fever in areas previously free of the disease, including cases in monkeys.

APPENDIXES

APPENDIX I
ASSOCIATIONS

ADOPTION

Adoption Resource Exchange for Single Parents, Inc. (ARESP)
8605 Cameron Street
Suite 220
Silver Spring, MD 29010
(301) 585-5836
http://www.aresp.org

A nonprofit organization offering a newsletter, information, referrals, and support to single parents interested in adoption.

Adoptive Families of America
33 Highway 100, N
Minneapolis, MN 55422
(800) 372-3300
http://www.adoptivefam.org

National nonprofit membership organization of 18,000 families and individuals and more than 250 adoptive parent support groups offers problem-solving help and information about the challenges of adoption to members of adoptive and prospective adoptive families; offers free "starter" kit, fact sheet, education, national magazine, aid to children, and advocacy.

American Academy of Adoption Attorneys
Box 33053
Washington, DC 20033-0053
http://www.adoptionattorneys.org

A national association of attorneys interested in the field of adoption law who promote adoption law reform and provide information on ethical adoption practices. Offers a newsletter, annual meetings, educational seminars, and directory.

Child Welfare League of America
440 First Street, NW
Suite 310
Washington, DC 20001
(202) 638-2952
http://www.cwla.org

Publishes the National Adoption Resource Directory, listing adoption agencies around the country.

Families Like Ours, Inc.
P.O. Box 3137
Renton, WA 98056
(425) 793-7911
http://www.familieslikeours.org

A national support group for gay and lesbian couples that provides information about adoption.

Family Pride Coalition
P.O. Box 34337
San Diego, CA 92163
(619) 296-0199
http://www.familypride.org

Organization dedicated to helping gay, lesbian, bisexual, and transgendered couples adopt; provides information, support, and referrals.

Latin American Parents Association
P.O. Box 339
Brooklyn, NY 11234
(718) 236-8689
http://www.lapa.com

Provides information about adopting babies from Latin America.

National Adoption Center
1218 Chestnut Street
Philadelphia, PA 19107

(800) TOADOPT (not in PA)
(215) 925-0200 (in PA)
http://www.adopt.org

Promotes adoption of children throughout the country (especially those with special needs).

National Adoption Information Clearinghouse

1400 Eye Street, NW
Suite 600
Washington, DC 20005
(202) 842-1919
http://www.calib.com/naic

Provides fact sheets, articles, and information about adoption, a computerized list of books, a directory of adoption agencies and other resources, and information on state and federal laws on adoption.

National Council for Adoption

1930 17th Street, NW
Washington, DC 20009
(202) 328-1200
http://www.ncfa-usa.org

An association of private adoption agencies that provides information, publications, and resource listings on adoption.

North American Council on Adoptable Children

970 Raymond Avenue
Suite #106
Saint Paul, MN 55114
(612) 644-3036
http://www.nacac.org

A national support group for adoptive parents that specializes in placing older, handicapped, and minority children.

AIDS

Elizabeth Glaser Pediatric AIDS Foundation

2950 31st Street
#125
Santa Monica, CA 90405

(310) 314-1459
(888) 499-HOPE
http://www.pedaids.org

The leading worldwide nonprofit organization dedicated to identifying, funding, and conducting pediatric HIV/AIDS research.

National Association of People with AIDS

1413 K Street, NW
Suite 700
Washington, DC 20005
(202) 898-0414
http://www.napwa.org

Nonprofit organization that advocates on behalf of all people living with HIV and AIDS in order to end the pandemic and the human suffering. The group is devoted to an ongoing mission to educate, inform, and empower all people living with HIV and AIDS.

ALBINISM

National Organization for Albinism and Hypopigmentation (NOAH)

P.O. Box 959
East Hampstead, NH 03826-0959
(800) 473-2310
(603) 887-2310
http://www.albinism.org

Nonprofit, tax-exempt organization that offers information and support to people with albinism, their families, and the professionals who work with them.

ALCOHOL ABUSE

National Clearinghouse for Alcohol and Drug Information (NCADI)

P.O. Box 2345
Rockville, MD 20847-2345
(800) 729-6686
(877) 767-8432 (español)
(301) 468-2600
(800) 487-4899 (TTY)
http://www.health.org

The world's largest resource for current information and materials concerning alcohol and substance abuse prevention, intervention, and treatment. NCADI is a service of the Center for Substance Abuse Prevention and offers a wide variety of free services, including NCADI Information Services Department, the NCADI Library, and Prevention Pipeline.

ALLERGY

Allergy & Asthma Network Mothers of Asthmatics

2751 Prosperity Avenue
Suite 150
Fairfax, VA 22031
(800) 878-4403
http://www.aanma.org

A national nonprofit network of families whose desire is to overcome, not cope with, allergies and asthma. AANMA advocates for patient access to specialty care and appropriate treatments, promotes the importance of a school nurse in every school, and supports children's rights to carry inhalers while at school after receiving appropriate training by medical professionals.

American Academy of Allergy, Asthma & Immunology

(800) 822-ASMA
http://www.aaaai.org

The largest professional medical specialty organization representing allergists, clinical immunologists, allied health professionals, and other physicians with a special interest in allergy. It was established in 1943 and includes more than 6,000 members.

Asthma and Allergy Foundation of America (AAFA)

1233 20th Street, NW
Suite 402
Washington, DC 20036
(202) 466-7643
http://www.aafa.org

A nonprofit patient organization dedicated to improving the quality of life for people with asthma and allergies and their caregivers, through education, advocacy, and research.

AAFA, founded in 1953, provides practical information, community-based services, support, and referrals through a national network of chapters and educational support groups. AAFA also sponsors research toward better treatments and a cure for asthma and allergic diseases.

Food Allergy & Anaphylaxis Network

10400 Eaton Place
Suite 107
Fairfax, VA 22030-2208
(800) 929-4040
http://www.foodallergy.org

Nonprofit group established in 1991 with more than 25,000 members worldwide, including families, dietitians, nurses, physicians, school staff, and representatives from government agencies and the food and pharmaceutical industries. FAAN serves as the communication link between the patient and others, raising public awareness, providing advocacy and education, and advancing research on behalf of all those affected by food allergies and anaphylaxis.

ANGELMAN SYNDROME

Angelman Syndrome Foundation

414 Plaza Drive
Suite 209
Westmont, IL 60559
(800) IF-ANGEL
(630) 734-9267
http://www.angelman.org

Foundation provides information on diagnosis, treatment, and management and offers support and advocacy.

ANOREXIA NERVOSA

See EATING DISORDERS.

ANXIETY DISORDERS

Anxiety Disorders Association of America

8730 Georgia Avenue
Suite 600
Silver Spring, MD 20910

(240) 485-1001

http://www.adaa.org

The ADAA promotes the prevention and cure of anxiety disorders and works to improve the lives of all people who suffer from them.

APHASIA

National Aphasia Association

156 Fifth Avenue

Suite 707

New York, NY 10010

(800) 922-4622

http://www.aphasia.org

A nonprofit organization that promotes public education, research, rehabilitation, and support services to assist people with aphasia and their families.

APNEA

See SLEEP DISORDERS.

APPEARANCE

See CRANIOFACIAL PROBLEMS.

APRAXIA

Apraxia-Kids Web site

http://www.avenza.com/~apraxia/index.html

Beginning as a listserv for parents of children with apraxia of speech, the site grew to became a forum for parents, therapists, and professionals all over the world.

Childhood Apraxia of Speech Association of North America (CASANA)

123 Eisele Road

Cheswick, PA 15024

(412) 767-6589

http://www.apraxia-kids.org

This nonprofit program of the Childhood Apraxia of Speech Association of North America (CASANA) includes the Apraxia-Kids Web site, message boards, listserv, and monthly internet newsletter. CASANA is dedicated to advocating for each child to have a voice.

ARTHRITIS

Arthritis Foundation

P.O. Box 7669

Atlanta, GA 30357-0669

(800) 283-7800

http://www.arthritis.org

The only national nonprofit organization that supports the more than 100 types of arthritis and related conditions with advocacy, programs, services, and research.

National Institute of Arthritis and Musculoskeletal and Skin Diseases

Information Clearinghouse

1 AMS Circle,

Bethesda, MD 20892-3675

(877) 226-4267

(301) 495-4484 (Voice)

(301) 565-2966 (TTY)

http://www.niams.nih.gov

This federal institute supports research into the causes, treatment, and prevention of arthritis and musculoskeletal and skin diseases, the training of basic and clinical scientists to carry out this research, and the dissemination of information on research progress in these diseases.

ASPERGER DISORDER/SYNDROME

Asperger's Disorder Home Page

http://www.aspergers.com

Web site offering list of U.S. specialists, bibliography, and links.

Asperger Syndrome Coalition of the United States

P.O. Box 351268

Jacksonville, FL 32235

(866) 4-ASPRGR

http://www.asperger.org

A national nonprofit support and advocacy organization for Asperger Syndrome and Related Disorders committed to providing the most up-to-date and comprehensive information on Asperger Syndrome and related conditions.

ASTHMA

Allergy & Asthma Network Mothers of Asthmatics

2751 Prosperity Avenue
Suite 150
Fairfax, VA 22031
(800) 878-4403
http://www.aanma.org

A national nonprofit network founded in 1985 whose desire is to overcome, not cope with, allergies and asthma. AANMA produces *Allergy & Asthma Today* magazine, *THE MA REPORT* newsletter and e-news updates, and operates a toll-free help line and community awareness programs.

American Academy of Allergy, Asthma & Immunology

611 East Wells Street
Milwaukee, WI 53202
(414) 272-6071
800-822-ASMA
http://www.aaaai.org

The largest professional medical specialty organization representing allergists, clinical immunologists, allied health professionals, and other physicians with a special interest in allergy. It was established in 1943 and includes more than 6,000 members.

Asthma and Allergy Foundation of America (AAFA)

1233 20th Street, NW
Suite 402
Washington, DC 20036
(202) 466-7643
http://www.aafa.org

A nonprofit patient organization dedicated to improving the quality of life for people with asthma and allergies and their caregivers, through education, advocacy, and research. AAFA, founded in 1953, provides practical information, community-based services, support, and referrals through a national network of chapters and educational support groups. AAFA also sponsors research toward better treatments and a cure for asthma and allergic diseases.

ATAXIA

Ataxia-Telangiectasia Children's Project

668 South Military Trail
Deerfield Beach, FL 33442
(800) 5-HELP-A-T
http://www.atcp.org

A nonprofit organization founded in 1993 by a Florida family with two young sons who have A-T. The A-T Children's Project was formed to raise funds through events and contributions from corporations, foundations, and friends, and used to support international scientific research aimed at finding a cure and improving the lives of all children with A-T.

The National Ataxia Foundation

2600 Fernbrook Lane
Suite 119
Minneapolis, MN 55477
(612) 553-0020
http://www.ataxia.org

Nonprofit organization with 45 chapters that supports research and offers information and educational programs.

ATTENTION DEFICIT HYPERACTIVITY DISORDER

Attention Deficit Disorder Web site

http://www.ADD.Idsite.com

Web site offering information on ADD, ADHD, ODD, and OCD for parents and teachers of affected children.

Attention Deficit Information Network, Inc.

475 Hillside Avenue
Needham, MA 02194
(781) 455-9895
http://www.addinfonetwork.com

Nonprofit organization that offers support and information to families of children with ADD, adults with ADD, and professionals.

Camps for Children and Adults with Attention Deficit Disorder

499 NW 70th Avenue
Suite 101

Plantation, FL 33317

(954) 587-3700

Call for state-by-state listing of special camps.

Children and Adults with Attention Deficit Disorder (CHADD)

8181 Professional Place

Suite 201

Landover, MD 20785

(301) 306-7070

http://www.chadd.org

Through family support and advocacy, public and professional education, and encouragement of scientific research, CHADD works to ensure that those with ADD reach their inherent potential. Local chapters hold regular meetings providing support and information.

National ADD Association (NADDA)

9930 Johnnycake Ridge Road

Suite 3E

Mentor, OH 44060

(800) 487-2282 (for information packet)

(440) 350-9595

http://www.add.org

National nonprofit organization focusing on needs of adults, young adults, and families with ADD, offering information, resources on treatment and research, as well as workplace, relationship, parenting, and educational information.

One ADD Place Web site

http://www.greatconnect.com/oneaddplace

Web site virtual neighborhood offering information on ADD/ADHD, including articles, products and services, and information on seminars, workshops, and links to other ADD-related Web sites.

AUTISM

Autism Network International

P.O. Box 448

Syracuse, NY 13210

(315) 476-2462

http://www.ani.autistics.org

Self-help group dedicated to supporting people with autism, offering peer support, tips, problem solving, and information and referrals.

Autism Research Institute

4182 Adams Avenue

San Diego, CA 92116

(619) 281-7165

http://www.autism-society.org

Research organization into autism, offering information to families by mail or phone.

Autism Society of America

7910 Woodmont Avenue

Suite 650

Bethesda, MD 20814-3015

(800)-3AUTISM, ext 150

(301)-657-0881

http://www.autism-society.org

A nonprofit organization that seeks to promote lifelong access and opportunities for persons within the autism spectrum and their families, to be fully included, participating members of their communities through advocacy, public awareness, education, and research related to autism.

Families for Early Autism Treatment

P.O. Box 255722

Sacramento , CA 95865

http://www.feat.org

Nonprofit organization of parents and professionals offering support and information.

National Alliance for Autism Research

414 Wall Street, Research Park

Princeton, NJ 08540

(888) 777-NAAR

(609) 430-9160

http://www.babydoc.home.pipeline.com/naar/naar.htm

Nonprofit organization dedicated to research and treatment.

AUTO SAFETY

National Safety Council

1121 Spring Lake Drive

Itasca, IL 60143

(630) 285-1121
http://www.nsc.org

The nation's leading advocate for safety and health, which aims to educate and influence society to adopt safety and health and environmental policies, practices, and procedures. The National Safety Council has been working for generations to protect lives and promote health with innovative programs. The Council is a nonprofit, nongovernmental, international public service organization dedicated to improving the safety, health, and environmental well-being of all people.

BED-WETTING

National Association for Continence (NAFC)
P.O. Box 8310
Spartanburg, SC 29305
(800) BLADDER
(864) 579-7900
http://www.nafc.org/site2/index.html

A national, private, nonprofit organization dedicated to being the leading source for public education and advocacy about the causes, prevention, diagnosis, treatments, and management alternatives for bed-wetting and incontinence.

National Kidney Foundation
30 East 33rd Street
Suite 1100
New York, NY 10016
(800) 622-9010
(212) 889-2210
http://www.kidney.org/misc/contact.cfm

Major voluntary health organization that seeks to prevent kidney and urinary tract diseases, provide information on bed-wetting, improve the health and well-being of individuals and families affected by these diseases, and increase the availability of all organs for transplantation.

BIPOLAR DISORDER
(MANIC DEPRESSION)

Anxiety Disorders Association of America
8730 Georgia Avenue
Suite 600
Silver Spring, MD 20910

(240) 485-1001
http://www.adaa.org

The ADAA promotes the prevention and cure of anxiety disorders and works to improve the lives of all people who suffer from them.

Depression and Bipolar Support Alliance
730 North Franklin Street
Suite 501
Chicago, IL 60610
(800) 826-3632
(312) 642-0049
http://www.dbsalliance.org

The nation's largest patient-directed, illness-specific organization, incorporated in 1986 and based in Chicago, representing the voices of the more than 23 million Americans living with depression and another 2.5 million living with bipolar disorder (manic depression). DBSA was formerly the National Depressive and Manic-Depressive Association.

BIRTH DEFECTS

Association of Birth Defect Children, Inc.
930 Woodcock Road
Suite 225
Orlando, FL 32803
(800) 313-ABDC
(407) 245-7035
http://www.birthdefects.org

A nonprofit organization that provides parents and expectant parents with information about birth defects and support services for their children. ABDC has a parent-matching program that links families who have children with similar birth defects. ABDC also sponsors the National Birth Defect Registry, a research project that studies associations between birth defects and exposures to radiation, medication, alcohol, smoking, chemicals, pesticides, lead, mercury, dioxin, and other environmental toxins.

Children's Craniofacial Association
12200 Park Central Drive
Suite 180
Dallas, TX 75251

(972) 566-5980
(800) 535-3643
http://www.ccakids.com

A nonprofit organization dedicated to improving the quality of life for people with facial differences and their families. CCA addresses the medical, financial, psychosocial, emotional, and educational concerns relating to craniofacial conditions. CCA's mission is to empower and give hope to facially disfigured children and their families. CCA envisions a world where all people are accepted for who they are, not how they look.

March of Dimes Birth Defects Foundation

1275 Mamaroneck Avenue
White Plains, NY 10605
(914) 428-7100
http://www.modimes.org

Nonprofit organization whose mission is to improve the health of babies by preventing birth defects and infant mortality.

BLINDNESS

American Council of the Blind

1155 15th Street, NW
Suite 1004
Washington, DC 20005
(800) 424-8666
(202) 467-5081
http://www.acb.org

The nation's leading membership organization of blind and visually impaired people, founded in 1961. The council strives to improve the well-being of all blind and visually impaired people by: serving as a representative national organization of blind people; elevating the social, economic, and cultural levels of blind people; improving educational and rehabilitation facilities and opportunities; cooperating with the public and private institutions and organizations concerned with blind services; and encouraging and assisting all blind persons to develop their abilities and conducting a public education program to promote greater understanding of blindness and the capabilities of blind people.

American Foundation for the Blind

11 Penn Plaza
Suite 300
New York, NY 10001
(800) AFB-LINE
(212) 502-7600
http://www.afb.org

Since 1921 the American Foundation for the Blind—to which Helen Keller devoted her life—has been eliminating barriers that prevent the 10 million Americans who are blind or visually impaired from reaching their potential. AFB is dedicated to addressing the most critical issues facing this growing population: independent living, literacy, employment, and technology.

Association for Education & Rehabilitation of the Blind & Visually Impaired

4600 Duke Street, #430
P.O. Box 22397
Alexandria, VA 22304
(703) 823-9690
http://www.aerbvi.org

The only international membership organization dedicated to helping professionals in all phases of education and rehabilitation of blind and visually impaired children and adults. It was formed in 1984 as the result of a consolidation between the American Association of Workers for the Blind and the Association for Education of the Visually Handicapped.

Helen Keller Services for the Blind (HKSB)

111 Middle Neck Road
Sands Point, NY 11050
(516) 944-8900
http://www.helenkeller.org

Nonprofit agency with a spectrum of special services that guide legally blind New Yorkers toward a life of independence and success. With its diverse services, HKSB often works one-on-one to teach, educate, and rehabilitate thousands of clients according to their individual needs. Its facilities throughout metropolitan New York serve residents of Brooklyn, Queens, Staten Island, and Nassau and Suffolk Counties. HKSB, founded in 1893 as the Industrial Home for the Blind, is one of the oldest continuously operated rehabilitation agencies in the United States. In 1986 the agency was renamed after Helen Keller.

National Association for the Visually Handicapped
22 West 21st Street
6th Floor
New York, NY 10010
(212) 889-3141

and

3201 Balboa Street
San Francisco, CA 94121
(415) 221-3201
http://www.navh.org

This nonprofit association works with millions of people worldwide coping with difficulties of vision impairment.

National Library Service for the Blind & Physically Handicapped
The Library of Congress
1291 Taylor Street, NW
Washington, DC 20011
(202) 707-5100 (Voice)
(202) 707-0744 (TTY)
http://www.loc.gov/nls

Through a national network of cooperating libraries, NLS administers a free library program of braille and audio materials circulated to eligible borrowers in the United States by postage-free mail.

BLOOD DISORDERS
American Association of Blood Banks
8101 Glenbrook Road
Bethesda, MD 20814-2749
(301) 907-6977
http://www.aabb.org

An international association of blood banks, including hospital and community blood centers, transfusion and transplantation services, and individuals involved in activities related to transfusion and transplantation medicine.

American Society of Hematology
1900 M Street, NW
Suite 200
Washington, DC 20036
(202) 776-0544
http://www.hematology.org

This group is committed to promoting and advancing a diffusion of information relating to the blood and blood diseases.

Leukemia & Lymphoma Society
1311 Mamaroneck Avenue
White Plains, NY 10605
(914) 949-5213
http://www.leukemia.org

The world's largest voluntary health organization dedicated to funding blood cancer research, education, and patient services. The society's mission is to cure leukemia, lymphoma, Hodgkin's disease, and myeloma, and to improve the quality of life of patients and their families. Since its founding in 1949, the society has provided more than $280 million for research specifically targeting blood-related cancers.

National Children's Leukemia Foundation
172 Madison Avenue
New York, NY 10016
(212) 686-2722
(800) GIVE-HOPE (out of state)
http://www.leukemiafoundation.org

One of the leading nonprofit organizations in the fight against leukemia and cancer for children and adults. The NCLF is established to support the unfortunate in various programs, to provide the cure for children and adults, and to ease the family's burden during their hospital stay. The 24-hour hotline (800) GIVE HOPE (800 448-3467) offers comprehensive information to any caller and provides referrals for initial testing, physicians, hospital admissions, and treatment options.

National Heart, Lung, and Blood Institute
NHLBI Health Information Center
Box 30105
Bethesda, MD 20824-0105

(301) 592-8573
(240) 629 3255 (TTY)
http://www.nhlbi.nih.gov

The NHLBI provides leadership for a national program in diseases of the heart, blood vessels, lung, and blood; blood resources; and sleep disorders. Since October 1997 the NHLBI has also had administrative responsibility for the NIH Woman's Health Initiative.

National Hemophilia Foundation

116 West 32nd Street
11th Floor
New York, NY 10001
(800) 42-HANDI
(212) 328-3700
http://www.hemophilia.org

Nonprofit organization established in 1948 to provide advocacy, education, research funds, and information.

Sickle Cell Disease Association of America, Inc.

200 Corporate Pointe
Suite 495
Culver City, CA 90230
(310) 216-6363
(800) 421-8453
http://www.sicklecelldisease.org

National nonprofit association formerly known as the National Association for Sickle Cell Disease (NASCD), founded in 1971 to provide an effective and coordinated community-based approach to sickle cell disease. Through three decades, SCDAA has demonstrated how community-based organizations can work with local and state government agencies to further national health-care objectives.

World Federation of Hemophilia

1425 René Lévesque Boulevard West
Suite 1010
Montréal, Quebec
Canada, H3G 1T7
(514) 875-7944
http://www.wfh.org

This Web site is an international nonprofit organization dedicated to introducing, improving, and maintaining care for persons with hemophilia and related disorders.

BRAIN INJURY/TUMORS

See also CANCER.

American Brain Tumor Association

2720 River Road
Des Moines, IA 60018
(847) 827-9910
(800) 886-2282 (Patient Services)
http://www.abta.org/

A nonprofit, independent organization not affiliated with any institution that serves individuals globally and awards funds to researchers throughout the United States and Canada. The group also offers a wide range of services to the public.

Brain Injury Association

105 North Alfred Street
Alexandria, VA 22314
(703) 236-6000
http://www.biausa.org

Organization offering advocacy, support services, and research.

Children's Brain Tumor Foundation

274 Madison Avenue
Suite 1301
New York, NY 10016
(212) 448-9494
http://www.cbtf.org

Group that seeks to improve treatment and outlook for children with brain and spinal cord tumors through research and treatment, education, and support.

Dana Alliance for Brain Initiatives

745 Fifth Avenue
Suite 700
New York, NY 10151

The Dana Alliance, a nonprofit organization of 150 neuroscientists, was formed to help provide information about the personal and public benefits of brain research.

National Brain Tumor Foundation

785 Market Street
Suite 1600
San Francisco, CA 94103
(415) 284-0208
(800) 934-2873
http://www.braintumor.org

Foundation that offers resources and support, plus research. Affected patients can receive referrals to a network of support groups.

National Institute of Neurological Disorders and Stroke

NIH Neurological Institute
P.O. Box 5801
Bethesda, MD 20824
(800) 352-9424

This federal institute conducts and supports research on many serious diseases affecting the brain.

BREAST-FEEDING

Adoptive Breastfeeding Resource Web site

http://www.fourfriends.com

This site was created in 1997 to serve the growing population of adoptive parents interested in adoptive breast-feeding. The site provides information about adoptive breast-feeding, message boards, profiles, ads, articles, and resources.

La Leche League

1400 North Meacham Road
Schaumburg, IL 60173
(847) 519-7730
http://www.lalecheleague.org/contact.html

La Leche League was founded to give information and encouragement, mainly through personal help, to all mothers who want to breast-feed their babies. While complementing the care of the physician and other health-care professionals, it recognizes the unique importance of one mother helping another to perceive the needs of her child and to learn the best means of fulfilling those needs.

BULIMIA

See EATING DISORDERS.

BURNS

International Shrine Headquarters

2900 Rocky Point Drive
Tampa, FL 33607
(813) 281-0300
(800) 237-5055 (U.S.)
(800) 361-7256 (Canada)
http://www.shrinershq.org

The Shrine of North America is an international fraternity of approximately 500,000 members throughout the United States, Mexico, Canada, and Panama. The Shrine's official philanthropy is Shriners Hospitals for Children, a network of 22 hospitals that provide expert, free orthopedic and burn care to children under 18. To refer a child that Shriners Hospitals might be able to help, call toll-free at the above numbers.

CANCER

Cancer Information Service

MSCC8322
National Cancer Institute, Room 3036A
6116 Executive Boulevard
Bethesda, MD 20892-8322
(800) 422-6237
(800) 332-8615 (TTY)
http://www.cancer.gov

An information service provided by the National Cancer Institute, with experts staffing phones to answer questions from the public about cancer.

Candlelighters Childhood Cancer Foundation

P.O. Box 498
Kensington MD 20895-0498
800-366-2223
(301) 962-3520
http://www.candlelighters.org

A national nonprofit membership organization whose mission is to educate, support, serve, and advocate for families of children with cancer, survivors of childhood cancer, and the professionals who care for them. The foundation was established in 1970 by concerned parents of children with cancer. Members include parents of children who are being treated or have been treated for cancer, children with and childhood survivors of cancer, immediate or extended family members, bereaved families, health-care professionals and educators. Candlelighters is a primary provider of essential programs and services required by families of children with cancer. Families whose children are diagnosed with cancer, who have financial constraints and need these resources, are encouraged to contact Candlelighters.

Childhood Brain Tumor Foundation

20312 Watkins Meadow Drive
Germantown, MD 20876
(301) 515-2900
(877) 217-4166 (toll-free)
http://www.childhoodbraintumor.org

Nonprofit group founded by families, friends, and physicians of children with brain tumors. Our mission is to raise funds for scientific research and heighten public awareness of this most devastating disease and to improve prognosis and quality of life for those that are affected.

Children's Brain Tumor Foundation

274 Madison Avenue
Suite 1301
New York, NY 10016
(212) 448-9494
(866) 228-HOPE (toll-free)
http://www.cbtf.org

The CBTF funds research on pediatric brain tumors and provides resources, newsletters, and a support group for parents.

Children's Oncology Camps of America

7 Richland Medical Park
Suite 203
Columbia, SC 29203
(803) 434-3503
http://www.coca-intl.org/

A listing of approximately 65 camps in the United States and other organizations elsewhere in the world that have camps for cancer kids.

National Childhood Cancer Foundation (NCCF)

440 East Huntington Drive
P.O. Box 60012
Arcadia, CA 91066-6012
(626) 447-1674
and
4600 East West Highway
#600
Bethesda, MD 20814-3457
(800) 458-6223 (U.S. and Canada)
(301) 718-0042
http://www.nccf.org

The foundation supports the work of the most prestigious childhood cancer treatment and research centers in North America, the Children's Oncology Group (COG). COG was formed by the merger of the four national pediatric cancer research organizations: the Children's Cancer Group, the Intergroup Rhabdomyosarcoma Study Group, the National Wilm's Tumor Study Group, and the Pediatric Oncology Group. The organization conducts clinical trials of new therapies for childhood cancer.

National Cancer Institute

NCI Public Inquiries Office
Suite 3036A
6116 Executive Boulevard, MSC8322
Bethesda, MD 20892-8322
http://www.cancer.gov

A component of the National Institutes of Health (NIH), the NCI was established under the National Cancer Act of 1937 as the federal government's principal agency for cancer research and training. The National Cancer Act of 1971 broadened the scope and responsibilities of the NCI and created the National Cancer Program. NCI coordinates the National Cancer Program, which conducts and supports research, training, health information dissemination, and other programs with respect to the cause, diagnosis, prevention, and treatment of cancer, rehabilitation from cancer, and the continuing care of cancer patients and the families of cancer patients.

National Foundation for Children's Pediatric Brain Tumors—Katie's Kids

P.O. Box 650039
Potomac Falls, VA 20165-0039
(877) KTS-KIDS
(703) 430-3813 (local)
http://www.katieskids.org

Katie's Kids' mission is to fund innovative and creative brain tumor research.

Pediatric Brain Tumor Foundation of the United States

302 Ridgefield Court
Asheville, NC 28806
(828) 665-6891
(800) 253-6530
http://www.pbtfus.org

The PBTFUS seeks to find the cause and cure of brain tumors in children by supporting medical research, increasing public awareness of the disease, and aiding in early detection and treatment of childhood brain tumors.

CEREBRAL PALSY

United Cerebral Palsy Association

1522 K Street, NW
Suite 1112
Washington, DC 20005
(800) 872-5827
(202) 776-0406
http://www.ucpa.org

Nonprofit group providing referral services, advocacy, research, and information.

Your Smile

http://wwwcpsmile.org

This Web site discusses dental care for children with cerebral palsy.

CHILD ABUSE AND NEGLECT

Child Abuse Prevention Network

http://wwwchild-abuse.com

The Internet nerve center for professionals in the field of child abuse and neglect, focusing on child maltreatment, physical abuse, psychological maltreatment, neglect, sexual abuse, and emotional abuse and neglect. The group provides unique and powerful tools for all workers to support the identification, investigation, treatment, adjudication, and prevention of child abuse and neglect. Originally launched as an outreach effort of the Family Life Development Center, the Child Abuse Prevention Network is sponsored by LifeNET, Inc.

Childhelp USA National Headquarters

15757 North 78th Street
Scottsdale, Arizona 85260
(480) 422-8212
http://www.childhelpusa.org

Childhelp USA is dedicated to meeting the physical, emotional, educational, and spiritual needs of abused and neglected children.

Child Welfare League

440 First Street, NW
Third Floor
Washington, DC 20001-2085
(202) 638-2952
http://www.cwla.org

An association of almost 1,200 public and private nonprofit agencies that assist more than 3.5 million abused and neglected children and their families each year with a wide range of services.

National Center for Missing and Exploited Children

Charles B. Wang International Children's Building
699 Prince Street
Alexandria, VA 22314
(703) 274-3900
(800) THE-LOST
http://www.missingkids.org

The nation's resource center for child protection, this private, nonprofit center provides help to parents, children, law enforcement, schools, and the community in recovering missing children and raising public awareness about ways to help prevent child abduction, molestation, and sexual exploitation. NCMEC has worked on more than 85,500 cases of missing and exploited children, helped recover more than 68,900 children, and raised its recovery rate from 60 percent in the 1980s to more than 93 percent today, thereby gaining national and international recognition as a major resource for missing and exploited children. The center was founded by John and Reve Walsh, whose six-year-old son Adam was abducted in 1981 and never found.

National Clearinghouse on Child Abuse and Neglect Information

330 C Street, SW
Washington, DC 20447
(800) 394-3366
(703) 385-7565
http://www.calib.com/nccanch

A huge database containing information on child maltreatment and prevention programs.

National Committee for the Prevention of Child Abuse

200 South Michigan Avenue
Suite 950
Chicago IL 60604
(312) 663-3520
(800) 55-NCPCA (for information on specific abuse topics)
http://www.childabuse.org

A nonprofit community of people dedicated to breaking the cycle of child abuse and neglect, serving and strengthening children and families.

National CASA (Court Appointed Special Advocate) Association

100 West Harrison
North Tower Suite 500
Seattle WA 98119
(800) 628-3233
http://www.nationalcasa.org

National nonprofit organization of trained community volunteers who speak for the best interests of abused and neglected children in court. The group began when a Seattle judge became concerned over making decisions about abused and neglected children's lives without sufficient information; soon judges across the country began using citizen advocates. In 1990 the U.S. Congress encouraged the expansion of CASA with passage of the Victims of Child Abuse Act. Today there are more than 900 CASA programs with 62,000 women and men serving as CASA volunteers. In addition to providing leadership for CASA programs across the country, the National CASA Association stages an annual conference, publishes a quarterly newsletter, and promotes CASA through public relations efforts.

Nation's Missing Children Organization

2432 West Peoria Avenue
Suite 1283
Phoenix, AZ 85029
(602) 944-1768
(800) 690-FIND
http://www.nmco.org

Nonprofit organization that offers a range of services to help missing and abused children.

Parents Anonymous

6733 South Sepulveda Boulevard
#270
Los Angeles, CA 90048
(800) 352-0386

Serves abusive parents. Call for nearest office.

CLEFT PALATE

AboutFace International

123 Edward Street
Suite 1003
Toronto, Ont. M5G 1E2 Canada
(800) 665-3223
http://www.aboutfaceinternational.org

AboutFace is an international organization that provides information and emotional support to individuals with facial differences and their families.

American Cleft Palate–Craniofacial Association

104 South Estes Drive
Suite 204
Chapel Hill, NC 27514
(919) 933-9044

(800) 24-CLEFT
http://www.cleftline.org

The ACPA is an international nonprofit association of more than 2,500 health-care professionals who are involved in the treatment and/or research of cleft lip, cleft palate, and other craniofacial anomalies.

Cleft Palate Foundation
104 South Estes Drive
Suite 204
Chapel Hill, NC 27514
(919) 933-9044
(800) 24-CLEFT
http://www.cleftline.org

A nonprofit organization dedicated to helping children affected by facial birth defects. Founded by the American Cleft Palate-Craniofacial Association in 1973, it is the public service arm of the professional association. CPF operates the CLEFTLINE, a toll-free service providing information to callers about clefts and other craniofacial anomalies. Callers can request information about cleft palate/craniofacial teams and parent-patient support groups in their local region. CPF also awards annual research grants to support investigation into the causes and treatments of facial birth defects.

Prescription Parents
45 Brentwood Circle
Needham, MA 02492
http://www.samizdat.com/pp1.html

Prescription Parents, a member of the National Cleft Palate Association, has a Web site for parents with information about cleft lip and palate and how to find or start a support group.

Wide Smiles
P.O. Box 5153
Stockton, CA 95205
(209) 942-2812
http://www.widesmiles.org

Wide Smiles offers support, inspiration, information, and networking for families dealing with the challenges associated with oral clefting.

COLITIS

Crohn's Colitis Foundation of America
386 Park Avenue South
17th Floor
New York, NY 10016
(800) 932-2423
http://www.ccfa.org

CCFA's mission is to cure and prevent Crohn's disease and ulcerative colitis through research, and to improve the quality of life of children and adults affected by these digestive diseases through education and support.

COMMUNICATION

See also DEAFNESS/HEARING LOSS; STUTTERING.

American Speech-Language-Hearing Association (ASHA)
10801 Rockville Pike
Rockville, MD 20852
(800) 498-2071 (voice)
301-897-5700 (TTY)
http://www.asha.org

Membership organization comprised of speech/language pathologists and audiologists that provides information and referrals to the public on speech, language, communication, and hearing disorders.

National Information Clearinghouse on Children Who Are Deaf-Blind
345 North Monmouth Avenue
Monmouth, OR 97361
(800) 438-9376 (voice)
(800) 854-7013 (TTY)
http://www.tr.wou.edu/dblink/

A federally funded information and referral service that identifies, coordinates, and disseminates free information related to children and youth who are deaf-blind (ages 0 to 21 years). Four organizations have pooled their expertise into a consortium-based clearinghouse, including American Association of the Deaf-Blind, Helen Keller National Center, and the Perkins School for the Blind.

National Institute on Deafness and Other Communication Disorders

Information Clearinghouse
1 Communication Avenue
Bethesda MD 20892-3456
(800) 241-1044
241-1055 (TTY)
http://www.nidcd.nih.gov

Part of the National Institutes of Health, NIDCD was established in 1988 and mandated to support biomedical and behavioral research and research training in the normal and disordered processes of hearing, balance, smell, taste, voice, speech, and language. The institute also supports research and training related to disease prevention and health promotion; addresses special biomedical and behavioral problems associated with people who have communication impairments or disorders; and supports efforts to create devices which substitute for lost and impaired sensory and communication function.

National Stuttering Association

4071 East La Palma Avenue
Suite A
Anaheim Hills, CA 92807
(800) 364-1677
(714) 630-7600
http://www.westutter.org

The nation's largest self-help organization for people who stutter.

CONSUMER PRODUCTS SAFETY

U.S. Consumer Product Safety Commission

4330 East-West Highway
Bethesda, Maryland 20814-4408
(301) 504-6816
800-638-2772 (consumer hotline: call to obtain product safety information and to report unsafe products, 24 hours a day, 7 days a week)
http://www.cpsc.gov

CPSC was created in 1972 by Congress under the Consumer Product Safety Act and began operating in 1973. CPSC is an independent federal regulatory agency that works to save lives and keep families safe by reducing the risk of injuries and deaths associated with consumer products. They do this by developing voluntary standards with industry, enforcing mandatory standards or banning consumer products, recalling products or arranging for their repair, conducting research on potential product hazards, informing and educating consumers.

CRANIOFACIAL PROBLEMS

American Cleft Palate–Craniofacial Association

104 South Estes Drive
Suite 204
Chapel Hill, NC 27514
(919) 933-9044
(800) 24-CLEFT
http://www.cleftline.org

The ACPA is an international nonprofit association of more than 2,500 health-care professionals who are involved in the treatment and/or research of cleft lip, cleft palate, and other craniofacial anomalies.

Children's Craniofacial Association

12200 Park Central Drive
Suite 180
Dallas, TX 75251
(972) 566-5980
(800) 535-3643
http://www.ccakids.com

A nonprofit organization dedicated to improving the quality of life for people with facial differences and their families. CCA addresses the medical, financial, psychosocial, emotional, and educational concerns relating to craniofacial conditions. CCA's mission is to empower and give hope to facially disfigured children and their families. CCA envisions a world where all people are accepted for who they are, not how they look.

FACES: The National Craniofacial Association

P.O. Box 11082
Chattanooga, TN 37401
(800) 332-2372

(423) 266-1632
http://www.faces-cranio.org

For 34 years, this nonprofit association has helped children with craniofacial disorders resulting from disease, accident, or birth. FACES provides resource files of specialized craniofacial centers and other relevant resources; financial aid to those needing to travel away from home for medical assistance; quarterly newsletters providing human interest stories as well as the latest research and information on craniofacial disorders.

Let's Face It USA
P.O. Box 29972
Bellingham, WA 98228-1972
(360) 676-7325
http://www.faceit.org

Nonprofit organization that can provide information and support on facial differences.

CRI DU CHAT SYNDROME

5p-Society
7108 Katella Avenue
#502
Stanton, CA 90680
(888) 970-0777
http://www.fivepminus.org

A nonprofit parent support group for families with a child who has 5p-syndrome, also known as cri du chat syndrome or cat cry syndrome. The organization tries to encourage communication among affected families and to educate others about the syndrome. The society was founded in 1986 by parents of children with 5p-syndrome.

CYSTIC FIBROSIS

Cystic Fibrosis Foundation
6931 Arlington Road
Bethesda, MD 20814
(800) 344-4823
http://www.cff.org

A nonprofit foundation established in 1955 to assure the cure and control of cystic fibrosis and to improve the quality of life for those with the dis-

ease. The foundation supports care centers and research, funds its own research centers, develops drugs, and supports a centralized lab.

DEAFNESS/HEARING LOSS

Alexander Graham Bell Association for the Deaf, Inc.
3417 Volta Place, NW
Washington, DC 20007
(202) 337-5220
http://www.agbell.org

An international membership organization and resource center on hearing loss and spoken language approaches and related issues. Founded in 1890 by Alexander Graham Bell, the association offers members a wide range of programs and services and provides information to all inquirers on a vast array of issues pertaining to hearing loss. The association's strength is in its diverse, collaborative membership of parents of children with hearing loss, educators, adults with hearing loss, and hearing health professionals.

American Society for Deaf Children
P.O. Box 3355
Gettysburg, PA 17325
(800) 942-2732 (voice/TTY)
(717) 334-7922 (T/TTY)
http://www.deafchildren.org

A nonprofit organization furthering the services of the International Association of Parents of the Deaf. ASDC was founded in 1967 as a parent-helping-parent organization; today it provides support, encouragement, and information to families raising children who are deaf or hard of hearing. ASDC supplies the information and support families request to ensure that their decisions and actions are based on up-to-date and accurate knowledge, and promotes a positive attitude toward signing and deaf culture.

Laurent Clerc National Deaf Education Center and Clearinghouse
KDES PAS-6, Gallaudet University
800 Florida Avenue, NE
Washington, DC 20002-3695

(202) 651-5051 (voice)
(202) 651-5052 (TT)
http://wwwclerccenter.gallaudet.edu

The Clerc Center has been mandated by Congress to develop, evaluate, and disseminate innovative curricula, instructional techniques and strategies, and materials. The aim of the Clerc Center is to improve the quality of education for deaf and hard of hearing children and youth from birth through age 21.The Center includes the Kendall Demonstration Elementary School and the Model Secondary School for the Deaf.

National Association of the Deaf

814 Thayer Avenue
Suite 250
Silver Spring, MD 20910
(301) 587-1788
(301) 587-1789 (TTY)
http://www.nad.org

The oldest and largest nonprofit organization safeguarding the accessibility and civil rights of 28 million deaf and hard-of-hearing Americans in education, employment, health care, and telecommunications. Programs and activities include grassroots advocacy and empowerment, captioned media, certification of American Sign Language professionals, certification of sign language interpreters, deafness-related information and publications, legal assistance, policy development and research, public awareness, and youth leadership development.

National Information Clearinghouse on Children Who Are Deaf-Blind

345 North Monmouth Avenue
Monmouth, OR 97361
(800) 438-9376 (voice)
(800) 854-7013 (TTY)
http://www.tr.wou.edu/dblink/

A federally funded information and referral service that identifies, coordinates, and disseminates free information related to children and youth who are deaf-blind (ages 0 to 21 years). Four organizations have pooled their expertise into a consortium-based clearinghouse, including American Association of the Deaf-Blind, Helen

Keller National Center, and the Perkins School for the Blind.

National Institute on Deafness and Other Communication Disorders

Clearinghouse
One Communication Avenue
Bethesda, MD 20892-3456
(800) 241-1044 (voice)
(800) 241-1055 (TT)
http://www.nidcd.nih.gov

Part of the National Institutes of Health, NIDCD was established in 1988 and mandated to support biomedical and behavioral research and research training in the normal and disordered processes of hearing, balance, smell, taste, voice, speech, and language. The institute also supports research and training related to disease prevention and health promotion; addresses special biomedical and behavioral problems associated with people who have communication impairments or disorders; and supports efforts to create devices which substitute for lost and impaired sensory and communication function.

Registry of Interpreters for the Deaf

333 Commerce Street
Alexandria, VA 22314
(703) 838-0030
(703) 838-0459 (TTY)
http://www.rid.org

A national membership organization of professionals who provide sign language interpreting/transliterating services for deaf and hard of hearing persons. Established in 1964 and incorporated in 1973, RID advocates for the increased quality, qualifications, and quantity of interpreters.

Self Help for Hard of Hearing People (SHHH)

7910 Woodmont Avenue
Suite 1200
Bethesda, MD 20814
(301) 657-2248 (voice)
(301) 657-2249 (TT)
http://www.shhh.org

The nation's foremost association representing 26 million people who are hard of hearing, enhancing their quality of life. SHHH was founded in 1979 as a consumer educational organization devoted to the welfare and interests of those who cannot hear well, their relatives, and friends. SHHH has 12,000 national members and 9,000 chapter members in all 50 states. As the voice for hard of hearing people, SHHH strives to improve the quality of hard of hearing people's lives through education, advocacy, and self-help.

DEATH AND DYING

Candlelighters Childhood Cancer Foundation

P.O. Box 498
Kensington, MD 20895
(301) 962-3520
(800) 366-2223
http://www.candlelighters.org

A national nonprofit membership organization whose mission is to educate, support, serve, and advocate for families of children with cancer, survivors of childhood cancer, and the professionals who care for them. The foundation was established in 1970 by concerned parents of children with cancer. Members include parents of children who are being treated or have been treated for cancer, children with and childhood survivors of cancer, immediate or extended family members, bereaved families, health-care professionals and educators. Candlelighters is a primary provider of essential programs and services required by families of children with cancer. Families whose children are diagnosed with cancer, who have financial constraints, and need these resources are encouraged to contact Candlelighters.

Children's Hospice International

901 North Pitt Street
Suite 230
Alexandria, VA 22314
(800) 2-4 CHILD
(703) 684-0330
http://www.chionline.org

A nonprofit organization was founded in 1983 to provide a network of support for children with life-threatening conditions. The hospice approach for children is a team effort that provides medical, psychological, social, and spiritual expertise and information in the United States and abroad. CHI is committed to the concept of care called "hospice," and recognizes the right and need for children and their families to choose health care and support whether in their own home, hospital, or hospice care facility.

Compassionate Friends, Inc.

P.O. Box 3696
Oak Brook, IL 60522
(630) 990-0010
(877) 969-0010 (toll-free)
http://www.compassionatefriends.org

A national nonprofit, self-help support organization that offers friendship and understanding to bereaved parents, grandparents, and siblings. There is no religious affiliation and there are no membership dues or fees.

DENTAL PROBLEMS

American Academy of Pediatric Dentistry

211 East Chicago Avenue
#700
Chicago, IL 60611-2663
(312) 337-2169
http://www.aapd.org

National professional organization for pediatric dentists.

American Dental Association

211 East Chicago Avenue
Chicago, IL 60611
(312) 440-2500
http://www.ada.org

The ADA provides information for dental patients and consumers.

Your Smile Web site

http://wwwcpsmile.org

This Web site discusses dental care for children with cerebral palsy.

DEPRESSION

See also POSTPARTUM DEPRESSION.

Anxiety Disorders Association of America

8730 Georgia Avenue
Suite 600
Silver Spring, MD 20910
(240) 485-1001
http://www.adaa.org

The ADAA promotes the prevention and cure of anxiety disorders and works to improve the lives of all people who suffer from them.

Depression and Bipolar Support Alliance

730 North Franklin Street
Suite 501
Chicago, Illinois 60610
(800) 826-3632
(312) 642-0049
http://www.dbsalliance.org

The nation's largest patient-directed, illness-specific organization, incorporated in 1986 and based in Chicago, representing the voices of the more than 23 million Americans living with depression and another 2.5 million living with bipolar disorder (manic depression). DBSA was formerly the National Depressive and Manic-Depressive Association.

DEVELOPMENTAL DISABILITIES

See also DOWN SYNDROME; FRAGILE X SYNDROME.

American Association of University Affiliated Programs for Persons with Developmental Disabilities

8630 Fenton Street
Suite 410
Silver Spring, MD 20910
(301) 588-8252
http://www.aauap.org

National association with sites at major universities and teaching hospitals that support the independence, integration, and inclusion of people with developmental disabilities and their families.

American Association on Mental Retardation

444 North Capitol Street, NW
Suite 846
Washington, DC 20001
(800) 424-3688
(202) 387-1968
http://www.aamr.org

National organization providing information, services, and support, plus advocacy.

Arc (formerly Association for Retarded Citizens)

500 East Border Street
Suite 300
Arlington, TX 76010
(800) 433-5255
(817) 261-6003
http://www.thearc.org

Volunteer organization committed to the welfare of all children and adults with mental retardation, offering information, books, and an annual conference.

Federation for Children with Special Needs

1135 Tremont Street
Suite 420
Boston, MA 02120
(617) 236-7210
(800) 331-0688
http://www.fcsn.org

A center for parents and organizations to work together on behalf of children with special needs and their families. Organized in 1975 as a coalition of parent groups representing children with a variety of disabilities, the federation operates a parent center in Massachusetts. The federation provides information, support, and assistance to parents of children with disabilities, their professional partners, and their communities.

National Fragile X Foundation

P.O. Box 190488
San Francisco, CA 94119
(800) 688-8765
(925) 938-9300
http://www.nfxf.org

Nonprofit organization that provides advocacy, consultation, information, research, newsletters, referrals, and education.

National Information Center for Children and Youth with Disabilities

P.O. Box 1492
Washington, DC 20013
(800) 695-0285 (voice/TTY)
(202) 884-8200 (voice/TTY)
http://www.nichcy.org/

The national information center that provides information on disabilities and disability-related issues. With a special focus is children and youth (birth to age 22), the Web site can provide information about specific disabilities, special education, and related services for children in school, individualized education programs, parent materials, disability organizations, professional associations, education rights, early intervention services for infants and toddlers, and transition to adult life.

National Institute for People with Disabilities

460 West 34th Street
New York, NY 10001
(212) 563-7474
http://www.yai.org

Nonprofit agency serving children and adults with developmental disabilities in New York, including information and referrals.

National Institute on Disability and Rehabilitative Research

Switzer Building
330 C Street, SW
Suite 3060 MES
Washington, DC 20202
(202) 205-8134
http://www.ed.gov/offices/OSERS/NIDRR/
nidrr.html

NIDRR conducts research and administers ADA technical assistance centers.

Office of Special Education and Rehabilitation Services

Switzer Building
330 C Street SW
Suite 3006
Washington, DC 20202

(202) 205-5465
http://www.ed.gov/offices/OSERS

Office supports programs that help in educating children with special needs and supports research. OSERS includes the Office of Special Education Programs, Rehabilitation Services Administration, and the National Institute on Disability and Rehabilitation Research.

Office of Special Education Programs

Switzer Building
330 C Street, SW
Suite 3086
Washington, DC 20202
(202) 205-5507

The OESP administers programs relating to education of all children, youth, and adults with disabilities through age 22.

Parents Helping Parents: The Parent-Directed Family Resource Center for Children with Special Needs

3041 Olcott Street
Santa Clara, CA 95054
(408) 727-5775
http://www.php.com

Founded by parents of children with special needs in 1976, PHP is one of the oldest and largest children's charities of its kind in the United States. Internationally, PHP is the leading consultation and assistance agency for others starting or operating parent-directed family resource centers.

Rehabilitation Services Administration

Switzer Building
330 C Street, SW
Suite 3026
Washington, DC 20202
(202) 205-5482
http://www.ed.gov/offices/OSERS/RSA/
rsa.html

RSA guides programs that help those with physical or mental disabilities get hired by providing counseling, health services, job training, and other support.

Special Olympics International

1325 G Street, NW
Suite 500
Washington, DC 20005
(202) 628-3630
http://www.specialolympics.org

The parent organization that administers the Special Olympics.

Voice of the Retarded

5005 Newport Drive
Suite 108
Rolling Meadows, IL 60008
(847) 253-6020

Organization that provides support, information, and advocacy with a large collection of research files.

DIABETES

American Diabetes Association

1660 Duke Street
Alexandria, VA 22314
(800) 232-3472
(703) 549-1500
http://www.diabetes.org

The nation's leading nonprofit health organization providing diabetes research, information, and advocacy. The ADA funds research, publishes scientific findings, and provides information and other services to people with diabetes, their families, healthcare professionals, and the public, and advocates for scientific research and for the rights of people with diabetes.

Juvenile Diabetes Research Foundation International

120 Wall Street
New York, NY 10005-4001
(800) 533-CURE
(212) 785-9500
http://www.jdf.org

The leading charitable funder and advocate of juvenile (type 1) diabetes research worldwide. The mission of JDRF is to find a cure for diabetes and its complications through the support of research.

National Diabetes Information Clearinghouse

One Information Way
Bethesda MD 20892
(301) 654-3327
http://www.niddk.nih.gov

Government organization that supports information and research into the care and treatment of diabetes.

National Institute of Diabetes and Digestive and Kidney Diseases

Information Clearinghouse
Three Information Way
Bethesda, MD 20892
(301) 654-4415
http://www.niddk.nih.gov

This federal institute conducts and supports research on many serious diseases affecting digestion and kidneys and on diabetes.

DIGESTIVE DISEASES

National Digestive Diseases Information Clearinghouse

Two Information Way
Bethesda, MD 20892
(301) 654-3327
http://www.niddk.nih.gov/health/digest/
nddic.htm

Federal clearinghouse that provides information on digestive diseases.

DISABILITIES

American Association of People with Disabilities

1819 H Street, NW
Suite 330
Washington, DC 20006
(800) 840-8844
(800) 235-7125
http://www.aapd-dc.org

Organization offering information and support for full implementation and enforcement of disability nondiscrimination laws.

Association for the Severely Handicapped

29 West Susquehanna Avenue
Suite 210
Baltimore, MD 21204
(410) 828-8274
http://www.tash.org

An international advocacy association of people with disabilities, their families, and others, with 38 chapters throughout the world. It actively promotes the full inclusion and participation of those with disabilities and seeks to eliminate physical and social obstacles that interfere with quality of life.

Association on Higher Education and Disability (AHEAD)

University of Massachusetts/Boston
100 Morrissey Boulevard
Boston, MA 02125-3393
(617) 287-3880
http://www.ahead.org

International, multicultural organization of professionals committed to full participation in higher education for persons with disabilities.

Children's Defense Fund

25 E Street, NW
Washington, DC 20001
(202) 628-8787
http://www.childrensdefense.org

A nonprofit research and advocacy organization that provides a strong voice for children who cannot speak for themselves, including children with disabilities. The organization has regional offices throughout the country.

Commission on Mental and Physical Disability Law

American Bar Association
740 15th Street, NW
Washington, DC 20005
(202) 662-1570
http://www.abanet.org/disability/home.html

This ABA-affiliated group is committed to justice for those with physical disabilities and maintains resources and references for helping the disability community.

Disability Rights Education and Defense Fund, Inc.

2212 Sixth Street
Berkeley, CA 94710
(510) 644-2555
http://www.dredf.org

A national law and policy center dedicated to protecting and helping people with disabilities through legislation, litigation, advocacy, technical help, and education.

Council for Exceptional Children

1110 North Glebe Road
Suite 300
Arlington, VA 22201
(703) 620-3360
(866) 915-5000 (TTY)
http://www.cec.sped.org/

A nonprofit association dedicated to aiding individuals with exceptionalities, students with disabilities, and gifted students. CEC provides opportunities for professional development, maintains 17 divisions offering specialized information, and publishes numerous journals and newsletters covering classroom techniques, government policies, and research. The council also sponsors conventions and conferences. Its misssion is to improve educational outcomes for indiviuals with exceptionalities. Founded in 1922.

Family Center for Technology and Disabilities

Academy for Educational Development (AED)
1825 Connecticut Avenue, NW
7th Floor
Washington, DC 20009-5721
(202) 884-8068
http://www.fctd.info

A resource designed to support organizations and programs that work with families of children and youth with disabilities, offering a range of information and services on the subject of assistive technologies.

Family Resource Center on Disabilities

Room 300
20 East Jackson Boulevard
Chicago, IL 60604
(800) 952-4199
(312) 939-3513

Coalition of parents, professionals, and volunteers dedicated to improving services for all children with disabilities.

National Association of Protection and Advocacy Systems

900 Second Street, NE
Suite 211
Washington, DC 20002
(202) 408-9514
http://www.protectionandadvocacy.com/
   napas.htm

A national membership organization for the federally mandated nationwide network of disability rights agencies, protection and advocacy systems, and client assistance programs.

National Clearinghouse on Women and Girls with Disabilities

114 East 32nd Street
Suite 701
New York, NY 10016
(212) 725-1803
http://www.onisland.com/eec

Clearinghouse that provides catalog of manuals, supplements, videos, and directories, many of which deal with sexual issues faced by women and girls with disabilities.

National Easter Seal Society

230 West Monroe Street
Suite 1800
Chicago, IL 60606
(800) 221-6827
(312) 726-6200
http://www.easter-seals.org

A nonprofit organization that has been helping individuals with disabilities and special needs and their families live better lives for more than 80 years. Whether helping someone improve physically or simply gain greater independence for everyday living, Easter Seals offers a variety of services to help people with disabilities address life's challenges and achieve personal goals.

National Information Center for Children and Youth with Disabilities

1875 Connecticut Avenue
8th floor
Washington, DC 20009
(800) 695-0285
http://www.aed.org/nichcy

An information clearinghouse that provides free information on disabilities and disability-related issues.

National Information Center for Children and Youth with Disabilities

P.O. Box 1492
Washington, DC 20013
(800) 695-0285
http://www.nichcy.org

Information clearinghouse that provides free information on disabilities and related issues, focusing on children and youth (birth to age 25). Free services include: personal responses, referrals, technical assistance, and information searches.

National Institute on Disability and Rehabilitative Research

Switzer Building
330 C Street, SW
Suite 3060 MES
Washington, DC 20202
(202) 205-8134
http://www.ed.gov/offices/OSERS/NIDRR/
   nidrr.html

NIDRR conducts research and administers ADA technical assistance centers.

National Library Service for the Blind and Physically Handicapped

500 East Remington Road
Suite 200
Schaumburg,IL 60173
(800) 331-2020

(800) 221-3004
(708) 843-2020

Voice mail system. Operators provide information on audiocassette, large print, and Braille books and magazines. Callers with learning disabilities must meet certain guidelines to use these services.

National Organization on Disability
910 16th Street, NW
Suite 600
Washington, DC 20006
(202) 293-5960
http://www.nod.org

National disability network group concerned with all disabilities of all ages.

National Parent Network on Disabilities
1130 17th Street, NW
Suite 400
Washington, DC 20036
(202) 434-8686
http://www.npnd.org

Membership advocacy organization open to all agencies, organizations, parent centers, parent groups, professionals, and individuals concerned with the quality of life for people with disabilities. Provides weekly e-mail newsletter with legislative news and more.

Protection and Advocacy
100 Howe Avenue
Suite 185-N
Sacramento, CA 95825
(800) 776-5746
http://www.pai-ca.org

Nonprofit agency that provides legal assistance to those with physical, developmental, and psychiatric disabilities. Services include information and referral to other help, peer and self-advocacy training, representation in administrative and judicial proceedings, investigation of abuse and neglect, and legislative advocacy.

Sibling Support Project
P.O. Box 5371 CL-09
Children's Hospital and Medical Center
Seattle, WA 98105

(206) 368-0371
http://www.chmc.org/department/sibsupp/
  default.htm

National program dedicated to interests of brothers and sisters of those with special health and developmental needs.

World Institute on Disability
510 16th Street
Suite 100
Oakland, CA 94612
(510) 763-4100
http://www.wid.org

Nonprofit public policy center dedicated to independence and inclusion of people with disabilities.

DIVORCE

Academy of Family Mediators
1500 South Highway 100
Suite 355
Golden Valley, MN 55416
(612) 525-8670

This organization helps families locate family mediators.

Children's Rights Council
6200 Editors Park Drive
Suite 103
Hyattsville, MD 20782
http://www.gocrc.com

Local chapters of the Children's Rights Council throughout the country deal with custody issues and divorce reform.

Divorce Online
NHLBI Information Center
P.O. Box 30105
Bethesda, MD 20824-0105
http://www.divorceonline.com

Divorce Online is for people involved in, or facing the prospect of, divorce.

Joint Custody Association
10606 Wilkins Avenue
Los Angeles, CA 90024
(310) 475-5352

This organization provides detailed information about joint custody.

Parents Without Partners
9907 Colesville Road
Silver Spring, MD 20910
(800) 647-7974
http://www.parentswithoutpartners.org

Parents Without Partners provides single parents and their children with an opportunity for enhancing personal growth, self-confidence, and sensitivity toward others by offering an environment for support, friendship, and the exchange of parenting techniques.

Stepfamily Foundation, Inc.
333 West End Avenue
New York, NY 10023
(212) 877-3244
http://www.stepfamily.org

Organization provides counseling, on the telephone and in person, and information to create a successful step relationship. Founded in 1975, the Stepfamily Foundation provides the vital training, information, and counseling to avoid the pitfalls which often stress these relationships.

DOMESTIC VIOLENCE

National Coalition Against Domestic Violence
P.O. Box 18749
Denver, CO 80218
(303) 839-1852
http://www.ncadv.org

A national information and referral center for the general public, media, battered women and their children, allied and member agencies and organizations. NCADV was formally organized in January 1978 when 100 battered women's advocates from all parts of the nation attended the U.S. Commission on Civil Rights hearing on battered women in Washington, DC, hoping to address common problems these programs usually faced in isolation. NCADV remains the only national organization of grassroots shelter and service programs for battered women. It is dedicated to the empowerment of battered women and their children and therefore is committed to the elimination of personal and societal violence in the lives of battered women and their children.

National CASA (Court Appointed Special Advocate) Association
100 West Harrison
North Tower Suite 500
Seattle, WA 98119
(800) 628-3233
http://www.nationalcasa.org

National nonprofit organization of trained community volunteers who speak for the best interests of abused and neglected children in court. The group began when a Seattle judge became concerned over making decisions about abused and neglected children's lives without sufficient information; soon judges across the country began using citizen advocates. In 1990 the U.S. Congress encouraged the expansion of CASA with passage of the Victims of Child Abuse Act. Today there are more than 900 CASA programs with 62,000 women and men serving as CASA volunteers. In addition to providing leadership for CASA programs across the country, the National CASA Association stages an annual conference, publishes a quarterly newsletter, and promotes CASA through public relations efforts.

National Domestic Violence Hotline
P.O. Box 161810
Austin, Texas 78716
(800) 799-SAFE (hotline)
(800) 787-3224 (TTY)
http://www.ndvh.org

Established by the Violence Against Women Act (VAWA) of 1994, featuring a database of more than 4,000 shelters and service providers across the United States, Puerto Rico, Alaska, Hawaii, and the U.S. Virgin Islands. The hotline provides information and is capable of setting up conference calls between battered women and their nearest shelter. Bilingual staff and a language line are available for non-English speakers.

DOWN SYNDROME

See also DEVELOPMENTAL DISABILITIES.

International Resource Center for Down Syndrome
1621 Euclid Avenue
Suite 514
Cleveland, OH 44115

(216) 621-5858
(800) 899-3039

Center provides research, information, education, and parental support.

National Down Syndrome Congress

1605 Chantilly Drive, NE
Suite 250
Atlanta, GA 30324
(800) 232-NDSC
(404) 633-1555
www.ndsccenter.org

National advocacy organization for Down syndrome, offering research, education, and resources.

National Down Syndrome Society

666 Broadway
Suite 810
New York, NY 10012
(800) 221-4602
(212) 460-9330
http://www.ndss.org

National organization that sponsors research and offers support, resources, information, and advocacy.

DRUG ABUSE

National Clearinghouse for Alcohol and Drug Information (NCADI)

P.O. Box 2345
Rockville, MD 20847-2345
(800) 729-6686
(877) 767-8432 (español)
(301) 468-2600
(800) 487-4899 (TTY)
http://www.health.org

The world's largest resource for current information and materials concerning alcohol and substance abuse prevention, intervention, and treatment. NCADI is a service of the Center for Substance Abuse Prevention and offers a wide variety of free services, including NCADI Information Services Department, The NCADI Library, and Prevention Pipeline.

DYSLEXIA

Hello Friend/Ennis William Cosby Foundation

Ennis William Cosby Foundation
P. O. Box 4061
Santa Monica, CA 90411
http://www.hellofriend.org

Nonprofit foundation dedicated to dyslexia resources and information for parents, students, and educators established by Drs. William H. and Camille O. Cosby in memory of their son Ennis. Ennis's common greeting, "Hello, Friend," inspired the name of the foundation. The foundation, formed in early 1997, is dedicated to being a friend to all people with dyslexia and language-based learning differences, recognizing and celebrating their gifts, opening the doors of learning to them, and helping them to reach their full potential. This foundation promotes: early recognition, compassionate understanding, and effective education.

The International Dyslexia Association (IDA)

Chester Building
8600 LaSalle Road
Suite 382
Baltimore, MD 21286-2044
(800) ABC-D123 (general information)
(410) 296-0232 (detailed information)
http://www.interdys.org

With 11,000 members in 45 branches around the world, IDA offers an international network that brings professionals in the field of dyslexia and parents together for a common purpose. The group offers informational meetings and support groups, referrals, journals, and publications regarding dyslexia.

Learning Disabilities Association

4156 Library Road
Pittsburgh, PA 15234
(412) 341-1515
http://www.ldanatl.org

The largest nonprofit volunteer organization for children with learning disabilities, with nearly 300 state and local affiliates in 50 states and Puerto

Rico. The association was formed in 1964 by a group of concerned parents on behalf of children with learning disabilities. LDA is devoted to defining and finding solutions for the broad spectrum of learning disabilities.

National Center for Learning Disabilities

381 Park Avenue South
Suite 1401
New York, NY 10016
(212) 545-7510 (toll-free)
(888) 575-7373
http://www.ncld.org

Develops training and educational materials for parents and practitioners including Every Child Is Learning, a training program to help preschool teachers and parents recognize the early warning signs of learning disabilities. NCLD provides national information and referrals, education, advocacy, quarterly newsletters, state-by-state resources, and videos about learning disabilities.

Recording for the Blind and Dyslexic, Inc.

20 Roszel Road
Princeton, NJ 08540
(800) 221-4792
(800) 803-7201
(609) 452-0606
http://www.rfbd.org

Operators provide information on more than 80,000 recorded textbooks and other classroom materials, from fourth grade through postgraduate levels, available for loan. Callers with learning disabilities are eligible to participate but must complete the certification requirements.

EATING DISORDERS

National Association of Anorexia Nervosa and Associated Disorders

P.O. Box 7
Highland Park, IL 60035
(847) 831-3438
http://www.anad.org

The oldest national nonprofit organization helping eating disorder victims and their families. In addition to its free hotline counseling, ANAD operates an international network of support groups for sufferers and families, and offers referrals to health-care professionals who treat eating disorders across the United States and in 15 other countries. ANAD publishes a quarterly newsletter and sends information packets customized to individual needs. It also provides speakers, programs, and presentations for schools, colleges, public health agencies, and community groups, and sponsors internships, organizes national conferences and local programs, and works to educate the general public. The association also promotes and develops research projects, fights insurance discrimination and dangerous advertising, and organizes advocacy campaigns to protect potential victims of eating disorders.

National Eating Disorders Association (formerly Eating Disorders Awareness and Prevention)

603 Stewart Street
Suite 803
Seattle, WA 98101
(800) 931-2237
(206) 382-3587
http://www.nationaleatingdisorders.org

Nonprofit organization dedicated to the prevention and treatment of eating disorders. The National Eating Disorders Association was founded in 2001, when Eating Disorders Awareness & Prevention (EDAP) joined forces with the American Anorexia Bulimia Association (AABA) to create the largest eating disorders prevention and advocacy organization in the world. Each organization has contributed years of valuable experience, unique programming, and the commitment of the field's most renowned clinicians, educators, and researchers to create a unified force in the fight against eating disorders. Headquartered in Seattle, Washington, with an office in New York, the National Eating Disorders Association is dedicated to eliminating eating disorders and body dissatisfaction. Through education, advocacy, and research the association serves as a national authority on eating disorders and related concerns and as a source for individuals with eating disorders, their loved ones, and their caregivers, promoting social attitudes that enhance healthy body image, and works to overcome the idealization of thinness that contributes to disordered eating.

EDUCATION

Department of Education
400 Maryland Avenue, SW
Washington, DC 20202
(800) USA-LEARN
http://www.ed.gov

Department administers more than 200 programs involving education.

Comprehensive Regional Assistance Centers

Sponsored by the U.S. Department of Education, the 15 Comprehensive Centers are part of an emerging network of organizations that support and assist states, districts, and schools in meeting the needs of children served under the Improving Americas Schools Act (1994).

HEATH Resource Center
The George Washington University
2121 K Street, NW
Suite 220
Washington, DC 20037
(800) 544-3284 (voice/TTY)
(202) 973-0904
http://www.heath.gwu.edu

HEATH (Higher Education and Adult Training for People with Handicaps) is a national clearinghouse that provides free information on postsecondary education and related issues for individuals with learning disabilities.

National Association for the Education of Young Children (NAEYC)
1509 16th Street, NW
Washington, DC 20036
(800) 424-2460

National membership organization that focuses on children from birth to age eight, offering an annual conference, a bimonthly journal, and a catalog of books, brochures, videos, and posters.

National Association for Private Schools for Exceptional Children
1522 K Street, NW
Suite 1032
Washington, DC 20005
(202) 408-3338
http://www.spedschools.com/napsec.html

Referral services for those interested in private special education in the United States, including publications and conferences.

National Head Start Association
1651 Prince Street
Alexandria, Virginia 22314
(703) 739-0875
http://www.nhsa.org

A not-for-profit membership organization representing the 835,000 children, upward of 170,000 staff, and 2,051 Head Start programs in America. NHSA provides a national forum for the continued enhancement of Head Start services for poor children ages birth to 5, and their families. It is the only national organization dedicated exclusively to the concerns of the Head Start community.

Office of Civil Rights
U.S. Department of Education, OCR
330 C. Street, SW
Suite 5000
Washington, DC 20202-1100
(202) 205-5413
http://www.ed.gov/offices/OCR

Agency ensures equal access to education and enforces civil rights. To file a formal civil rights complaint (a Section 504 complaint), contact this office or the regional office servicing your area.

Office of Educational Research and Improvement
555 New Jersey Avenue, NW
Washington, DC 20208
(202) 219-1385
http://www.ed.gov/offices/OERI

Provides support for educational research and statistics and offers a variety of services. Its agencies include the National Center for Educational Statistics, the National Institute on Early Childhood

Development and Education, the National Institute on the Education of at Risk Students, and the National Institute on Student Achievement, Curriculum, and Assessment.

Office of Special Education and Rehabilitation Services

Switzer Building
330 C Street, SW
Suite 3006
Washington, DC 20202
(202) 205-5465
http://www.ed.gov/offices/OSERS

Office supports programs that help in educating children with special needs and supports research. OSERS includes the Office of Special Education Programs, the Rehabilitation Services Administration, and the National Institute on Disability and Rehabilitation Research.

Office of Special Education Programs

Switzer Building
330 C Street, SW
Suite 3086
Washington, DC 20202
(202) 205-5507

The OSEP administers programs relating to education of all children, youth, and adults with disabilities through age 22.

Parent Advocacy Coalition for Educational Rights

4826 Chicago Avenue South
Minneapolis, MN 55417
(612) 827-2966
http://www.pacer.org

Parent-to-parent organization with lots of resources for parents of children with disabilities, including training programs for parents and youth, technical assistance, and advocacy.

EPILEPSY

American Epilepsy Society

342 North Main Street
West Hartford, CT 06117-2507

(860) 586-7505
http://www.aesnet.org

The American Epilepsy Society promotes research and education for professionals dedicated to the prevention, treatment, and cure of epilepsy. The Web site offers information, articles, information about prescription drug assistance, and publications.

Epilepsy Foundation

4351 Garden City Drive
Landover, MD 20785-7223
(301) 459-3700
http://www.efa.org

A national, charitable organization founded in 1968 as the Epilepsy Foundation of America, the only such organization wholly dedicated to the welfare of people with epilepsy. The EF mission is to work for children and adults affected by seizures through research, education, advocacy, and service.

Epilepsy International

http://www.epiworld.com

This site is a worldwide resource center for epilepsy information.

FETAL ALCOHOL SYNDROME/EFFECT

FASCETS (Fetal Alcohol Syndrome Consultation, Education, and Training Services)

P.O. Box 83175
Portland, OR 97283
(503) 621-1271
http://www.fascets.org

FASCETS is dedicated to contributing to prevention of fetal alcohol syndrome/alcohol-related neurodevelopmental disorders (FAS/ARND) and other birth defects resulting from prenatal alcohol and other drug exposure.

FAS Family Resource Institute

P.O. Box 2525
Lynnwood, WA 98036
(253) 531-2878
(800) 999-3429 (in Washington)
http://www.accessone.com/~delindam

The mission of this nonprofit corporation is to identify, understand, and care for individuals disabled by prenatal alcohol exposure and to prevent this disability in future generations.

National Organization of Fetal Alcohol Syndrome
216 G Street, NE
Washington, DC 20002
(202) 785-4585
http://www.nofas.org

A nonprofit organization founded in 1990 and dedicated to eliminating birth defects caused by alcohol consumption during pregnancy and improving the quality of life for those individuals and families affected. NOFAS, the only national organization focusing solely on FAS, takes a multicultural approach to prevention and healing. It is committed to raising public awareness of FAS (the leading known cause of mental retardation) and to developing and implementing innovative ideas in prevention, intervention, education, and advocacy in communities throughout the nation.

FOOD SAFETY

See also ALLERGY.

Food and Drug Administration (FDA)
5600 Fishers Lane
Rockville, MD 20857
(888) 463-6332
http://www.fda.gov

The FDA regulates drugs and medical devices to ensure that they are safe and effective. This government agency provides a number of publications for consumers.

FDA Office of Seafood
1110 Vermont Avenue, NW
Suite 110
Washington, DC 20005
(800) 332-4010
(202) 205-4314

Meat and Poultry Hotline
800-535-4555 (nationwide)
(202) 720-3333 (Washington, DC area)
(800) 256-7072 (TDD/TTY)

Food Safety and Inspection Service
South Building, Room 1175
1400 Independence Avenue, SW
Washington, DC 20250
(202) 720-7943
http://www.fsis.usda.gov

For help with meat, poultry, and egg products:
USDA Meat and Poultry Hotline
(800) 535-4555
(202) 720-3333 (Washington, DC area)
(800) 256-7072 (TDD/TTY)

For help with restaurant food problems
call the local Health Department

For help with nonmeat or poultry food products (such as cereal):
Food and Drug Administration (FDA)
5600 Fishers Lane
Rockville, MD 20857
(301) 472-4750

Turkey hotline
(800) 535-4555

Seafood hotline
(800) FDA-4010

FOSTER PARENTS

National Foster Parent Association
P.O. Box 81
Alpha, Ohio 45301-0081
(800) 557-5238
http://www.nfpainc.org

A nonprofit, volunteer organization established in 1972 and designed to bring together foster parents, agency representatives, and the community who wish to work together to improve the foster care system and enhance the lives of all children and families.

FRAGILE X SYNDROME

National Fragile X Foundation
P.O. Box 190488
San Francisco, CA 94119
(800) 688-8765
(925) 938-9300
http://www.nfxf.org

Nonprofit organization that provides advocacy, consultation, information, research, newsletters, referrals, and education.

GAY AND LESBIAN PARENTS

Families Like Ours, Inc.
P.O. Box 3137
Renton, WA 98056
(425) 793-7911
http://www.familieslikeours.org

A national support group for gay and lesbian couples that provides information about adoption.

Family Pride Coalition
P.O. Box 34337
San Diego, CA 92163
(619) 296-0199
http://www.familypride.org

Organization dedicated to helping gay, lesbian, bisexual, and transgendered couples adopt; provides information, support, and referrals.

GENERAL

American Academy of Pediatrics (AAP)
141 Northwest Point Boulevard
Elk Grove Village, IL 60007-1098
(847) 434-4000
http://www.aap.org

The AAP is committed to the health and well-being of infants, adolescents, and young adults. The Web site offers news articles and tips on health for families.

American College of Obstetricians and Gynecologists
409 12th Street SW
P.O. Box 96920
Washington, DC 20090
http://www.acog.org

Founded in 1951 in Chicago, Illinois, ACOG is the nation's leading group of professionals providing health care for women. Now based in Washington, DC, it is a private nonprofit membership organization working primarily in four areas: Serving as a strong advocate for quality health care for women, maintaining the highest standards of clinical practice and continuing education, promoting patient education and stimulating patient understanding of and involvement in medical care, and increasing awareness among its members and the public of the changing issues facing women's health care. Web site offers information on numerous health issues and includes a "physician finder."

American Medical Association
515 North State Street
Chicago, IL 60610
(312) 464-5000
http://www.ama-assn.org

Primary professional organization for the nation's physicians.

GIFTED CHILDREN

American Association for Gifted Children at Duke University
Box 90270
Durham, NC 27708-0270
(919) 783-6152
http://www.aagc.org

The nation's oldest advocacy organization for gifted children was established in the late 1940s. AAGC has published materials for the educational research community, for people in the medical profession, and for parents and teachers of gifted children. It tries to foster a better understanding of the needs and capabilities of gifted children, to encourage research in the field of education and nurturing of gifted children, and to accomplish and encourage other initiatives relating to the development of gifted children. For many years, AAGC has had a role in the Presidential Scholars Program, which recognizes 141 outstanding high school graduates each year, awarding scholarships for the Presidential Scholars.

The National Research Center on the Gifted and Talented
University of Connecticut
2131 Hillside Road, Unit 3007
Storrs, CT 06269-3007
(860) 486-4676
http://www.gifted.uconn.edu/nrcgt.html

A collaborative research effort aimed at solving specific problems and providing practical options and programs for parents and educators working with gifted children.

GOVERNMENT ORGANIZATIONS

Centers for Disease Control and Prevention
1600 Clifton Rd.
Atlanta, GA 30333
(404) 639-3534
(800) 311-3435
http://www.cdc.gov

The mission of the CDC is to promote health and quality of life by preventing and controlling disease, injury, and disability.

Federal Trade Commission
Consumer Response Center
CRC-240
Washington, DC 20580
(877) FTC-HELP or (877) 382-4357 (toll free)
(202) 326-2502 (TTY)
http://www.ftc.gov

The FTC enforces consumer protection laws, offers publications to guide consumers, and collects information about fraudulent claims.

Food and Drug Administration
5600 Fishers Lane
Rockville, MD 20857
(301) 472-4750
http://www.fda.gov

The FDA regulates drugs and medical devices to ensure that they are safe and effective. This government agency provides a number of publications for consumers.

Head Start Bureau
Administration on Children, Youth and Families
U.S. Department of Health & Human Services
P.O. Box 1182
Washington, DC 20013
http://www.acf.dhhs.gov/programs/hsb/

Federal administrator of the Head Start program.

Maternal Child and Health Bureau
18-05 Parklawn Building
5600 Fishers Lane
Rockville, MD 20857
(301) 443-2170
http://www.mchb.hrsa.gov

This U.S. government agency is charged with promoting and improving the health of mothers and children. MCHB seeks a nation where there is equal access for all to quality health care in a supportive, culturally competent, family, and community setting. Divisions include children with special needs, child adolescent and family health, perinatal systems, and women's health.

National Center for Complementary and Alternative Medicine
NCCAM Clearinghouse
P.O. Box 7923
Gaithersburg, MD 20898
(888) 644-6226 (toll-free)
(866) 464-3615 (TTY)
http://www.nccam.nih.gov

One of the 27 institutes and centers that make up the National Institutes of Health (NIH), whose mission is to support rigorous research on complementary and alternative medicine (CAM), to train researchers in CAM, and to provide information about which CAM modalities work, which do not, and why. Information specialists at the NCCAM Clearinghouse can answer questions about the center and complementary and alternative medicine.

National Information Center for Children and Youth with Disabilities
P.O. Box 1492
Washington, DC 20013
(800) 695-0285 (voice/TTY)

(202) 884-8200 (voice/TTY/phones answered "live" 9:30 A.M. to 6:30 P.M. EST)
http://www.nichcy.org/

The national information center that provides information on disabilities and disability-related issues. With a special focus is children and youth (birth to age 22), the Web site can provide information about specific disabilities, special education and related services for children in school, individualized education programs, parent materials, disability organizations, professional associations, education rights, early intervention services for infants and toddlers, and transition to adult life.

National Institute of Allergy and Infectious Diseases
National Institutes of Health
Building 31, Room 7A32
9000 Rockville Pike
Bethesda, MD 20892
(301) 496-5717

Federal institute that supports research and information on allergies and infectious diseases.

National Institute of Child Health and Human Development
Building 31, Room 2A32
9000 Rockville Pike
Bethesda, Maryland 20892-2425
(301) 496-5133
http://www.nichd.nih.gov

Institute that supports research into the health of children and offers information on a wide variety of topics relevant to children and maternal health.

National Organization for Rare Disorders (NORD)
P.O. Box 1968
Danbury, CT 06813-1968
(800) 999-6673
(203) 744-0100 (voice)
(203) 797-9590 (TTY)
http://www.rarediseases.org

A unique federation of voluntary health organizations dedicated to helping people with rare "orphan" diseases and assisting the organizations that serve them. NORD is committed to the identification, treatment, and cure of rare disorders through programs of education, advocacy, research, and service. For almost 20 years, NORD has served as the primary nongovernmental clearinghouse for information on rare disorder and provides referrals, support groups, and other sources of assistance. NORD is a nonprofit, voluntary health agency that exists to serve rare-disease patients and their families.

Office of Civil Rights
U.S. Department of Education, OCR
330 C. Street, SW
Suite 5000
Washington, DC 20202-1100
(202) 205-5413
http://www.ed.gov/offices/OCR

Agency ensures equal access to education and enforces civil rights. To file a formal civil rights complaint (a Section 504 complaint), contact this office or the regional office servicing your area.

GRANDPARENTING

The Foundation for Grandparenting
108 Farnham Road
Ojai, CA 93023
http://www.grandparenting.org

A nonprofit organization trying to raise grandparent consciousness and promote the importance of grandparenting as a role and function that both gives important meaning and empowerment to later life and benefits all family members. In addition, the foundation promotes aspects of grandparenting as a role for all elders, whether or not they have biological grandchildren.

GROUP B STREP INFECTIONS

Group B Strep Association
P.O. Box 16515
Chapel Hill, NC 27516
http://www.groupbstrep.org

A nonprofit organization formed in 1990 by parents whose babies were victims of GBS infections. The association works to create increased public awareness; as a result, in 1996 the Centers for Disease Control, the American College of Obstetrics and Gynecology, and the American Academy of Pediatrics issued aggressive guidelines for prenatal screening and prevention of GBS disease.

GROWTH DISORDERS

Human Growth Foundation
997 Glen Cove Avenue
Glen Head, N.Y. 11545
(800) 451-6434
http://www.hgfound.org

A voluntary nonprofit organization whose mission is to help children with disorders of growth and growth hormone through research, education, support, and advocacy. Members include parents and friends of children with growth problems, and interested health professionals.

Little People of America
P.O. Box 65030
Lubbock, TX 79464
(888) LPA-2001
http://www.lpaonline.org

A nonprofit organization that provides support and information to people of short stature and their families. The Web site offers resources pertaining to dwarfism and LPA, medical data, instructions on how to join an e-mail discussion group, and links to numerous other dwarfism-related sites.

Little People's Research Fund
80 Sister Pierre Drive
Towson, MD 21204
800-232-LPRF (toll-free)
http://www.lprf.org

The only health organization in the world supporting the research for the special medical needs of Little People—people affected with skeletal dysplasia.

MAGIC Foundation (Major Aspects of Growth Disorders in Children)
6645 West North Avenue
Oak Park, IL 60302

(800) 361-4423
(708) 383-0808
http://www.magicfoundation.org

A national nonprofit organization created to provide support services for the families of children afflicted with a wide variety of chronic and/or critical disorders, syndromes, and diseases that affect a child's growth. Established in 1989 by five families of children with growth disorders, MAGIC has grown to be the leading organization of growth disorders in this country. MAGIC covers more than 100 different types of growth disorders, 11 specific divisions, and educational/supportive services worldwide.

HANDICAPPED CHILDREN

See also DISABILITIES.

National Information Center for Children and Youth with Disabilities
P.O. Box 1492
Washington, DC 20013
(800) 695-0285
(202) 884-8200 (voice/TTY)
http://www.nichcy.org/

Provides information on disabilities and disability-related issues for families, educators, and professionals related to children and youth.

HEADACHE

American Headache Society
19 Mantua Road
Mount Royal, NJ 08061
(856) 423-0043
http://www.ahsnet.org

A professional society of health-care providers dedicated to the study and treatment of headache and face pain. Founded in 1959, AHS brings together physicians and other health providers from various fields and specialties to share concepts and developments about headache and related conditions.

National Headache Foundation
820 North Orleans
Suite 217
Chicago, IL 60610

(888) NHF-5552

http://www.headaches.org

A nonprofit foundation dedicated to educating headache sufferers and health-care professionals about headache causes and treatments.

HEAD INJURY

Brain Injury Association

105 North Alfred Street

Alexandria, VA 22314

(800) 444-6443

http://www.biausa.org

The only nonprofit organization working on behalf of individuals with brain injury and their families.

Brain Trauma Foundation

523 East 72nd Street

8th Floor

New York, NY 10021

(212) 772-0608

http://www.braintrauma.org

A nonprofit organization dedicated to improving the outcome of brain trauma patients nationwide.

Head Injury Hotline

212 Pioneer Building

Seattle, WA 98104

(206) 621-8558

http://www.headinjury.com

A nonprofit clearinghouse founded and operated by head injury activists since 1985.

HEALTH SERVICES

HRSA Information Center

Parklawn Building

5600 Fishers Lane

Rockville, MD 20857

(888) 275-4772

http://www.ask.hrsa.gov

Federal agency that can provide publications and resources on health-care services for low-income, uninsured individuals and those with special health-care needs. Publications available in Spanish; Spanish speaker on staff.

National Health Information Center

P.O. Box 1133

Washington, DC 20013-1133

(800) 336-4797

(301) 565-4167

http://www.health.gov/nhic/

A federal health information referral service that puts health professionals and consumers who have health questions in touch with those organizations that are best able to provide answers. NHIC was established in 1979 by the Office of Disease Prevention and Health Promotion (ODPHP), Office of Public Health and Science, and the Office of the Secretary, U.S. Department of Health and Human Services.

HEARING PROBLEMS

See DEAFNESS.

HEART PROBLEMS

American Heart Association

7272 Greenville Avenue

Dallas, TX 75231

(800) 242-8721

http://www.americanheart.org

A nonprofit association trying to reduce disability and death from cardiovascular diseases and stroke, and to provide credible heart disease and stroke information for effective prevention and treatment.

Children's Health Information Network

1561 Clark Drive

Yardley, PA 19067

(215) 493-3068

http://www.tchin.org

The Children's Health Information Network is an international organization that provides reliable information, support services, and resources to families of children with congenital heart defects and acquired heart disease, adults with congenital heart defects, and the professionals who work with them.

National Heart, Lung, and Blood Institute

NHLBI Health Information Center

P.O. Box 30105

Bethesda, MD 20824-0105

(301) 592-8573
(240) 629-3255 (TTY)
http://www.nhlbi.nih.gov

The NHLBI provides leadership for a national program in diseases of the heart, blood vessels, lung, and blood; blood resources; and sleep disorders. Since October 1997 the NHLBI has also had administrative responsibility for the NIH Woman's Health Initiative.

HELICOBACTER PYLORI

Helicobacter Foundation
P.O. Box 7965
Charlottesville, VA 22906-7965
http://www.helico.com

The foundation was started by Dr. Barry J. Marshall in early 1994 and is dedicated to providing the latest information about *Helicobacter pylori,* its diagnosis, treatment, and clinical correlations.

HEMOPHILIA

See BLOOD DISORDERS.

HEPATITIS

American Liver Foundation
75 Maiden Lane
Suite 603
New York, NY 10038
(800) GOLIVER or (800) 465-4837
http://www.liverfoundation.org

A national nonprofit organization dedicated to the prevention, treatment, and cure of hepatitis and other liver diseases through research, education, and advocacy on behalf of those at risk of, or affected by, liver disease.

Children's Liver Alliance Web site
http://www.liverkids.org.au

Hepatitis Foundation International
30 Sunrise Terrace
Cedar Grove, NJ 07009-1423
(973) 239-1035
(800) 891-0707
http://www.hepfi.org

Nonprofit organization dedicated to the eradication of viral hepatitis. The foundation provides education, training programs, and material for the public, patients, health educators, and medical professionals, and supports hepatitis research, provides a patient telephone support network and a hotline, maintains a database of hepatitis support groups, and hosts a Web site.

Hepatitis Information Network
http://www.hepnet.com

Helpful Web site all about hepatitis.

HYDROCEPHALUS

Hydrocephalus Association
875 Market Street
Suite 705
San Francisco, CA 94102
(415) 732-7040
http://www.hydroassoc.org

Nonprofit organization that promotes the understanding of hydrocephalus and disseminates information and support.

National Hydrocephalus Foundation
400 North Michigan Avenue
Suite 1102
Chicago, IL 60611-4102
(815) 467-6548

Nonprofit organization founded in 1980 to familiarize the public with hydrocephalus and to combat stigma, disseminate information, counsel parents, create a consumer group, obtain health insurance covering this disease, and form local chapters to help accomplish these goals.

INTERNET SAFETY

American Library Association
50 East Huron
Chicago, IL 60611
(800) 545-2433
http://www.ala.org/alsc/parents.links.html

This site has a listing of links for parents about safe surfing online resources.

Family Education Network
http://www.familyeducation.com

Visit this site to learn more about blocking, filtering, and monitoring and tracking software.

KAWASAKI DISEASE

Kawasaki Disease Foundation
6 Beechwood Circle
Boxford, MA 01921
(978) 887-9357
http://www.kdfoundation.org

The only nonprofit organization of parents, patients, and professionals dedicated to advancing Kawasaki disease issues and focusing on awareness, support, and research.

KIDNEY PROBLEMS

American Association of Kidney Patients
3505 Frontage Road
Suite 315
Tampa, FL 33607
(800) 749-2257
(415) 455-4575
(415) 455-0491 (TTY)
http://www.aakp.org

The AAKP serves kidney patients and their families by helping them cope with the emotional, physical, and social impact of kidney failure.

National Institute of Diabetes & Digestive & Kidney Diseases
Information Clearinghouse
3 Information Way
Bethesda, MD 20892
(301) 654-4415
http://www.niddk.nih.gov

Federal institute that conducts and supports basic and clinical research into kidney diseases among others.

National Kidney Foundation
30 East 33rd Street
New York, NY 10016

(212) 889-2210
http://www.kidney.org

A major voluntary health organization that seeks to prevent kidney and urinary tract diseases, improve the health and well-being of individuals and families affected by these diseases, and increase the availability of all organs for transplantation.

Nephron Information Center Web site
http://www.nephron.com

The Nephron Information Center offers information about how the kidneys work, transplants, and links to other Web sites.

Polycystic Kidney Research Foundation
4901 Main Street
Suite 200
Kansas City, MO 64112
(816) 931-2600
(800) 753-2873
http://www.pkdcure.org

The only nonprofit organization worldwide that works for improving clinical treatment and discovering a cure for PKD. The organization works to develop funding for peer-approved biomedical research projects and advocates for the importance of PKD research conducted by the National Institutes of Health (NIH).

LEAD POISONING

Environmental Protection Agency
Safe Drinking Water Hotline
(800) 426-4791

For information on laboratories certified to test for lead in water.

National Center for Lead-Safe Housing
205 American City Building
Columbia, MD 21044
(410) 964-1230

For information about lead in housing.

National Lead Information Center
8601 Georgia Avenue
Suite 503

Silver Spring, MD 20910
(800) 424-5323
(800) LEAD-FYI or (800) 532-3394
http://www.epa.gov/lead/nlic.htm

Materials about lead poisoning are available in Spanish and English.

LEARNING DISABILITIES

Council for Exceptional Children and the Division for Learning Disabilities
1920 Association Drive
Reston, VA 22091-1589
(800) 328-0272
(703) 620-3660
Council for Exceptional Children:
  http://www.cec.sped.org
Division for Learning Disabilities:
  http://www.dldcec.org

An international professional association with more than 52,000 members focused on advancing the education of exceptional children (both the disabled and the gifted). DLD is the division of the CEC that focuses on the special needs of individuals with learning disabilities. This membership organization has 17 specialized divisions including the Division of Learning Disabilities, which is dedicated to the field of learning disabilities. CEC conducts an annual conference and publishes a newsletter and magazines.

Council for Learning Disabilities
P.O. Box 40303
Overland Park, KS 66204
(913) 492-2546
http://www.cldinternational.org

The CLD is an international organization of and for professionals who establish standards of excellence and promote innovative strategies for research and practice through collaboration and advocacy. Membership organization of and for professionals who establish standards of excellence and promote innovative strategies for research and practice through collaboration and advocacy.

Federation for Children with Special Needs
1135 Tremont Street
Suite 420
Boston, MA 02120

(617) 236-7210
(800) 331-0688
http://www.fcsn.org

Nonprofit federation designed to provide support for children with special needs.

Learning Disabilities Association of America
4156 Library Road
Pittsburgh, PA 15234
(888) 300-6710
http://www.ldanatl.org

National nonprofit membership organization with more than 60,000 members and 600 state and local affiliates in 50 states, Washington, DC, and Puerto Rico. Members gather for education, networking, and advocacy; conduct an annual conference, and offer information and various publications.

Learning Resources Network
1550 Hayes Drive
Manhattan, KS 66502
(800) 678-5376
http://www.lern.org

Organization providing information and support about learning disabilities and those who teach adult education.

LD On-Line
http://www.ldonline.org

A to Z database on all aspects of learning disabilities and children.

National Center for Learning Disabilities
381 Park Avenue South
Suite 1401
New York, NY 10016
(888) 575-7373 (for general information)
(212) 545-7510 (for detailed information)
http://www.ncld.org

Develops training and educational materials for parents and practitioners including Every Child Is Learning, a training program to help preschool teachers and parents recognize the early warning signs of learning disabilities. NCLD seeks to raise public awareness and understanding, furnish national information and referrals, and arrange educational programs and legislative advocacy. NCLD provides educational tools to heighten understanding of learning disabilities, including the annual publications called "Their World," quarterly newsletters, informative articles, specific state-by-state resource listings, and informative videos regarding learning disabilities.

Nonverbal Learning Disorders Association

2446 Albany Avenue
West Hartford, CT 06117
(860) 570-0217
http://www.nlda.org

A nonprofit corporation dedicated to research, education, and advocacy for nonverbal learning disorders.

Nonverbal Learning Disorder on the Web

http://www.NLDontheweb.org

Schwab Foundation for Learning

1650 South Amphlett Boulevard
Suite 300
San Mateo, CA 94402
(800) 230-0988
http://www.schwablearning.org

Group that provides services to parents and educators to help students with learning differences succeed. Services include a lending library and Bridges To Reading, a step-by-step guide to understanding, identifying, and addressing reading problems.

LEUKEMIA

Leukemia & Lymphoma Society

1311 Mamaroneck Avenue
White Plains, NY 10605
(914) 949-5213
http://www.leukemia.org

The world's largest voluntary health organization dedicated to funding blood cancer research, education, and patient services. The society's mission is to cure leukemia, lymphoma, Hodgkin's disease, and myeloma and to improve the quality of life of patients and their families. Since its founding in

1949, the society has provided more than $280 million for research specifically targeting blood-related cancers.

National Children's Leukemia Foundation

172 Madison Avenue
New York, NY 10016
(212) 686-2722
(800) GIVE-HOPE (out of state)
http://www.leukemiafoundation.org

One of the leading nonprofit organizations in the fight against leukemia and cancer for children and adults that was established to support the unfortunate in various programs. NCLF's main objective is to provide the cure for children and adults, and to ease the family's burden during their hospital stay. Through a 24-hour hotline the organization offers comprehensive information to any caller and provides referrals for initial testing, physicians, hospital admissions, and treatment options.

LIVER DISORDERS

See HEPATITIS.

LOWE SYNDROME

Lowe Syndrome Association

222 Lincoln Street
West Lafayette, IN 47906
(765) 743-3634
http://www.medhelp.org/lowesyndrome

Voluntary health organization of parents, professionals, and others to provide information and support and to support research and treatments.

LUPUS

Lupus Foundation of America, Inc.

1300 Piccard Drive
Suite 200
Rockville, MD 20850-4303
(301) 670-9292
http://www.lupus.org

The only nationwide voluntary organization exclusively serving the entire lupus community, including patients, their families, physicians, researchers, and the general public. The mission is to educate and support those affected by lupus and find the cure. The LFA was incorporated as a nonprofit health agency in 1977. Since its establishment the LFA has remained a grassroots, volunteer-driven organization.

LYME DISEASE

American Lyme Disease Foundation
293 Route 100
Somers, New York 10589
(914) 277-6970
http://aldf.com

This nonprofit foundation supports research and plays a key role in providing reliable and scientifically accurate information to the public and health-care provider.

Lyme Disease Association, Inc.
P.O. Box 1438
Jackson, NJ 08527
(888) 366-6611
http://www.lymediseaseassociation.org

Major nonprofit organization dedicated to Lyme disease education, prevention, and research. In its search for a cure for chronic Lyme, the LDA has funded dozens of research projects coast to coast and sponsored several national medical conferences, including the first to focus on the problems of children with Lyme disease.

Lyme Disease Foundation
One Financial Plaza
18th Floor
Hartford, CT 06103
860-525-2000 (24-Hour Hotline)
(800) 886-LYME
http://www.lyme.org

A major nonprofit organization dedicated to finding solutions for tick-borne disorders. The LDF works with businesses, patients, government, and the medical community to find solutions to tick-borne disorders.

Lyme Disease Network
43 Winton Road
East Brunswick, NJ 08816
http://www.lymenet.org

Nonprofit foundation dedicated to public education of the prevention and treatment of Lyme disease and other tick-borne illnesses. Founded in 1991, the network has maintained its Internet presence since 1994.

MANIC DEPRESSION (BIPOLAR DISORDER)

Depression and Bipolar Support Alliance
730 North Franklin Street
Suite 501
Chicago, IL 60610
(800) 826-3632
(312) 642-0049
http://www.dbsalliance.org

The nation's largest patient-directed, illness-specific organization, incorporated in 1986 and based in Chicago, representing the voices of the more than 23 million Americans living with depression and another 2.5 million living with bipolar disorder (manic depression.) DBSA was formerly the National Depressive and Manic-Depressive Association.

MARFAN SYNDROME

National Marfan Foundation
22 Manhasset Avenue
Port Washington, NY 11050
(800) 8-MARFAN
(516) 883-8712
http://www.marfan.org/publications.html

A nonprofit organization founded in 1981 by people who have Marfan syndrome and their families.

MENTAL HEALTH

American Academy of Child and Adolescent Psychiatry
3615 Wisconsin Avenue, NW
Washington, DC 20016-3007
(202) 966-7300
http://www.aacap.org

The leading national nonprofit professional medical association dedicated to treating and improving the quality of life for children, adolescents, and families affected by mental disorders. Established in 1953, its members actively research, evaluate, diagnose, and treat psychiatric disorders. The AACAP widely distributes information on mental illnesses; advances efforts in prevention of mental illnesses, and assures proper treatment and access to services for children and adolescents.

American Psychiatric Association

1000 Wilson Boulevard
Suite 1825
Arlington, VA
22209-3901
(703) 907-7300
http://www.psych.org

A medical specialty society that works to ensure humane care and effective treatment for everyone with mental disorder, mental retardation, or substance-related disorders.

American Psychological Association

750 First Street, NE
Washington, DC 20002-4242
(800) 374-2721
(202) 336-5510
http://www.apa.org

A scientific and professional organization that represents psychology in the United States with more than 155,000 members—the largest association of psychologists worldwide.

Center for Mental Health Services

Room 17-99
5600 Fishers Lane
Rockville, MD 20857
http://www.mentalhealth.org

Federal agency that provides information and resources on mental health including database of community resources, extensive catalog, events, and more. The goal of this agency is to provide the treatment and support services needed by adults with mental disorders and children with serious emotional problems.

Federation of Families for Children's Mental Health

1101 King Street
Suite 420
Alexandria, VA 22314

(703) 684-7710
http://www.ffcmh.org

A nonprofit group working for mental health rights of children.

National Institute of Mental Health (NIMH)

5600 Fishers Lane
Rockville, MD 20857
(301) 443-4513
http://www.nimh.nih.gov

Foremost mental health research organization in the world.

MENTAL ILLNESS

National Alliance for the Mentally Ill (NAMI)

Colonial Place Three
2107 Wilson Boulevard
Suite 300
Arlington, VA 22201-3042
(800) 950-6264
(703) 524-7600
(703) 516-7991 (TTY)
http://www.nami.org

Nonprofit organization dedicated to supporting individuals with mental illness and their families.

National Association for the Dually Diagnosed (NADD)

132 Fair Street
Kingston, NY 12401
(800) 331-5362
(845) 331-4336
http://www.thenadd.org

Nonprofit organization to support those with both mental illness and mental retardation.

MENTAL RETARDATION

See DEVELOPMENTAL DISABILITIES; DOWN SYNDROME; FRAGILE X SYNDROME.

MISSING CHILDREN

See also CHILD ABUSE.

Federal Bureau of Investigation Web site

http://www.fbi.gov/kids/kids.htm

Visit the FBI Web site for Internet safety tips for kids and parents and other safety information.

National Center for Missing and Exploited Children

699 Prince Street
Alexandria, VA 22314
(703) 274-3900
(800) THE-LOST
http://www.missingkids.org

The nation's resource center for child protection, this private, nonprofit center provides help to parents, children, law enforcement, schools, and the community in recovering missing children and raising public awareness about ways to help prevent child abduction, molestation, and sexual exploitation. NCMEC has worked on more than 85,500 cases of missing and exploited children, helped recover more than 68,900 children, and raised its recovery rate from 60 percent in the 1980s to more than 93 percent today, thereby gaining national and international recognition as "the" resource for missing and exploited children. The center was founded by John and Reve Walsh, whose six-year-old son Adam was abducted in 1981 and never found.

Nation's Missing Children Organization

2432 West Peoria Avenue
Suite 1283
Phoenix, AZ 85029
(602) 944-1768
(800) 690-FIND
http://www.nmco.org

Nonprofit organization that offers a range of services to help missing and abused children.

MULTIPLE BIRTHS

The Center for Study of Multiple Births (CSMB)

333 East Superior Street
Suite 464
Chicago, IL 60611
(312) 266-9093
http://www.multiplebirth.com/

Promotes and advances the health of women and children (particularly multiples) through education, research, and public service; offers resources, articles, research, news, and events.

Mothers of SuperTwins (MOST)

P.O. Box 951
Brentwood, NY 11717-0627
(631) 859-1110
http://www.mostonline.org

An international nonprofit organization involving a network of families with triplets, quadruplets, and more that provides information, resources, empathy, and good humor during pregnancy and after birth.

The National Organization of Mothers of Twins Clubs, Inc. (NOMOTC)

P.O. Box 23188
Albuquerque, NM 8792-1188
(505) 275-0955

A support group for parents of multiples offering information, publications, research, referrals, special needs, and links.

The Triplet Connection

P.O. Box 99571
Stockton, CA 95209
(209) 474-0885
http://www.tripletconnection.org

A nonprofit organization for multiple-birth families that provides vital information to those expecting triplets, quadruplets, quintuplets, or more, as well as encouragement, resources, and networking opportunities for families who have larger multiples.

MULTIPLE SCLEROSIS

National Multiple Sclerosis Society

733 Third Avenue
New York, NY 10017
(800) 624-8236
http://www.nmss.org

National nonprofit organization that supports more MS research and serves more people with MS than any other MS organization in the world. Programs for everyone affected by MS are available in every local chapter. Information about MS and referrals to area professionals and resources, including referral to chapter-affiliated self-help groups, are free to all as are emergency equipment loans. National information specialists research difficult questions if the local staff is unable to answer. Free and nominal-fee programs may include education, counseling, and recreational events.

MUNCHAUSEN BY PROXY

AsherMeadow Web site

http://www.ashermeadow.com

This Web site offers news, statistics, a bookstore, and more about this syndrome.

Dr. Marc Feldman's Munchausen Syndrome, Factitious Disorder, and Munchausen by Proxy Page

http://wwwourworld.compuserve.com/
  homepages/Marc_Feldman_2/

Web site of a psychiatrist and author specializing in Munchausen Syndrome and other factitious disorders.

Munchausen by Proxy Survivors Network

http://www.mbpsnetwork.com

This site was created in recognition of the victims of Munchausen by Proxy Syndrome.

MUSCULAR DYSTROPHY

Muscular Dystrophy Association

3300 East Sunrise Drive
Tucson, AZ 87518
http://www.mdausa.org

A voluntary health agency dedicated to conquering MD and supporting patients and their families with the condition.

NEONATAL DEATH

See DEATH AND DYING.

NEUROFIBROMATOSIS

National Neurofibromatosis Foundation

95 Pine Street
16th Floor
New York, NY 10005
(800) 323-7938
http://www.nf.org

A nonprofit medical foundation, dedicated to improving the health and well-being of individuals and families affected by the neurofibromatoses (NF).

OBSESSIVE-COMPULSIVE DISORDER

Obsessive-Compulsive Foundation

337 Notch Hill Road
North Branford, CT 06471
(203) 315-2190
http://www.ocfoundation.org

OCF educates the public and professional communities about OCD and related disorders, provides assistance to families, and supports research of the causes and effective treatments of these disorders.

OCCUPATIONAL THERAPY

American Occupational Therapy Association

4720 Montgomery Lane
P.O. Box 31220
Bethesda, MD 20824-1220
(301) 652-2682
(800) 377-8555 (TDD)
http://www.aota.org

The AOTA Web site provides national and regional news and information about occupational therapy and related issues.

National Organization on Disability

910 Sixteenth Street, NW
Suite 600
Washington, DC 20006
(202) 293-5960
http://www.nod.org

This Web site provides information, programs, publications, and more for people with disabilities and their families.

OT Kids Web site
http://www.alaska.net/~otkids

This Web site offers information on occupational therapy, therapy activities, and the different ways OT can benefit children.

PARENTING

Center on Positive Behavioral Interventions and Supports
1761 Alder Street
1235 University of Oregon
Eugene, OR 97403-5262
(541) 346-2505
http://www.pbis.org

MUMS, National Parent-to-Parent Network
150 Custer Court
Green Bay, WI 54301-1243
(920) 336-5333
(877) 336-5333 (parents only)
http://www.netnet.net/mums

Zero to Three
(formerly National Center for Clinical Infant Programs)
2000 M Street, NW
Suite 200
Washington, DC 20036
(800) 899-4301 (for publications)
(202) 638-1144
http://www.zerotothree.org

PHYSICAL THERAPY

American Physical Therapy Association
1111 North Fairfax Street
Alexandria, VA 22314
(800) 999-2782
(703) 684-2782 (voice)
(703) 683-6748 (TTY)
http://www.apta.org

This site provides information on almost every aspect of physical therapy, from therapists in each state to current research.

Pediatric Physical Therapy Web site
http://www.pediatricphysicaltherapy.com

This site is designed for pediatric physical therapists but has helpful resources and information about current research in the field.

Youth Sports Network Web site
http://www.ysn.com/

Youth Sports Network offers links to several sports-related Web sites for kids and teens.

POSTPARTUM DEPRESSION

Depression After Delivery
91 East Somerset Street
Raritan, NJ 08869
(800) 944-4773
http://www.depressionafterdelivery.com

DAD was formed to provide support for women with postpartum depression. It has expanded its focus to include education, information, and referral for women and families coping with mental health issues associated with childbearing, both during pregnancy and postpartum.

Postpartum Education for Parents
P.O. Box 6154
Santa Barbara, CA 93160
http://www.sbpep.org

PEP was founded by a group of mothers to offer each other support after the births of their children. PEP is a nonprofit corporation staffed by trained parent volunteers.

Postpartum Support International Web page
http://www.chss.iup.edu/postpartum/

PSI is an international network that focuses on postpartum mental health and social support.

POST-TRAUMATIC STRESS DISORDER (PTSD)

National Center for PTSD
VA Medical Center (116D)
215 North Main Street
White River Junction, VT 05009
(802) 296-6300
http://www.ncptsd.org

PTSD Alliance
(877) 507-PTSD (toll-free)
http://www.ptsdalliance.org/home2.html

A group of professional and advocacy organizations that have joined forces to provide educational resources to individuals diagnosed with PTSD and their loved ones; those at risk for developing PTSD; and medical, health-care, and other professionals.

PRADER-WILLI SYNDROME

Prader-Willi Syndrome Association
5700 Midnight Pass Road
Suite 6
Sarasota, FL 34242
(800) 926-4797
(941) 312-0400
http://www.pwsausa.org

Organization providing information, education, and support services to members.

PROGERIA

Progeria Research Foundation
P.O. Box 3453
Peabody, MA 01961-3453
http://www.progeriaresearch.org

Nonprofit foundation that supports research, promotes education and awareness, and supports fund-raising.

PSORIASIS

National Psoriasis Foundation
6600 SW 92nd Avenue
Suite 300
Portland, OR 97223
(503) 297-1545
(503) 244-7404
http://www.psoriasis.org

The world's largest nonprofit organization dedicated to educating, serving, and empowering people with psoriasis and psoriatic arthritis. For more than 35 years, the foundation has made a significant difference in the way psoriasis and psoriatic arthritis are treated and perceived. Its mission is to improve patients' quality of life, promote awareness and understanding, ensure access to treatment, and support research that will lead to effective management and, ultimately, a cure.

RABIES

CDC Division of Viral and Rickettsial Diseases
(404) 639-1075

RESPIRATORY DISEASE

American Lung Association
1740 Broadway
New York, NY 10019
http://www.lungusa.org

The oldest voluntary health organization in the United States that was founded in 1904 to fight tuberculosis. Today ALA fights lung disease in all its forms, with special emphasis on asthma, tobacco control, and environmental health.

National Heart, Lung, and Blood Institute
NHLBI Health Information Center
P.O. Box 30105
Bethesda, MD 20824-0105
(301) 592-8573
(240) 629-3255 (TTY)
E-mail: nhlbiinfo@rover.nhlbi.nih.gov
http://www.nhlbi.nih.gov

The NHLBI provides leadership for a national program in diseases of the heart, blood vessels, lung, and blood; blood resources; and sleep disorders. Since October 1997 the NHLBI has also had administrative responsibility for the NIH Woman's Health Initiative.

RETT SYNDROME

International Rett Syndrome Association
9121 Piscataway Road
Suite 2B
Clinton, MD 20735
(800) 818-7388
(301) 856-3334
http://www.rettsyndrome.org

Promoting research and offering information, advocacy, referrals to support groups, genetic counseling, and other services.

Rett Syndrome Research Foundation (RSRF)
4600 Devitt Drive
Cincinnati OH 45246
http://www.rsrf.org

Promoting research and offering information, advocacy, referrals to support groups, genetic counseling, and other services.

REYE'S SYNDROME
National Reye's Syndrome Foundation
P.O. Box 829
Bryan, OH 43506
(800) 233-7393
(419) 636-2679
http://www.reyessyndrome.org

Nonprofit citizen group dedicated to public relations, support, and research into eradicating Reye's syndrome.

SAFETY ISSUES
See also AUTO SAFETY; CONSUMER PRODUCTS; FOOD; INTERNET SAFETY.

American Red Cross Web site
http://www.redcross.org

The Web site of the American Red Cross provides first aid and safety information.

Brady Center to Prevent Gun Violence
1225 I Street, NW
Suite 1100
Washington, DC 20005
http://www.bradycenter.com

The largest national, nonpartisan, grassroots organization leading the fight to prevent gun violence, the Brady Campaign and the Brady Center are dedicated to creating an America free from gun violence, where all Americans are safe at home, at school, at work, and in their communities. The Brady Campaign and the Brady Center believe that a safer America can be achieved without banning all guns, and they work to enact and enforce sensible gun laws, regulations, and public policies through grassroots activism, electing pro-gun-control public officials and increasing public awareness of gun violence. The Brady Center works to reform the gun industry and educate the public about gun violence through litigation and grassroots mobilization and also works to enact and enforce sensible regulations to reduce gun violence, including regulations governing the gun industry.

Food and Drug Administration
5600 Fishers Lane
Rockville, MD 20857
(888) 463-6332 (toll-free)
http://www.fda.gov

The FDA regulates drugs and medical devices to ensure that they are safe and effective. This government agency provides a number of publications for consumers.

National Center for Injury Prevention and Control
Mailstop K65
4770 Buford Highway, NE
Atlanta, GA 30341-3724
(770) 488-1506
http://www.cdc.gov/ncipc

A division of the Centers for Disease Control and Prevention that works to reduce morbidity, disability, mortality, and costs associated with injuries.

National Safe Kids Campaign
1301 Pennsylvania Avenue, NW
Suite 1000
Washington, DC 20004
(202) 662-0600
http://www.safekids.org

The first and only national nonprofit organization dedicated solely to the prevention of unintentional childhood injury—the number one killer of children ages 14 and under. More than 300 state and local SAFE KIDS coalitions in all 50 states, the District of Columbia, and Puerto Rico compose the Campaign.

National Safety Council
1121 Spring Lake Drive
Itasca, IL 60143-3201
(630) 285-1121
http://www.nsc.org

The nation's leading advocate for safety and health, which aims to educate and influence society to adopt safety, health, and environmental policies, practices, and procedures. The National Safety Council has been working for generations to protect lives and promote health with innovative programs. The Council is a nonprofit, nongovernmental, international public service organization dedicated to improving the safety, health, and environmental well-being of all people.

U.S. Consumer Product Safety Commission Web site
http://www.cpsc.gov

This federal agency collects information about consumer goods and issues recalls on unsafe or dangerous products.

SCOLIOSIS

National Scoliosis Foundation
5 Cabot Place
Stoughton MA 02072
(800) 673-6922
http://www.scoliosis.org

A patient-led nonprofit organization dedicated since 1976 to helping children, parents, adults, and health-care providers to understand the complexities of spinal deformities such as scoliosis.

Scoliosis Association, Inc.
P.O. Box 811705
Boca Raton, FL 33481
(800) 800-0669
http://www.scoliosis-assoc.org

A nonprofit, volunteer nonmedical organization that since 1974 has been helping those with scoliosis by providing information, support groups, and other help.

Scoliosis Research Society
6300 North River Road
Suite 727

Rosemont, IL 60018-4226
(847) 698-1627
http://www.srs.org

The Web site provides patients and their parents with a better understanding of scoliosis and its diagnosis and management.

SEXUALLY TRANSMITTED DISEASES

American Social Health Association
P.O. Box 13827
Research Triangle Park, NC 27709
(919) 361-8400
http://www.ashastd.org

Nonprofit association established in 1914 to deliver accurate, medically reliable information about STDs. Public and college health clinics across the United States order ASHA educational pamphlets and books to give to clients and students, and community-based organizations depend on ASHA to help communicate about risk, transmission, prevention, testing, and treatment.

National Center for HIV, STD and TB Prevention
1108 Corporate Square
Atlanta, GA 30329
(404) 639-8040
http://www.cdc.gov/nchstp/od/nchstp.html

Government center that provides information and support for a variety of infectious diseases, including STDs and HIV.

SHAKEN BABY SYNDROME

See also CHILD ABUSE.

National Center on Shaken Baby Syndrome
http://www.dontshake.org

This Web site provides national information, support, and resources for shaken baby syndrome.

Shaken Baby Alliance
P.O. Box 150734
Ft. Worth, TX 76108
(877) 6-END-SBS or (877) 636-3727
http://www.shakenbaby.com

The Shaken Baby Alliance provides support for families and offers information on prevention.

SICKLE-CELL DISEASE

See also BLOOD DISEASES.

Sickle Cell Disease Association of America, Inc.

200 Corporate Pointe
Suite 495
Culver City, CA 90230
(310) 216-6363
(800) 421-8453
http://www.sicklecelldisease.org

This nonprofit organization is dedicated to providing support and information about sickle cell disease.

National Heart, Lung, and Blood Institute Web site

http://www.nhlbi.nih.gov

The NHLBI provides leadership for a national program in diseases of the heart, blood vessels, lung, and blood; blood resources; and sleep disorders.

The Sickle Cell Information Center Web page

http://www.emory.edu/PEDS/SICKLE

The mission of this site is to provide patient and professional education, news, research updates, and sickle cell resources.

SICK SCHOOL SYNDROME

Environmental Protection Agency

1200 Pennsylvania Avenue, NW
Washington, DC 20460
http://www.epa.gov

Government agency whose mission is to protect human health and safeguard the natural environment.

SKIN DISORDERS

American Academy of Dermatology

930 North Meacham Road
P.O. Box 4014
Schaumburg, IL 60168-4014
(847) 330-0230
http://www.aad.org

This Web site provides patients with up-to-date information on the treatment and management of disorders of the skin, hair, and nails.

Foundation for Ichthyosis and Related Skin Types

650 North Cannon Avenue
Suite 17
Lansdale, PA 19446
(800) 545-3286
(215) 631-1411
http://www.scalyskin.org

National Institute of Arthritis and Musculoskeletal and Skin Diseases

Information Clearinghouse
1 AMS Circle
Bethesda, MD 20892-3675
(877) 226-4267
(301) 495-4484 (voice)
(301) 565-2966 (TTY)
http://www.niams.nih.gov

SLEEP DISORDERS

American Academy of Sleep Medicine

Westbrook Corporate Center
Suite 920
Westchester, IL 60154
(708) 492-0930
http://www.aasmnet.org

AASM strives to increase awareness of sleep disorders in public and professional communities.

American Sleep Apnea Association

1424 K Street, NW
Suite 302
Washington, DC 20005
(202) 293-3650
http://www.sleepapnea.org

An organization dedicated to reducing injury, disability, and death from sleep apnea and to enhancing the well-being of those affected by this common disorder.

Narcolepsy and Cataplexy Foundation of America

445 East 68th Street
New York, NY 10021
(212) 570-5506

Nonprofit foundation that can provide medical referrals and referrals for nonmedical services, information, and support for individuals interested in narcolepsy or cataplexy.

National Sleep Foundation
1522 K Street, NW
Suite 500
Washington, DC 20005
(202) 347-3471
http://www.sleepfoundation.org

SPEECH PROBLEMS

See COMMUNICATION; STUTTERING.

SPINA BIFIDA

Spina Bifida Association of America
4590 MacArthur Boulevard, NW
Suite 250
Washington, DC 20007
(800) 621-3141
(202) 944-3285
http://www.sbaa.org

A nonprofit organization dedicated to publicizing developments in medicine, education, and legislation; supporting research, promoting treatment; and encouraging the training of competent professionals. SBAA publishes brochures, reports, and educational videotape programs for parents and health professionals, plus a 35-mm slide presentation on the abilities and potential of people with spina bifida.

Spinabifida.net
http://www.spinabifida.net

This site offers information about spina bifida, hydrocephalus, physical disabilities, children with special needs, latex allergies, teens with physical challenges, folic acid, plus personal stories of people with spina bifida.

SPINAL INJURIES

Christopher Reeve Paralysis Association
500 Morris Avenue
Springfield, NJ 07081

(800) 225-0292
(973) 379-2690
http://www.christopherreeve.org

Nonprofit association committed to funding research to develop treatments and cures for paralysis caused by spinal cord injury and other central nervous system disorders. The foundation also vigorously works to improve the quality of life for people living with disabilities through its grants program, paralysis resource center, and advocacy efforts. In addition, CRPA has awarded more than $2.5 million in grants to organizations that help people with disabilities live more independently and in a manner that is dictated by their abilities and not their disabilities.

National Spinal Cord Injury Association
6701 Democracy Boulevard
Suite 300-9
Bethesda, MD 20817
(301) 588-6959
http://www.spinalcoRoadorg

Nonprofit association established in 1948 to help the 7,800 individuals who sustain a spinal cord injury each year, and the 400,000 persons living with spinal cord injuries. The NSCIA has many chapters throughout the United States.

Spinal Network
3911 Princeton Drive
Santa Rosa, CA 95405-7013
(707) 577-8796
(800) 548-2673
http://www.spinalcordinjury.org

A nonprofit organization dedicated to facilitating access to quality health care by providing information and referral services to spinal-cord-injured individuals and their families.

STEPFAMILIES

Stepfamily Association of America, Inc.
650 J Street
Suite 205
Lincoln, NE 68508
(800) 735-0329
http://www.saafamilies.org

A national nonprofit organization dedicated to providing support and guidance to families with children from previous relationships. SAA provides information, education, support, and advocacy for stepfamilies and those who work with them.

Stepfamily Foundation, Inc.
333 West End Avenue
New York, NY 10023
(212) 877-3244

STREPTOCOCCUS INFECTION
Group B Strep Association
P.O. Box 16515
Chapel Hill, NC 27516
http://www.groupbstrep.org

A nonprofit organization formed in 1990 by parents whose babies were victims of GBS infections. The association works to create increased public awareness; as a result, in 1996 the Centers for Disease Control, the American College of Obstetrics and Gynecology, and the American Academy of Pediatrics issued aggressive guidelines for prenatal screening and prevention of GBS disease.

STURGE-WEBER
Sturge-Weber Syndrome Foundation
P.O. Box 418
Mount Freedom, NJ 07970
(800) 627-5482
(973) 895-4445
http://www.sturge-weber.com

Nonprofit foundation incorporated in 1987 for parents, professionals, and others concerned with Sturge-Weber syndrome; in 1992 the mission was expanded to include support for individuals with capillary vascular malformations (Port-Wine Stain or PWS) and Klippel Trenaunay (KT).

STUTTERING
See also COMMUNICATION.

National Center for Stuttering
200 East 33rd Street
Suite 17C
New York, NY 10016

(800) 221-2483
http://www.stuttering.com

Center that offers information, a hotline, treatment, continuing education, and research.

Stuttering Foundation of America
3100 Walnut Grove Road
Suite 603
P.O. Box 11749
Memphis, TN 38111-0749
http://www.stutteringhelp.org

The Stuttering Foundation of America provides free online resources, services, and support to those who stutter and their families, as well as support for research into the causes of stuttering.

Stuttering Home Page
http://www.stutteringhomepage.com

This site offers information about speech disorders through chat rooms, articles, and awareness.

SUDDEN INFANT DEATH SYNDROME
American SIDS Institute
2480 Windy Hill Road
Suite 380
Marietta, GA 30067
(770) 612-1030
(800) 232-SIDS
http://www.sids.org

National nonprofit health-care organization founded in 1983 that is dedicated to the prevention of sudden infant death and the promotion of infant health through an aggressive, comprehensive, nationwide program of research about the cause and prevention of SIDS, clinical services assisting pediatricians in the medical management of high-risk infants, education about prevention methods aimed at the public and medical community, and crises phone counseling, grief literature, and referrals.

SUICIDE
American Foundation for Suicide Prevention
120 Wall Street
22nd Floor
New York, NY 10005

(888) 333-AFSP
(212) 363-3500
http://www.afsp.org

This organization provides research, education, and current statistics regarding suicide; links to other suicide and mental health sites are offered.

American Association of Suicidology

2459 South Ash Street
Denver, CO 80222
(303) 692-0985
(202) 237-2280
http://www.suicidology.org

Organization provides information on current research, prevention, ways to help a suicidal person, and surviving suicide. A list of crisis centers is available.

Boys Town

(800) 448-3000 (crisis hotline)
(800) 545-5771
http://www.boystown.org

This organization cares for troubled children—both boys and girls—and for families in crisis. Their hotline staff is trained to handle calls and questions about violence and suicide.

SUPPORT

STARBRIGHT Foundation

11835 West Olympic Boulevard
Suite 500
Los Angeles, CA 90064
(310) 479-1212
http://www.starbright.org

Foundation dedicated to projects that empower seriously ill children to combat the medical and emotional challenges. STARBRIGHT projects address the pain, fear, loneliness, and depression that can be as damaging as the sickness itself. Through the efforts of STARBRIGHT chairmen Steven Spielberg and General H. Norman Schwarzkopf, a computer network is available where hospitalized children and teens can interact with a community of peers and help each other cope with the day-to-day realities of living with illness.

TAY-SACHS DISEASE

National Tay Sachs and Allied Diseases Association

2001 Beacon Street
Suite 204
Brookline, MA 02146
(800) 906-8723
http://www.ntsad.org

Nonprofit association dedicated to the treatment and prevention of Tay-Sachs, Canavan, [Canavan disease is related to Tay-Sachs and belongs to a group of diseases known as leukodystrophies, characterized by myelin defects. Children with Canavan disease have an enzyme deficiency that leads to myelin destruction. Children with Canavan disease eventually become blind, usually dying in infancy or early childhood], and related diseases, and to provide information and support services to individuals and families affected by these diseases, as well as the public at large. Strategies for achieving these goals include public and professional education, research, genetic screening, family services, and advocacy.

TOURETTE'S SYNDROME

Tourette's Syndrome Association

4240 Bell Boulevard
Suite 205
Bayside, NY 11361
(718) 224-2999
(800) 237-0717
http://www.tsa.mgh.harvard.edu

TSA is a volunteer organization working to find the cause of and cure for Tourette's syndrome. It has books, pamphlets, and videos about the condition and related topics, and there are state chapters and local support groups for people with or affected by Tourette's syndrome.

TUBEROUS SCLEROSIS

Tuberous Sclerosis Alliance

801 Roeder Road
Suite 750
Silver Spring, MD 20910
(800) 225-6872
http://www.tsalliance.org

A national nonprofit health organization dedicated to finding a cure for the many aspects of tuberous sclerosis complex. The Alliance was founded in 1974 by four mothers to provide fellowship, generate awareness, pursue more knowledge, and provide hope to those that shared the common bond of tuberous sclerosis.

VACCINE INJURY

National Vaccine Injury Compensation Program
(800) 338-2382
http://www.hrsa.gov/osp/vicp

Program administered by the federal government that provides for compensation for anyone injured by a required vaccine.

National Vaccine Injury Information Center
421-E Church Street
Vienna, VA 22180
(703) 938-DPT3
(800) 909-SHOT
http://www.909shot.com

A national nonprofit educational organization founded in 1982, the oldest and largest national organization advocating reformation of the mass vaccination system.

VIOLENCE

Center for the Prevention of School Violence Web site
http://www.ncsu.edu/cpsv

Established in 1993, the center serves as a primary point of contact for dealing with school violence.

Join Together
(617) 437-1500
http://www.jointogether.org

Join Together, a project of the Boston University School of Public Health, is a national resource for communities working to reduce substance abuse and gun violence.

Parents and Children Together to Stop Violence (PACT) Web site
http://pact.aol.com/mynews/teenpact.adp

Teens can visit this site to sign a pact to stop violence.

School Violence Web page
http://www.uncg.edu/edu/ericcass/violence/index.htm

School Violence offers school safety information and resources for parents.

VISUAL PROBLEMS

See BLINDNESS.

VON HIPPEL–LANDAU

Von Hippel–Lindau Family Alliance
171 Clinton Road
Brookline, MA 02445
(800) 767-4845
(617) 277-5667
http://www.vhl.org

Nonprofit group that provides information for families and physicians about this disorder, and local self-help support groups for families affected with VHL. Local family support chapters exist in many U.S. states.

APPENDIX II
CAMPS FOR KIDS WITH CANCER

GENERAL INFORMATION

Children's Oncology Camping Association International

http://www.coca-intl.org

A listing of approximately 65 camps in the United States and other organizations elsewhere in the world that have camps for cancer kids.

Camp Quality USA

Email: info@campqualityusa.com
http://www.campqualityusa.org

A summer camping experience and year-round support program for children with cancer.

CONNECTICUT

Hole in the Wall Gang Camp

565 Ashford Center Road
Ashford, CT 06278
(860) 429-3444
E-mail: ashford@holeinthewallgang.org
http://www.holeinthewallgang.org

A camp in Northeast Connecticut, founded by actor Paul Newman, that offers camping experiences to children with cancer and blood diseases.

FLORIDA

Boggy Creek Camp

30500 Brantley Branch Road
Eustis, FL 32736
(352) 483-4200
E-mail: info@boggycreek.org
http://www.boggycreek.org

A camp in central Florida that serves children with different types of medical needs.

BaseCamp Candlelighters Children's Cancer Foundation

7501 Glenmoor Lane
Winter Park, FL 32792-9061
E-mail: email@basecampccf.com
http://www.basecampccf.com

A camp in Central Florida for children with cancer.

MAINE

Camp Sunshine

35 Acadia Road
Casco, ME 04015
(207) 655-3800
E-mail: info@campsunshine.org
http://www.campsunshine.org

A camp that offers weeklong camping for the entire family who has a child with cancer. There are workshops, recreational activities, and medical support available.

MARYLAND

Camp Fantastic–Special Love Program

117 Youth Development Court
Wincester, VA 22602
(888) 930-2707
http://www.speciallove.org/progrmfr.html

A summer camping program, as well as other weekend programs throughout the year.

MONTANA

Camp Make a Dream
Children's Oncology Camp Foundation
P.O. Box 1450
Missoula, MT 59806
(406) 549-5987
http://www.campdream.org

A camp with programs for cancer kids, siblings, teens, and young adult camp experiences.

NEW YORK

Camp Simcha
(212) 465-0949
http://www.chailifeline.org/camp_simcha.asp

A kosher camp in New York for Jewish children with cancer.

APPENDIX III
TOLL-FREE HEALTH HOTLINES

Acne Help Line
(800) 222-SKIN
(800) 221-SKIN (in California)

AIDS
See National AIDS Hot Line

AIDS Clinical Trials Information Service
(800) 874-2572 (English and Spanish)
(800) 243-7012 (TDD)

American Academy of Facial Plastic and Reconstructive Surgery
(800) 332-FACE

American Academy of Pediatrics (AAP)
(800) 421-0589

American Council of the Blind
(800) 424-8666

American Diabetes Association
(800) 232-3472

American Kidney Fund
(800) 638-8299 (in Maryland)
(800) 492-8361

American Liver Foundation
(800) 223-0179

American Paralysis Association
(800) 225-0292

American Parkinson's Disease Association
(800) 233-2732

American Social Health Association
(800) 982-5803

American Society for Dermatologic Surgery
(800) 441-ASDS

American Society of Plastic and Reconstructive Surgeons
(800) 635-0635

American Trauma Society (ATS)
(800) 556-7890

American Tuberous Sclerosis Association
(800) 446-1211

Anorexia Nervosa/Bulimia Hotline
(847) 831-3438

Arthritis Medical Center
(800) 327-3027
(305) 739-3202 (in Ft. Lauderdale)

Better Hearing Institute
(800) 424-8576

Bulimia and Anorexia Self Help
(800) 762-3334
(314) 768-3838 (in St. Louis)

Cancer Information Service
(800) 4-CANCER
(800) 638-6070 (in Alaska)

Centers for Disease Control STD National Hotline
(800) 227-8922

Consumer Product Safety Commission
(800) 638-2772
(800) 492-8363 (in Maryland)
(800) 638-8333 (in Alaska and Hawaii)

Cystic Fibrosis Foundation
(800) 344-4823

Deafness Research Foundation
(800) 535-3323

Dial-a-Hearing Screen Test
(800) 222-EARS
(800) 345-3277 (in Pennsylvania)

Epilepsy Foundation of America
(800) EFA-1000
(301) 459-1000 (in Maryland)

Gallaudet College (National Information Center on Deafness)
(800) 672-6720

Head Injury Hotline
(206) 621-8558

Institute of Logopedics (multiply handicapped children)
(800) 835-1043

Juvenile Diabetes Foundation (JDF)
(800) 223-1138

Living Bank (organ and body donations)
(800) 528-2971

Medic Alert Foundation International (emergency medical identification system)
(800) 344-3226

Metro-Help National Runaway Switchboard
(800) 621-4000
(800) 972-6004 (in Illinois)

National AIDS Clearinghouse
(800) 458-5231 (English and Spanish)
(800) 243-7012 (TDD)

National AIDS Hot Line
(800) 342-2437 (24 hours)
(800) 344-7432 (Spanish)
(800) 243-7889 (TDD)

National Alliance of Blind Students
(800) 424-8666

National Association for Hearing and Speech Action (NAHSA)
(800) 638-8255

National Association for Sickle Cell Disease
(800) 421-8453

National Association for the Education of Young Children
(800) 424-2460

National Center for Missing and Exploited Children
(800) 843-5678

National Center for Stuttering
(800) 221-2483
(212) 532-1460 (in New York City)

National Children's Leukemia Foundation
(800) GIVE-HOPE
(800) 448-3467

National Cocaine Hot Line
(800) 262-2463

National Domestic Violence Hotline
(800) 799-SAFE or (800) 799-7233

National Down Syndrome Congress
(800) 446-3835
(800) 232-NDSC (in Illinois)

National Down Syndrome Society
(800) 221-4602

National Federation of Parents for Drug-Free Youth
(800) 554-5437

National Gay Task Force
(800) 221-7044

National Health Information Clearinghouse
(800) 336-4797

National Hearing Aid Society
(800) 521-5247

National Information Center for Orphan Drugs and Rare Diseases
(800) 336-4797

National Institute on Drug Abuse
(800) 662-4357

National Jewish Hospital and Research Center/National Asthma Center
(800) 222-5864

National Neurofibromatosis Foundation
(800) 323-7938

National Parkinson Foundation
(800) 327-4545

National Pesticide Telecommunications
  Network
(800) 858-7378

National Rehabilitation Information Center
(800) 34-NARIC

National Retinitis Pigmentosa Foundation
(800) 638-2300

National Reye's Syndrome Foundation
(800) 233-7393
(800) 231-7393 (in Ohio)

National Sexually Transmitted Disease
  Hotline
(800) 227-8922

National Sudden Infant Death Syndrome
  Foundation
(800) 221-SIDS

National Vaccine Injury Compensation
  Program
(800) 338-2382

Recording for the Blind (RFB)
(800) 221-4792

Runaway Hot Line
(800) 231-6946
(800) 392-3552 (in Texas)

Safe Drinking Water Hotline
(800) 426-4791

Sexually Transmitted Disease Hot Line
(800) 227-8922

Smallpox Vaccination Hotline
(888) 246-2675

Spina Bifida Association of America
(800) 621-3141

Sudden Infant Death Syndrome Hot Line
(800) 221-7437
(301) 459-3388 (in Maryland)

APPENDIX IV
HANDLING EMERGENCIES

Every parent at one time or another agonizes over this question: *Is this serious enough to call the doctor?* On the one hand, parents hate to bother the pediatrician over what might be a routine matter. On the other hand, a baby is so vulnerable. This situation is made even harder by the fact that it seems the baby always gets sick in the middle of the night.

Problems such as earache, flu, colds, or a slight fever are not emergencies and can be managed by the pediatrician during regular office hours. Parents should talk to the doctor *before* a child gets sick and find out whom to call or see when the doctor is not available.

THIS IS AN EMERGENCY

For babies: The doctor should be called right away if an infant has *any* of the following signs. If the doctor is not available, the emergency room should be the first stop if the baby:

- is lethargic
- refuses to eat
- has sleeping problems
- has diarrhea or vomiting
- has a fever over 101°F
- has unusual chest motion or sucking in of the spaces between the ribs or under the chest during breathing
- has severe stridor (a crowing sound when breathing in) or severe wheezing (whistling sound when breathing out)
- has tense or bulging fontanel (the soft spot on the side of an infant's head) when sitting upright and quiet
- has signs of severe dehydration including:
  - dry mouth
  - sunken eyeballs
  - failure to urinate for more than eight hours
  - sunken soft spot on the head
  - irritability and extreme listlessness
  - doughy, wrinkled skin

For children: The doctor should be called right away if a child has *any* of the following signs. If the doctor is not available, the emergency room should be the first stop if the child:

- cannot be awakened
- has trouble making eye contact
- is choking
- has seizures (convulsions)
- has severe breathing difficulty
- has very rapid or very labored breathing
- makes a grunting sound with breathing
- has severe stridor (a crowing sound when breathing in) or severe wheezing (whistling sound when breathing out)
- has severe difficulty inhaling because of anxiety, fear, refusal to swallow, or drooling
- has a stiff neck, in a very sick child
- has a rash caused by broken blood vessels in a child who seems sick (tiny red dots that do not disappear when skin is pressed, or larger blood spots that look like bruises)
- has a convulsion with or without fever if a child has never had convulsions before
- has severe lethargy, sleeplessness, or listlessness
- has extreme unexplained irritability
- has a fever of more than 105°F
- has an unusual cry (such as a weak or whimpering constant cry or a high-pitched cry)

- had a head injury in which the child lost consciousness even briefly and has not returned to the usual level of awareness, has vomited more than twice after the injury, or has abnormal pupils
- had a near-drowning episode, even if the child is awake and breathing
- has abnormal bleeding, vomiting, bloody diarrhea, or excessive bruising
- has had suspected poisoning, even if the child is still conscious and breathing easily
- has signs of severe dehydration including:
  ○ dry mouth
  ○ sunken eyeballs
  ○ failure to urinate for more than eight hours (or 12 hours for an older child)
  ○ sunken soft spot on the head
  ○ irritability and extreme listlessness
  ○ doughy, wrinkled skin

CALL A DOCTOR IN AN HOUR OR TWO

In the following situations, a child may need some kind of medical evaluation in a few hours:

- mild breathing difficulty (mild wheezing or whistling noise when the child breathes out or in) or mild stridor (a crowing sound when the child breathes in, without color change or other signs of distress)
- unusual behavior such as:
  ○ lethargy
  ○ listlessness
  ○ clumsy movements
  ○ refusal to eat or drink in 12 to 24 hours
  ○ unusual irritability, and persistent crying, severe or prolonged vomiting or diarrhea
  ○ signs of mild dehydration, such as severe reduction in the amount of urine, sticky mouth and lips, and listlessness or irritability
  ○ persistent pain anywhere in the body (headache, abdominal pain, earache, sore throat, or bone pain)
  ○ head injury, in which the child lost consciousness but now seems normal or nearly normal

○ suspected broken bone when the person can be easily moved
○ fever over 103°F with other symptoms that suggest a serious illness
○ signs of a possible serious infection

MAKE AN APPOINTMENT WITHIN 24 HOURS

Parents probably should call the doctor to make an appointment in 24 hours for their child if:

- the child does not seem to be recovering from a minor illness or injury after several days
- a very young baby suffers with severe congestion (especially if it interferes with feeding or sleeping)
- a fever lasts longer than three days without other symptoms of a specific illness
- there is persistent or recurring pain, mild to moderate breathing problems, or persistent vomiting or diarrhea
- there is loss of appetite for more than a week or if the child does not seem quite right
- there is blood in the stool

PREPARING FOR EMERGENCIES

The best time to prepare for an emergency is *before* it happens. *Every* member of the family should know what to do in a serious situation. Any child over age four should know how to place a call for help.

List emergency numbers One of the best ways to be prepared is to gather all the emergency numbers in one place. During an emergency, it is easy for parents to become so upset they get disoriented. If all important phone numbers are readily available by the phone, things will be much easier. A laminated emergency phone numbers list is a good idea. Each entry should be printed clearly with a pen with dark-colored ink. The list should include:

- 911 or other emergency medical services (Most places have 911 service, but some rural communities may have another emergency number. Check your telephone book.)
- national poison control number: 1 (800) 222-1222
- hospital emergency room

- fire department
- police department
- pediatrician
- parent(s) work and cell phone numbers
- neighbors (at least two)
- relatives (at least two)

Calling the doctor When calling the doctor about a problem with a child's health, the parent should give both parents' names and child's name (particularly if last names are different). If this is not a life-threatening situation, parents should write down questions to ask the doctor before calling to avoid having to call back to ask other questions.

Parents should be prepared with the answers to all of the following questions, because either the nurse or the doctor will ask them:

When did the problem start? Be as specific as possible: yesterday morning, two nights ago, a week ago today.

What are the symptoms? Parents should list the symptoms in the order they occurred, as briefly and succinctly as possible.

How severe are the symptoms? Parents should be as specific as possible:

- She has had a fever of 104°F for the past two hours.
- He has vomited six times in the last five hours.
- She seems lethargic ever since she fell out of the tree house.

Is it getting worse? The doctor needs to know how the symptoms are progressing. For example: "After she fell off the horse we thought she was okay, but then she seemed to get sleepy and did not respond clearly when I asked her questions."

What have you done so far? The doctor wants to know what first aid actions have been taken. If the child has taken ibuprofen every six hours and it has not touched the fever, this can be important.

How does the child look? Parents may not think to mention it right away, but physical appearance can help in a diagnosis: "He seems pale and his skin has a bluish tinge" or "The baby's head seems to be bulging a bit at the top."

Does the child have a chronic disease? If the doctor has a large practice, he or she may not remember that the child has diabetes or asthma.

Does your child take medication routinely? Sometimes medications can have side effects that may just be appearing now, or that may interact with something the pediatrician is about to prescribe.

Does the child have any allergies? The doctor needs to know if a child is allergic to certain antibiotics or other drugs, but other allergies could be important, too. Report any problems with insects, food, milk, or other substances.

How much does your child weigh? This is especially important if the child sees the pediatrician only once a year for a well-child checkup. Children grow constantly, and since medication is given based on weight, an accurate measurement is important.

IF THE CHILD GETS WORSE

If the doctor has not called back and the child is getting worse, parents should not wait for the doctor to return a call. Parents should call the doctor again if the situation changes and explain the situation, letting the receptionist or nurse know that a doctor—*any* doctor—needs to come to the phone right away.

APPENDIX V
TYPICAL CHILDHOOD INFECTIONS AND DISEASES

COMMON CHILDHOOD INFECTIONS

acute ear infection
adenovirus
bronchiolitis
candidiasis (diaper rash, thrush, vaginal
    yeast infection)
common cold
croup
diphtheria
eye infections
fungal infections (ringworm, jock itch,
    athlete's foot)
head lice
influenza (flu)
measles
meningitis
pneumocystis carinii
pneumonia
respiratory syncytial virus
scarlet fever
strep throat (group A streptococci infections)
swimmer's ear
tuberculosis
urinary tract infections
varicella (chicken pox)
whooping cough

PARASITIC INFESTATIONS

giardiasis
head lice
lice
malaria
pinworm
scabies
toxocariasis
toxoplasmosis
trichomoniasis

SEXUALLY TRANSMITTED DISEASES

chlamydia
genital warts
gonococcal infections
herpes simplex
HIV and AIDS
lice
pelvic inflammatory disease
scabies
trichomoniasis

SKIN INFECTIONS AND RASHES

cellulitis
chicken pox
eczema
fifth disease
herpes simplex
impetigo
Lyme disease
measles
Rocky Mountain spotted fever
roseola
rubella (german measles)
scabies
scarlet fever
toxic shock syndrome
warts

STOMACH AND INTESTINAL INFECTIONS

appendicitis
campylobacter infections
food poisoning
giardiasis
Helicobacter pylori infection
pinworms
rotavirus
salmonellosis
shigellosis

APPENDIX VI
CHILDREN'S HOSPITALS IN THE UNITED STATES

MAJOR HOSPITAL WEB SITES

ARKANSAS

Arkansas Children's Hospital
Little Rock, AR
http://www.archildrens.org

Provides information about the hospital and health care for children, parents, professionals, and the community.

ARIZONA

Phoenix Children's Hospital
Phoenix, AZ
http://www.phxchildrens.com

Health and safety information for parents of infants, children, and teens; care tips for childhood illnesses and injuries; pediatric medical specialty clinics; kids' page; and consumer health library.

CALIFORNIA

Children's Hospital and Health Center
San Diego, CA
http://www.chsd.org

A full-service pediatric health center.

Children's Hospital Los Angeles
Los Angeles, CA
http://www.ChildrensHospitalLA.org

Includes a heart institute, cancer and blood diseases, and research institute.

Children's Hospital Central California
Madera, CA
http://www.childrenscentralcal.org

Pediatric care facility.

Children's Hospital of Orange County
Orange, CA
http://www.chochospital.org

Center of a regional pediatric health care system dedicated to serving the needs of infants, children, and adolescents, including preventive medical care, education, and state-of-the-art pediatric biomedical research.

**Children's Recovery Center
of Northern California**
Campbell, CA
http://www.pedisubacute.com

Providing health care to meet the unique medical and developmental needs of children.

**Lucile Salter Packard Children's
Hospital**
San Francisco and Palo Alto, CA
http://www.lpch.org

Part of the Stanford Health Care System of the University of California–San Francisco (UCSF)

Mattel Children's Hospital at UCLA
Los Angeles, CA
http://www.pediatrics.medsch.ucla.edu

Pediatric care at the Mattel Children's Hospital at the University of California–Los Angeles

University Children's Medical Group
Los Angeles, CA
http://www.ucmg.org

Multispecialty pediatric medical group, including world-renowned physicians.

COLORADO

The Children's Hospital
Denver, CO
http://www.thechildrenshospital.org

Affiliated with the University of Colorado Health Sciences Center, providing information on clinical departments and pediatric subspecialties.

CONNECTICUT

Connecticut Children's Medical Center
Hartford, CT
http://www.ccmckids.org

Pediatric health care services, teaching and research for children from birth to age 18.

Yale–New Haven Children's Hospital
New Haven, CT
http://www.ynhh.org/ynhch/ynhch.html

Located in southern Connecticut, this 900-bed tertiary care facility serves as the primary teaching hospital for the Yale University School of Medicine.

DELAWARE

The Alfred I. duPont Hospital for Children
Wilmington, DE
http://www.nemours.org/no/aidhc

A full-service children's hospital operated by the Nemours Foundation.

FLORIDA

All Children's Hospital
St. Petersburg, FL
http://www.allkids.org

A regional referral center for children with some of the most challenging medical problems.

Arnold Palmer Hospital for Children and Women
Orlando, FL
http://www.arnoldpalmerhospital.org

A 281-bed hospital dedicated to caring for the health care needs of children and women.

Joe DiMaggio Children's Hospital
Hollywood, FL
http://www.jdch.com

Regional provider of children's services offering inpatient and outpatient medical/surgical services and a level III neonatal ICU and pediatric ICU.

Miami Children's Hospital
Miami, FL
http://www.mch.com

Renowned Miami children's hospital.

GEORGIA

Medical College of Georgia Children's Medical Center
Augusta, GA
http://www.mcghealth.org/cmc

A top pediatric trauma center caring for critically ill or injured children.

Scottish Rite Children's Medical Center
Atlanta, GA
http://www.scottishritechildrens.org

Offers pediatric health care information on illness, injury, health, parenting, and safety of infants, children, and adolescents.

ILLINOIS

Children's Memorial Hospital
Chicago, IL
http://www.childrensmemorial.org

Information for patients, parents, and staff, as well as child advocacy, research, residency program, and sites for kids.

Hope Children's Hospital
Oak Lawn, IL
http://www.advocatehealth.com/hope

A children's specialty hospital staffed by more than 140 pediatricians representing more than 30 specialties.

Lutheran General Children's Hospital
Park Ridge, IL
http://www.advocatehealth.com/lgch

This hospital is designed to meet the unique health care needs of children with 185 pediatricians and pediatric subspecialists on staff in virtually every medicinal and surgical specialty.

University of Chicago Children's Hospital
Chicago, IL
http://peds-www.bsd.uchicago.edu

Renowned children's hospital in Chicago.

University of Illinois Medical Center, Department of Pediatrics/Child and Adolescent Center
Chicago, IL
http://www.uillinoismedcenter.org/
    content.cfm/peds

Provides complete child-centered care from infancy through the teen years. Includes on-line library and visitor information.

IOWA
Children's Hospital of Iowa
Iowa City, IA
http://www.vh.org/VCH

Information for health care providers and parents, fact sheets on common ailments, and pages for kids.

LOUISIANA
Children's Hospital
New Orleans, LA
http://www.chnola.org

The regional children's medical center for Louisiana: a 188-bed pediatric medical center offering a full range of inpatient and outpatient care.

MARYLAND
Johns Hopkins Children's Center
Baltimore, MD
http://www.hopkinschildrens.org

Acute care hospital for children, including faculty, residency program, links, clinical, and referral information.

University of Maryland Medicine's Children's Hospital
Baltimore, MD
http://www.umm.edu/pediatrics

Statewide resource for critically ill children; provides 17 divisions to address complicated pediatric problems.

MASSACHUSETTS

Children's Hospital
Boston, MA
http://www.childrenshospital.org

Pediatric teaching hospital of Harvard Medical School, rated the number-one pediatric medical center in the United States for more than 10 years.

Franciscan Children's Hospital and Rehabilitation Center
Boston, MA
http://www.fchrc.org

The largest pediatric rehabilitation hospital in New England.

MICHIGAN
Children's Hospital of Michigan
Detroit, MI
http://www.chmkids.org

Specialty in pediatric medicine, surgery, health research, and education.

MINNESOTA
Fairview Childrens Hospital
Minneapolis, MN
http://www.fairviewchildrens.org

Providing state-of-the-art care for children and meeting the unique needs of children.

Gillette Children's Hospital
St. Paul, MN
http://www.gillettechildrens.org

Specialty care for children and young adults with cerebral palsy.

MISSOURI

Children's Mercy Hospitals and Clinics
Kansas City, MO
http://www.childrens-mercy.org

Exclusive pediatric medical center and health care network, with all staff trained specifically to work with children.

Pediatric Cardiology at St. Louis
   Children's Hospital
St. Louis, MO
http://peds.wustl.edu/div/cardiology

The Division of Pediatric Cardiology offers care for all forms of congenital and acquired heart disease in the pediatric age range.

NEW YORK

Center for Children
New York, NY
http://www.nyuhjdcenterforchildren.org

Located at the Hospital for Joint Diseases, the center provides medical treatment of disabled children through a comprehensive outpatient facility.

Child Life Services
New York, NY
http://www.med.nyu.edu/childlife

Located in the Tisch Hospital at New York University (NYU) Medical Center, the unit serves children with a wide array of illnesses and provides specialized care in cardiology, hematology, neurology, oncology, and reconstructive and general surgeries.

Children's Hospital of Buffalo
Buffalo, NY
http://www.chob.edu

The Western New York regional center for specialized pediatric care, with a special "Kid's Department" to help children with a scary trip to the hospital.

Strong Children's Hospital
Rochester, NY
http://www.urmc.rochester.edu/sch

Part of the Department of Pediatrics at Strong Memorial Hospital of the University of Rochester.

OHIO

Children's Hospital
Columbus, OH
http://www.childrenscolumbus.com

Specialties in surgical, neurosciences, rehabilitation, burns, dialysis, and bone marrow units serving infants to adolescents.

Cincinnati Children's Hospital Medical
   Center
Cincinnati, OH
http://www.cincinnatichildrens.org

Nonprofit, specialty pediatric hospital serving infants through adolescents.

Children's Hospital Medical Center
   of Akron
Akron, OH
http://www.akronchildrens.org

Web site provides information for parents, "virtual visit," patient greetings, teen health resources, and doctor finder.

Children's Medical Center of Dayton
Dayton, OH
http://www.cmc-dayton.org

Cares for children of all ages from newborns to teenagers. Information for parents, teens, physicians, and event calendar.

Rainbow Babies and Children's Hospital
Cleveland, OH
http://www.uhrainbow.com

The pediatric hospital of University Hospitals of Cleveland, dedicated solely to the comprehensive care of children. General information, staff directory, and information for parents, families, and healthcare professionals.

OREGON

Legacy Emanuel Children's Hospital
Portland, OR
http://www.legacyhealth.org/findus/hospitals/
  ech/ech.ssi

Serving Oregon, southwest Washington, Alaska, and Idaho, it provides virtually all medical specialties in a state-of-the-art child-focused environment.

PENNSYLVANIA

Children's Hospital of Pittsburgh
Pittsburgh, PA
http://www.chp.edu

This is the only free-standing hospital in western Pennsylvania dedicated solely to the care of infants, children, and young adults.

Children's Hospital of Philadelphia
Philadelphia, PA
http://www.chop.edu/index.html

Providing comprehensive inpatient and outpatient care for children from birth through age 19.

Children's Institute
Pittsburgh, PA
http://amazingkids.org/index.html?cState=tci

Rehabilitation facility offering several rehabilitation programs, including special education, programs for learning disabilities and Prader-Willi syndrome, and special needs adoption.

Penn State Children's Hospital
Hershey, PA
http://www.hmc.psu.edu/childrens

Part of Pennsylvania State University's College of Medicine.

**Penn State Children's Hospital—
  Heart Group**
Hershey, PA
http://www.hmc.psu.edu/childrensheartgroup

A team of experienced pediatric cardiovascular physicians, working together to provide heart care for children.

RHODE ISLAND

Pediatric Surgery at Hasbro
Providence, RI
http://bms.brown.edu/pedisurg/pedisurg.html

Surgical care for infants, children, and adolescents, including congenital anomalies, tumors, trauma, endoscopy, and laparoscopy.

**Women and Infants Hospital
  of Rhode Island**
Providence, RI
http://www.womenandinfants.com

Health care facilities for women, as well as primary care and specialized services for women and newborn children.

SOUTH CAROLINA

MUSC Children's Hospital
Charleston, SC
http://www.musckids.com

Children's hospital named by *Child* magazine as one of the nation's top 10 in 2001.

TENNESSEE

East Tennessee Children's Hospital
Knoxville, TN
http://www.etch.com

Pediatric specialty hospital.

Le Bonheur Children's Medical Center
Memphis, TN
http://www.lebonheur.org

Comprehensive children's medical facility.

Vanderbilt Children's Hospital
Nashville, TN
http://www.vanderbiltchildrens.com

Provides information, services, research, and events.

Vanderbilt Children's Hospital Division of Pediatric Cardiology
Nashville, TN
http://peds.mc.vanderbilt.edu/car

Provides the highest level of cardiac care for children and young adults from throughout the United States.

TEXAS

Children's Medical Center of Dallas
Dallas, TX
http://www.childrens.com

This hospital has a pediatric emergency center, intensive care unit, and wide spectrum of services; its Web site offers online health tips for kids and parents.

Cook Children's Medical Center
Fort Worth, TX
http://www.CookChildrens.org

Cares for ill and injured children from Fort Worth and 90 counties in north-central and west Texas.

Texas Children's Hospital—Pediatric Health Care
Houston, TX
http://www.texaschildrenshospital.org

The largest pediatric facility in the United States, offering treatment of cancer, diabetes, and premature births and surgical and transplant services.

VIRGINIA

Children's Hospital
Richmond, VA
http://childrenshosp-richmond.org

Private, nonprofit, specialty pediatric hospital that serves children from birth through the age of 21.

Children's Hospital of the King's Daughters
Hampton Roads, VA
http://www.chkd.org

Providing a variety of services to benefit the health and well-being of the region's children.

Children's Medical Center
Charlottesville, VA
http://galen.med.virginia.edu/~smb4v/
    cmchome.html

Dedicated to the health and well-being of the region's children.

WASHINGTON

Children's Hospital and Regional Medical Center
Seattle, WA
http://www.seattlechildrens.org

Pediatric referral center serving children in Washington, Alaska, Montana, and Idaho.

Sacred Heart Children's Hospital
Spokane, WA
http://www.shmcchildren.org

A nonprofit, Catholic-sponsored children's hospital, affiliated with network facilities throughout the western states.

WASHINGTON, D.C.

Children's Hospital

Washington, D.C.

http://www.dcchildrens.com

Specializes in pediatric care and family-oriented health care since 1870.

Children's National Medical Center

Washington, D.C.

http://www.cnmc.org

Includes specialty centers for cardiovascular care, neurology, cancer, and blood disorders.

WISCONSIN

Children's Hospital of Wisconsin

Milwaukee, WI

http://www.chw.org

Pediatric specialists in congenital heart disease; heart, lung, and bone marrow transplantation; pain management; and other diagnoses and treatment.

University of Wisconsin Children's Hospital

Madison, WI

http://www.uwchildrenshospital.org

Complete children's medical and surgical center within University of Wisconsin Hospital and Clinics.

SHRINERS HOSPITALS FOR CHILDREN

CALIFORNIA

Shriners Hospital—Los Angeles

(orthopedic)

3160 Geneva Street

Los Angeles, CA 90020

(213) 388-3151

Shriners Hospital—Northern California

(orthopedic, burn, and spinal cord injury)

2425 Stockton Boulevard

Sacramento, CA 95817

(916) 453-2000

CANADA

Shriners Hospital—Canada

(orthopedics)

1529 Cedar Avenue

Montreal, Quebec, H3G 1A6

(514) 842-4464

FLORIDA

Shriners Hospital—Tampa

(orthopedic)

12502 North Pine Drive

Tampa, FL 33612-9499

(813) 972-2250

HAWAII

Shriners Hospital—Honolulu

(orthopedic)

1310 Punahou Street

Honolulu, HI 96826-1099

(808) 941-4466

ILLINOIS

Shriners Hospital—Chicago

(orthopedics and spinal cord injury)

2211 North Oak Park Avenue

Chicago, IL 60707

(773) 622-5400

KENTUCKY

Shriners Hospital—Lexington

(orthopedic)

1900 Richmond Road

Lexington, KY 40502

(859) 266-2101

LOUISIANA

Shriners Hospital—Shreveport
(orthopedic)
3100 Samford Avenue
Shreveport, LA 71103
(318) 222-5704

MASSACHUSETTS

Shriners Hospital—Boston
(burn)
51 Blossom Street
Boston, MA 02114
(617) 722-3000

Shriners Hospital—Springfield
(orthopedic)
516 Carew Street
Springfield, MA 01104
(413) 787-2000

MINNESOTA

Shriners Hospital—Twin Cities
(orthopedic)
2025 East River Parkway
Minneapolis, MN 55414
(612) 596-6100

MISSOURI

Shriners Hospital—St. Louis
(orthopedic)
2001 South Lindbergh Boulevard
St. Louis, MO 63131-3597
(314) 432-3600

OHIO

Shriners Hospital—Cincinnati
(burn)
3229 Burnet Avenue
Cincinnati, OH 45229-3095
(513) 872-6000

OREGON

Shriners Hospital—Portland
(orthopedic)
3101 Southwest Sam Jackson Park Road
Portland, OR 97239
(503) 241-5090
http://www.shcc.org

PENNSYLVANIA

Shriners Hospital—Erie
(orthopedic)
1645 West 8th Street
Erie, PA 16505
(814) 875-8700

Shriners Hospital—Philadelphia
(orthopedic and spinal cord injury)
3551 North Broad Street
Philadelphia, PA 19140
(215) 430-4000

SOUTH CAROLINA

Shriners Hospital—Greenville
(orthopedic)
950 West Faris Road
Greenville, SC 29605-4277
(864) 271-3444

TEXAS

Shriners Hospital—Galveston
(burn)
815 Market Street
Galveston, TX 77550-2725
(409) 770-6600

Shriners Hospital—Houston
(orthopedic)
6977 Main
Houston, TX 77030-3701
(713) 797-1616

UTAH

Shriners Hospital—Intermountain
(orthopedic)
Fairfax Road at Virginia Street
Salt Lake City, UT 84103
(801) 536-3500

WASHINGTON

Shriners Hospital—Spokane
(orthopedic)
911 West Fifth Avenue
Spokane, WA 99204-2901
(509) 455-7844

APPENDIX VII
POISON CONTROL CENTERS

The U.S. poison emergency phone number is (800) 222-1222, and anyone who calls this number—24 hours a day, seven days a week—will be connected to a poison expert. Anyone experiencing a poison emergency or who has a question about a poison or about poison prevention should call right away. The U.S. nationwide poison control number is connected to a network of 62 poison centers around the United States, and callers are connected automatically to a local poison center expert in their area, selected according to the area code and exchange of the phone number from which the call originates.

Cell phone calls also will reach a poison center. Depending on the cell phone carrier, however, the caller might reach a poison center in their local area or in the "home" area of the cell phone company, but either poison center can help. Old numbers for local poison centers presently still work, but families should post and learn the new number.

Poison centers certified by the American Association of Poison Control Centers (AAPCC) are printed in italics.

Poison control centers in Canada are also listed.

ALABAMA

Alabama Poison Center
2503 Phoenix Drive
Tuscaloosa, AL 35405
(800) 462-0800

Regional Poison Control Center
Children's Hospital
1600 7th Avenue South
Birmingham, AL 35233
(800) 292-6678

ALASKA

(serviced by Oregon Poison Center)
Oregon Poison Center
Oregon Health Sciences University
3181 Southwest Sam Jackson Park Road
CB550
Portland, OR 97201
(800) 452-7165

ARIZONA

Arizona Poison and Drug Info Center
Arizona Health Sciences Center
Room 1156
1501 North Campbell Avenue
Tucson, AZ 85724
(800) 362-0101

Banner Poison Control Center
Good Samaritan Regional Medical Center
1111 East McDowell
Phoenix, AZ 85006
(800) 222-1222

ARKANSAS

Arkansas Poison and Drug Information Center
College of Pharmacy, University of Arkansas for Medical Sciences
4301 West Markham
Mail Slot 522-2
Little Rock, AR 72205
(800) 641-3805 (TDD/TTY)

CALIFORNIA

California Poison Control System—Fresno/Madera Division
Children's Hospital Central California
9300 Valley Children's Place
MB 15
Madera, CA 93638-8762
(800) 972-3323 (TDD/TTY)

California Poison Control System— Sacramento Division
UC Davis Medical Center
2315 Stockton Boulevard
Sacramento, CA 95817
(800) 972-3323 (TDD/TTY)

California Poison Control System— San Diego Division
University of California—San Diego Medical Center
200 West Arbor Drive
San Diego, CA 92103-8925
(800) 972-3323 (TDD/TTY)

California Poison Control System— San Francisco Division
UCSF Box 1369
San Francisco, CA 94143-1369
(800) 972-3323 (TDD/TTY)

COLORADO

Rocky Mountain Poison and Drug Center
777 Bannock Street
Mail Code 0180
Denver, CO 80204-4028
(303) 739-1123 (TDD/TTY)

CONNECTICUT

Connecticut Poison Control Center
University of Connecticut Health Center
263 Farmington Avenue
Farmington, CT 06030-5365
(800) 343-2722

DELAWARE

The Poison Control Center
Children's Hospital of Philadelphia
34th and Civic Center Boulevard
Philadelphia, PA 19104-4303
(215) 590-8789 (TDD/TTY)

DISTRICT OF COLUMBIA

National Capital Poison Center
3201 New Mexico Avenue, NW
Suite 310
Washington, DC 20016
(800) 222-1222 (TDD/TTY)

FLORIDA

Florida Poison Information Center—Jacksonville
655 West Eighth Street
Jacksonville, FL 32209
(800) 222-1222 (TDD/TTY)
(800) 282-3171 (FL only)

Florida Poison Information Center—Miami
University of Miami
Department of Pediatrics
P.O. Box 016960 (R-131)
Miami, FL 33101
(800) 222-1222

Florida Poison Information Center—Tampa
Tampa General Hospital
P.O. Box 1289
Tampa, FL 33601
(800) 222-1222

GEORGIA

Georgia Poison Center
Hughes Spalding Children's Hospital
Grady Health System
80 Jesse Hill Jr. Drive, SE
P.O. Box 26066
Atlanta, GA 30335-3801
(404) 616-9287 (TDD/TTY)

HAWAII

(serviced by Rocky Mountain Poison and Drug Center)

Rocky Mountain Poison and Drug Center
777 Bannock Street
Mail Code 0180
Denver, CO 80204-4028
(303) 739-1127 (TDD/TTY)

IDAHO

(serviced by Rocky Mountain Poison and Drug Center)

Rocky Mountain Poison and Drug Center
777 Bannock Street
Mail Code 0180
Denver, CO 80204-4028
(303) 739-1127 (TDD/TTY)

INDIANA

Indiana Poison Center
Methodist Hospital
Clarian Health Partners
I-65 at 21st Street
Indianapolis, IN 46206-1367
(317) 962-2336 (TDD/TTY)

ILLINOIS

Illinois Poison Center
222 South Riverside Plaza
Suite 1900
Chicago, IL 60606
(312) 906-6136 (TDD/TTY)

IOWA

Iowa Statewide Poison Control Center
St. Luke's Regional Medical Center
2910 Hamilton Boulevard
Suite 101
Sioux City, IA 51104
(800) 222-1222

KANSAS

Mid-America Poison Control Center
University of Kansas Medical Center
3901 Rainbow Boulevard
Room B-400
Kansas City, KS 66160-7231
(913) 588-6639 (TDD/TTY)

KENTUCKY

Kentucky Regional Poison Center
P.O. Box 35070
Louisville, KY 40232-5070
(800) 222-1222

LOUISIANA

Louisiana Drug and Poison Information Center
University of Louisiana at Monroe
700 University Avenue
Monroe, LA 71209
(800) 222-1222

MAINE

Northern New England Poison Center
22 Bramhall Street
Portland, ME 04102
Emergency Phone: (800) 222-1222
(877) 299-4447 (TDD/TTY)
(207) 871-2879 (ME only)

MARYLAND

Maryland Poison Center
University of Maryland at Baltimore
School of Pharmacy
20 North Pine Street
PH 772
Baltimore, MD 21201
(410) 706-1858 (TDD/TTY)

National Capital Poison Center
3201 New Mexico Avenue, NW
Suite 310
Washington, DC 20016
(800) 222-1222 (TDD/TTY)

MASSACHUSETTS

*Regional Center for Poison Control
and Prevention Serving Massachusetts
and Rhode Island*
300 Longwood Avenue
Boston, MA 02115
(888) 244-5313 (TDD/TTY)

MICHIGAN

*Children's Hospital of Michigan Regional Poison
Control Center*
4160 John R. Harper Professional Office
Building
Suite 616
Detroit, MI 48201
(800) 356-3232 (TDD/TTY)

*DeVos Children's Hospital Regional
Poison Center*
1840 Wealthy Southeast
Grand Rapids, MI 49506-2968
(800) 222-1222 (TDD/TTY)

MINNESOTA

Hennepin Regional Poison Center
Hennepin County Medical Center
701 Park Avenue
Mail Code RL
Minneapolis, MN 55415
(612) 904-4691 (TDD/TTY)

MISSISSIPPI

Mississippi Regional Poison Control Center
University of Mississippi Medical Center
2500 North State Street
Jackson, MS 39216
(800) 222-1222

MISSOURI

Missouri Regional Poison Center
7980 Clayton Road
Suite 200
St. Louis, MO 63117
(314) 612-5705 (TDD/TTY)

MONTANA

Rocky Mountain Poison and Drug Center
777 Bannock Street
Mail Code 0180
Denver, CO 80204-4028
(303) 739-1127 (TDD/TTY)

NEBRASKA

Nebraska Regional Poison Center
8200 Dodge Street
Omaha, NE 68114
(800) 222-1222

NEVADA

*(Northern Nevada serviced
by Oregon Poison Center)*

Oregon Poison Center
Oregon Health Sciences University
3181 Southwest Sam Jackson Park Road
CB550
Portland, OR 97201
(800) 222-1222

*(Clark County serviced by
Rocky Mountain Poison and Drug Center)*

*Rocky Mountain Poison
and Drug Center*
777 Bannock Street
Mail Code 0180
Denver, CO 80204-4028
(303) 739-1127 (TDD/TTY)

NEW HAMPSHIRE

**New Hampshire Poison Information
Center**
**Dartmouth-Hitchcock
Medical Center**
One Medical Center Drive
Lebanon, NH 03756
(800) 222-1222

NEW JERSEY

New Jersey Poison Information and Education System
University of Medicine and Dentistry at New Jersey
65 Bergen Street
Newark, NJ 07107-3001
(973) 926-8008 (TDD/TTY)

NEW MEXICO

New Mexico Poison and Drug Info Center
Health Science Center Library
Room 130
University of New Mexico
Albuquerque, NM 87131-1076
(800) 222-1222

NEW YORK

Central New York Poison Center
750 East Adams Street
Syracuse, NY 13210
(800) 222-1222

Finger Lakes Regional Poison and Drug Information Center
University of Rochester Medical Center
601 Elmwood Avenue
Box 321
Rochester, NY 14642
(585) 273-3854 (TDD/TTY)

Long Island Regional Poison and Drug Information Center
Winthrop University Hospital
259 First Street
Mineola, NY 11501
(516) 663-2650 or (516) 542-2323

New York City Poison Control Center
NYC Bureau of Labs
455 First Avenue
Room 123, Box 81
New York, NY 10016
(212) 689-9014 (TDD/TTY)

Western New York Poison Center
Children's Hospital of Buffalo
219 Bryant Street
Buffalo, NY 14222
(800) 222-1222

NORTH CAROLINA

Carolinas Poison Center
Carolinas Medical Center
5000 Airport Center Parkway
Suite B
Charlotte, NC 28208
(800) 222-1222

NORTH DAKOTA
(serviced by Minnesota Poison Center)

Hennepin Regional Poison Center
Hennepin County Medical Center
701 Park Avenue
Minneapolis, MN 55415
(612) 904-4691 (TDD/TTY)

OHIO

Central Ohio Poison Center
700 Children's Drive
Room L032
Columbus, OH 43205
(614) 228-2272 (TDD/TTY)

Cincinnati Drug and Poison Information Center
3333 Burnet Avenue
Vernon Place
Third Floor
Cincinnati, OH 45229-9004
(800) 253-7955 (TDD/TTY)

Greater Cleveland Poison Control Center
11100 Euclid Avenue
Cleveland, OH 44106-6010
(800) 222-1222

OKLAHOMA

Oklahoma Poison Control Center
Children's Hospital at OU Medical Center
940 Northeast 13th Street
Room 3510
Oklahoma City, OK 73104
(405) 271-1122 (TDD/TTY)

OREGON

Oregon Poison Center
Oregon Health Sciences University
3181 SW Sam Jackson Park Road
CB550
Portland, OR 97201
(800) 222-1222

PENNSYLVANIA

Pittsburgh Poison Center
Children's Hospital of Pittsburgh
3705 Fifth Avenue
Pittsburgh, PA 15213
(800) 222-1222

The Poison Control Center
Children's Hospital of Philadelphia
34th and Civic Center Boulevard
Philadelphia, PA 19104-4303
(215) 590-8789 (TDD/TTY)

PUERTO RICO

Puerto Rico Poison Center
San Jorge Children's Hospital
Calle San Jorge #252
Santurce, PR 00912
(800) 222-1222

RHODE ISLAND

*Regional Center for Poison Control
   and Prevention Serving Massachusetts
   and Rhode Island*
300 Longwood Avenue
Boston, MA 02115
(888) 244-5313 (TDD/TTY)

SOUTH CAROLINA

Palmetto Poison Center
College of Pharmacy
University of South Carolina
Columbia, SC 29208
(800) 222-1222

SOUTH DAKOTA
(serviced by Minnesota Poison Control Center)

Hennepin Regional Poison Center
Hennepin County Medical Center
701 Park Avenue
Minneapolis, MN 55415
(612) 904-4691 (TDD/TTY)

TENNESSEE

Middle Tennessee Poison Center
501 Oxford House
1161 21st Avenue South
Nashville, TN 37232-4632
(615) 936-2047 (TDD/TTY)

TEXAS

Central Texas Poison Center
Scott and White Memorial Hospital
2401 South 31st Street
Temple, TX 76508
(800) 222-1222

North Texas Poison Center
Parkland Memorial Hospital
5201 Harry Hines Boulevard
Dallas, TX 75235
(800) 222-1222

Southeast Texas Poison Center
University of Texas Medical Branch
3.112 Trauma Building
Galveston, TX 77555-1175
(800) 222-1222

South Texas Poison Center
University of Texas Health Science Center—
  San Antonio
Department of Surgery
Mail Code 7849
7703 Floyd Curl Drive
San Antonio, TX 78229-3900
(800) 222-1222

Texas Panhandle Poison Center
1501 South Coulter
Amarillo, TX 79106
(800) 222-1222

West Texas Regional Poison Center
Thomason Hospital
4815 Alameda Avenue
El Paso, TX 79905
(800) 222-1222

UTAH

Utah Poison Control Center
585 Komas Drive
Suite 200
Salt Lake City, UT 84108
(800) 222-1222

VERMONT

Northern New England Poison Center
22 Bramhall Street
Portland, ME 04102
(877) 299-4447 (TDD/TTY)
(207) 871-2879 (VT only)

VIRGINIA

Blue Ridge Poison Center
Jefferson Park Place
1222 Jefferson Park Avenue
Charlottesville, VA 22903
(800) 222-1222

Virginia Poison Center
Medical College of Virginia Hospitals
Virginia Commonwealth University
  Health System
P.O. Box 980522
Richmond, VA 23298-0522
(800) 222-1222

WASHINGTON

Washington Poison Center
155 Northeast 100th Street
Suite 400
Seattle, WA 98125-8011
(206) 517-2394 (TDD/TTY)
(800) 572-0638 (TDD, WA only)

WEST VIRGINIA

West Virginia Poison Center
3110 MacCorkle Ave, S.E.
Charleston, WV 25304
(304) 388-9698 (TDD/TTY)

WISCONSIN

Children's Hospital of Wisconsin
  Poison Center
P.O. Box 1997
Mail Station 677A
Milwaukee, WI 53201-1997
(414) 266-2542 (TDD/TTY)

WYOMING
(serviced by Nebraska Poison Control)

Nebraska Regional Poison Center
8200 Dodge Street
Omaha, NE 68114
(800) 222-1222

CANADA POISON CONTROL CENTERS

ALBERTA

Poison and Drug Information Service
Foothills Medical Centre
1403 29th Street, NW
Calgary, AB T2N 2T9
(800) 332-1414 (Alberta only)
(403) 670-1212

BRITISH COLUMBIA

British Columbia Drug and Poison
 Information Centre
St. Paul's Hospital
1081 Burrard Street
Vancouver, BC V6Z 1Y6
(800) 567-8911
(604) 682-5050

MANITOBA

Provincial Poison Information Centre
Children's Hospital Health Services Centre
840 Sherbrook Street
Winnipeg, MB R3A 1S1
(204) 787-2591
(204) 787-2444

NEW BRUNSWICK

Poison Control Centre
Moncton Hospital
135 McBeal Avenue
Moncton, NB E1C 6Z8
(506) 857-5555
(506) 857-5353

NEWFOUNDLAND AND LABRADOR

Provincial Poison Control Centre
Dr. Charles A. Janeway Child Health Centre
710 Janeway Place
St. John's, NL A1A 1R8
(709) 722-1110

NORTHWEST TERRITORIES

Emergency Department
Stanton Yellowknife Hospital
550 Byrne Road
Yellowknife, NT X1A 2N1
(867) 669-4100

NOVA SCOTIA

IWK Regional Poison Centre—
 IWK Health Centre
5850 University Avenue
P.O. Box 3070
Halifax, NS B3J 3G9
(800) 565-8161
(902) 470-8161

NUNAVUT

Baffin Regional Hospital
P.O. Box 200
Iqaluit, NU X0A 0H0
(867) 979-7350

ONTARIO

Ontario Regional Poison Centre
Children's Hospital of Eastern Ontario
401 Smyth Road
Ottawa, ON K1H 8LI
(800) 267-1373
(613) 737-1100

PRINCE EDWARD ISLAND

IWK Regional Poison Centre—
 IWK Health Centre
5850 University Avenue
Halifax, NS B3J 3G9
Canada
(800) 565-8161

QUEBEC

Centre Antipoison du Québec/Quebec Poison Control Center
Le Centre Hospitalier de l'Université Laval
Aile "L," 1er étage
1050 Chemin Sainte-Foy
Quebec, QC G1S 4L8
(800) 463-5060

SASKATCHEWAN

Emergency Department
Regina General Hospital
1440 14th Avenue
Regina, SK S4P 0W5
Canada
(800) 667-4545
(306) 766-4545

YUKON

Emergency Department
Whitehorse General Hospital
5 Hospital Road
Whitehorse, YT Y1A 3H7
(403) 667-8726

GLOSSARY

adrenal glands A pair of small glands, one located on top of each kidney, that produce steroid hormones, adrenaline, and noradrenaline to help control heart rate, blood pressure, and other important body functions.

antibody A protein that is manufactured by white blood cells to identify, neutralize, or destroy bacteria, viruses, and other harmful microorganisms.

antigen A substance that can trigger an immune response, causing the production of an antibody as part of the body's defense against infection. Many antigens are not found naturally in the body; they include microorganisms, toxins, and tissues from another person used in an organ transplant.

brain stem Composed of midbrain, pons, and medulla; contains reticular activating system and other key centers.

calcium A mineral that makes bones and teeth strong, helps muscles work, and aids in proper blood clotting.

carbohydrate Sugars and starches that are the most efficient source of food energy. The most basic carbohydrate is a simple sugar (such as glucose or fructose), which serves as a building block for complex carbohydrates (starchy foods like pastas, whole grains, and potatoes).

cell The basic structural unit of all life. All living matter is composed of cells.

central nervous system (CNS) The brain and spinal cord; one of the two major divisions of the nervous system. The CNS is the control network for the entire body.

cerebrospinal fluid (CSF) The fluid that fills the areas surrounding the brain and spinal cord.

chromosome An H-shaped structure inside the cell nucleus made up of tightly coiled strands of genes. Each chromosome is numbered (in humans, from 1 through 46) and contains DNA, sequences of which make up genes.

cognitive The process of knowing in the broadest sense, including perception, memory, and judgment.

cognitive abilities Mental abilities such as judgment, memory, learning, comprehension, and reasoning.

complete blood count (CBC) The number of red blood cells, white blood cells, and platelets in a sample of blood.

corticosteroid A group of drugs based on the structure of cortisone (a hormone produced by the adrenal glands) with anti-inflammatory properties.

DNA One of two nucleic acids (the other is RNA) found in the nuclei of all cells. DNA contains genetic information on cell growth, division, and cell function.

echolalia Repetition of words or phrases.

endocrine glands Glands that manufacture and secrete hormones into the blood. Endocrine glands include the pituitary, thyroid, parathyroid, and adrenal glands, the ovaries and testes, placenta, and part of the pancreas.

enzyme A protein that promotes essential functions involved in cell growth and metabolism.

folate Also called folic acid, this B vitamin helps the body make nucleic acids (RNA and DNA), amino acids, and red blood cells.

gene The biological unit of heredity. Each gene is located at a specific spot on a particular chromosome and is made up of a string of chemicals arranged in a certain sequence along the DNA molecule.

gram-negative bacteria   A type of bacteria that resists the chemical stain used in Gram's method of identifying microorganisms for characterization purposes.

gram-positive bacteria   A type of bacteria that retains the violet color of the stain used in Gram's method of identifying microorganisms for characterization purposes.

hemoglobin   A protein in red blood cells that carries oxygen from the lungs to the body's tissues.

hormones   Chemical messengers secreted by endocrine glands to regulate the activity of target cells that play a role in sexual development, calcium and bone metabolism, growth, and many other activities.

hypothalamus   A brain structure composed of many nuclei with different functions, including regulation of activities of internal organs, monitoring information from the autonomic nervous system, and controlling the pituitary gland.

iron   A mineral that is an important part of hemoglobin, the blood's oxygen-carrying molecule. Iron also helps the body resist infection and use energy from food.

larynx   Also called the "voice box," this is the part of the throat containing the vocal cords.

lymph gland   Also known as a lymph node, this tissue mass contains lymphocytes that filter the lymphatic fluid.

lymphatic system   The tissues and organs (including the bone marrow, spleen, thymus, and lymph glands) that produce and store cells that fight infection and the network of channels that carry lymph.

lymphocyte   A type of white blood cell that helps produce antibodies and other substances that fight infection and diseases.

mast cell   A type of white blood cell.

meninges   The membranes that cover and protect the brain and spinal cord.

metabolism   The chemical and physiological process by which the body builds and maintains itself, and by which it breaks down food and nutrients to produce energy.

peptide   Any compound consisting of two or more amino acids, the building blocks of proteins.

pharynx   The throat area that starts behind the nose and ends at the top of the trachea (windpipe) and esophagus.

platelet   A type of blood cell that helps prevent bleeding by causing blood clots to form.

protein   A major component of all body tissue that helps the body grow and repair itself. Protein is also a necessary component of hormones, enzymes, and hemoglobin.

red blood cell   A cell (also called an erythrocyte) that carries oxygen to all parts of the body.

strabismus   Weakness of eye muscles that allows eyes to cross.

tactile   The ability to receive and interpret stimuli through contact with the skin.

thyroid gland   A gland located beneath the larynx that produces thyroid hormone and helps regulate growth and metabolism.

ventricles   Four natural cavities in the brain that are filled with cerebrospinal fluid.

virus   The smallest known type of infectious agent, causing diseases that range from mild (such as warts) to extremely serious (rabies, AIDS, and probably some types of cancer).

white blood cell   A blood cell that does not contain hemoglobin, including lymphocytes, neutrophils, eosinophils, macrophages, and mast cells. These cells are made by bone marrow and help the body fight infection and other diseases.

BIBLIOGRAPHY

Abbott, M. B., and Levin, R. H. "What's New: Newly Approved Drugs for Children," *Pediatrics in Review* 24, no. 7 (July 2003): 240–243.

Ablin, A. R., ed. *Supportive Care of Children with Cancer*. Baltimore: Johns Hopkins University Press, 1997.

Abramson, J. S., McMillan, J. A., Baltimore, R. S. "The U.S. Smallpox Vaccination Plan," *Pediatrics* 111, no. 6 (June 2003): 1,431–1,432.

Adzick, N. S., and Nance, M. L. "Pediatric Surgery," *New England Journal of Medicine* 342 (2000): 1,651.

Aicardi, J. *Diseases of the Nervous System in Childhood*. 2nd ed. London: MacKeith, 1998.

American Academy of Allergy, Asthma, and Immunology. *Pediatric Asthma: Promoting Best Practice Guide for Managing Asthma in Children*. Milwaukee: American Academy of Allergy, Asthma, and Immunology, 1999.

American Academy of Child and Adolescent Psychiatry. "Practice Parameters for the Assessment and Treatment of Children and Adolescents with Depressive Disorders," *Journal of the American Academy of Child and Adolescent Psychiatry* 37 (1998): 63S.

———. "Practice Parameters for the Assessment and Treatment of Children with Bipolar Disorder," *Journal of the American Academy of Child and Adolescent Psychiatry* 36 (1997): 157S.

———. "Practice Parameters for the Assessment and Treatment of Children with Conduct Disorder," *Journal of the American Academy of Child and Adolescent Psychiatry* 36 (1997): 122S.

———. "Practice Parameters for the Assessment and Treatment of Children with Anxiety Disorders," *Journal of the American Academy of Child and Adolescent Psychiatry* 36 (1997): 69S.

———. "Practice Parameters for the Assessment and Treatment of Children with OCD," *Journal of the American Academy of Child and Adolescent Psychiatry* 37, no. 10 (1998): 27S.

———. "Practice Parameters for the Assessment and Treatment of Children and Adolescents with Post-Traumatic Stress Disorder," *Journal of the American Academy of Child and Adolescent Psychiatry* 37 (1998): 4S.

American Academy of Pediatrics. *Guidelines for Perinatal Care*. 4th ed. American Academy of Pediatrics, 1997.

———. "Clinical Practice Guideline: Diagnosis and Evaluation of the Child with Attention-Deficit Hyperactivity Disorder," *Pediatrics* 105 (2000): 1,117–1,119.

———. *Improving Access to Children's Health Insurance in the United States: Health Insurance Status of Children Through Age 18 in the United States—2000* Projections. Elk Grove Village, Ill.: American Academy of Pediatrics, 2000.

American Academy of Pediatrics Committee on Adolescents: "Suicide and Suicide Attempts in Adolescents," *Pediatrics* 105, no. 4 (2000): 871–874.

American Academy of Pediatrics Committee on Infectious Diseases: "Report of the Committee on Infectious Diseases, 26th edition," *Red Book 2003*. Elk Grove Village, Ill.: American Academy of Pediatrics, 2003.

———. "Poliomyelitis Prevention: Revised Recommendations for Use of Inactivated and Live Oral Poliovirus Vaccines," *Pediatrics* 103 (1999): 171.

———. "Policy Statement: Recommendations for the Prevention of Pneumococcal Infections, Including the Use of Pneumococcal Conjugate

Vaccine (Prevnar), Pneumococcal Polysaccharide Vaccine, and Antibiotic Prophylaxis," *Pediatrics* 106 (2000): 362.

American Academy of Pediatrics Committee on Infectious Disease and Committee of Fetus and Newborn. "Revised Guidelines for Prevention of Early-Onset Group B Strep (GBS) Infection," *Pediatrics* 99 (1997): 489.

American Academy of Pediatrics Committee on Injury, Violence, and Poison Prevention. "Prevention of Drowning in Infants, Children, and Adolescents," *Pediatrics* 112, no. 2 (August 2003): 437–439.

American Academy of Pediatrics Committee on Nutrition. "Iron Fortification of Infant Formulas," *Pediatrics* 104 (1999): 119.

———. "Prevention of Pediatric Overweight and Obesity," *Pediatrics* 112, no. 2 (August 2003): 424–430.

American Academy of Pediatrics Committee on Pediatric AIDS. "Evolution and Medical Treatment of the HIV-Exposed Infant," *Pediatrics* 99 (1997): 909.

American Academy of Pediatrics Committee on Practice and Ambulatory Medicine. "Recommendations for Preventive Pediatric Health Care," *Pediatrics* 105 (2000): 645.

American Academy of Pediatrics Committee on Substance Abuse. "Marijuana, a Continuing Concern for Pediatricians," *Pediatrics* (1999): 982.

———. "Tobacco's Toll: Implications for the Pediatrician," *Pediatrics* (2001): 794.

American Academy of Pediatrics Task Force on Infant Sleep Positions and Sudden Infant Death Syndrome. "Concepts of Sudden Infant Death Syndrome: Implications for Infant Sleeping Environment and Sleep Position," *Pediatrics* 105 (2000): 650.

American Academy of Pediatrics Task Force on Newborn and Infant Hearing. "Newborn and Infant Hearing Loss, Detection and Intervention," *Pediatrics* 103 (1999): 527.

American Diabetes Association. "Standards of Medical Care for Patients with Diabetes Mellitus," *Diabetes Care* 21 (1998): 523.

———. "Type 2 Diabetes in Children and Adolescents," *Diabetes Care* 23 (2000): 381.

American Psychiatric Association. *Diagnostic and Statistical Manual of Mental Disorders—IV–TR.* Washington, D.C.: American Psychiatric Association, 2000.

Anderson, Elizabeth, and Emmons, Pauline. *Unlocking the Mysteries of Sensory Dysfunction.* Arlington, Tex.: Future Horizons, 1996.

Anderson, M. "Annotation: Conceptions of Intelligence," *Journal of Child Psychology and Psychiatry* 42, no. 3 (March 2001): 287–298.

Arnon, S. S., et al. "Botulinum Toxin as a Biological Weapon; Weapon; Medical and Public Health Management; Small Pox as a Biological Weapon, Medical and Public Health Management," *Journal of the American Medical Association* 285 (2001): 1,059.

Ash, L. R., and Orihel, T. C. *Atlas of Human Parasitology.* 4th ed. Chicago: American Society of Clinical Pathologists, 1997.

Avery, G. B., et al., eds. *Neonatology: Pathophysiology and Management of the Newborn.* 5th ed. Philadelphia: Lippincott, Williams & Wilkins, 1999.

Baird, G., et al. "Current Topic: Screening and Surveillance for Autism and Pervasive Developmental Disorders," *Archives of Disabled Child* 84 (2001): 468–475.

Bakalian, S., and Lewis, C. W. "Question from the Clinician: Fluoridated Water," *Pediatrics in Review* 24, no. 2 (February 2003): 70.

Ball, S., Becker, T., Boys, M., et al. "Early Screening for Dyslexia—a Collaborative Pilot Project," *International Journal of Language and Communication Disorders* 36 (Suppl., 2001): 75–79.

Baltimore, R. S. "Early-Onset Neonatal Sepsis in the Era of Group B Strep Prevention," *Pediatrics* 108 (2001): 1,094.

Barkley, R. A. *Attention Deficit Hyperactivity Disorder: A Clinical Workbook.* 2nd ed. New York: Guilford, 1998.

Barlow, W. E., Davis, R. L., Glasser, J. W., et al. "The Risk of Seizures after Receipt of Whole-Cell Pertussis or Measles, Mumps, and Rubella Vaccine," *New England Journal of Medicine* 345 (2001): 656.

Barnard, N. D. "The Milk Debate Goes on and on and on!" *Pediatrics* 112, no. 2 (August 2003): 448.

Barr, R. G. "Colic and Crying Syndromes in Infants," *Pediatrics* 102 (1998): 1,282.

Batshaw, Mark L. *Children with Disabilities.* 4th ed. Baltimore: Paul H. Brookes Publishing, 1997.

Bauchner, H., Pelton, S. I., Kelein, J. O. "Parents, Physicians and Antibiotic Use," *Pediatrics* 103 (1999): 395.

Beardslee, W. R., Gladstone, T. R., Wright, E. J., et al. "A Family-Based Approach to the Prevention of Depressive Symptoms in Children at Risk: Evidence of Parental and Child Change," *Pediatrics* 112, no. 2 (August 2003): e119–131.

Beers, N. S. "Managing Temper Tantrums," *Pediatrics in Review* 24, no. 2 (February 2003): 70–71.

Bell-Dolan, D., and Brazeal, T. "Separation Anxiety Disorder, Overanxious Disorder, and School Refusal," *Child and Adolescent Psychiatric Clinics of North America* 2 (1993): 563.

Benoit, D. "Phenomenology and Treatment of Failure to Thrive," *Child and Adolescent Psychiatric Clinic of North America* 2 (1993): 61.

Block, Mary Ann. *No More Ritalin: Treating ADHD Without Drugs.* New York: Kensington Publishing Co., 1997.

Boone, K. B., Swerdloff, R. S., Miller, B. L., et al. "Neuropsychological Profiles of Adults with Klinefelter Syndrome," *Journal of the International Neuropsychological Society* 7, no. 4 (May 2001): 56.

Bluestone, C. D. "Clinical Course, Complications and Sequelae of Acute Oritis Media," *Pediatric Infectious Disease* 19 (2000): S37.

Bond, G. R. "Snake, Spider and Scorpion Envenomation in North America," *Pediatrics in Review* 20 (1999): 147.

Bowman, U. W., et al. "Psychological Aspects of Turner Syndrome," *Journal of Psychosomatic Obstetrics and Gynaecology* 19 (1998): 1.

Boyles, Nancy S., and Contadino, Darlene. *Parenting a Child with Attention Deficit Hyperactivity Disorder.* Los Angeles: Lowell House, 1996.

———. *The Learning Differences Sourcebook.* New York: NTC Contemporary, 1998.

Braun, M., et al. "Infant Immunization with Acellular Pertussis Vaccines in the U.S.: Assessment of the First Two Years' Data from the Vaccine Adverse Event Reporting System," *Pediatrics* 106 (2000): 51.

Brenner, R. A. "Prevention of Drowning in Infants, Children, and Adolescents," *Pediatrics* 112, no. 2 (August 2003): 440–445.

Brenningstall, G. N. "Breath Holding Spells," *Pediatric Neurology* 14 (1996): 91.

Brunstein, C. G., and McGlave, P. B. "The Biology and Treatment of Chronic Myelogenous Leukemia," *Oncology.* 15 (2001): 23.

Burack, J. A., Hodapp, R. M., and Zigler, E., eds. *Handbook of Mental Retardation and Development.* London: Cambridge University Press, 1999.

Burchett, S. K., and Pizzo, P. A. "HIV Infection in Infants, Children, and Adolescents," *Pediatrics in Review* 24, no. 6 (June 2003): 186–194.

Burks, A. W., and Sampson, H. A. "Anaphylaxis and Food Allergy," *Clinical Review of Allergy and Immunology* 17 (1999): 339.

Burks, W. "Skin Manifestations of Food Allergy," *Pediatrics* 111 (June 2003): 1,617–1,624.

Burstein, G. R., and Murray, P. J. "Diagnosis and Management of Sexually Transmitted Diseases among Adolescents," *Pediatrics in Review* 24, no. 4 (April 2003): 119–127.

Busse, W. W., and Lemanske, R. F. "Asthma," *New England Journal of Medicine* 344 (2001): 350.

Cahall, Jeanne S. *Stages of Reading Development.* 2nd ed. New York: Harcourt Brace College Publishers, 1996.

Campbell, Linda. *Teaching and Learning Through Multiple Intelligences.* Needham Heights, Mass: Allyn & Bacon, 1996.

Caulfield, P. "Dental Caries: A Transmissible and Infectious Disease Revisited: A Position Paper," *Pediatric Dentistry* 19 (1997): 491.

Centers for Disease Control and Prevention. "Youth Risk Behavior Surveillance United States, 2001," *Morbidity and Mortality Weekly Report: CDC Surveillance Summaries* 51/SS-4 (2002): 1–64.

Cherry, J. D. "Risks to Children of Health Care Personnel Receiving Smallpox Vaccination,"

Pediatric Infectious Disease Journal 22, no. 6 (June 2003): 574–575.

Chien, J. W., and Johnson, J. L. "Viral Pneumonias," *Postgraduate Medicine* 107 (2000): 67.

Cieslak, T. J., and Henretig, F. M. "Bioterrorism," *Pediatric Annals* 32, no. 3 (March 2003): 154–165.

Clark, R. F., et al. "Clinical Presentation and Treatment of Black Widow Spider Envenomation: A Review of 163 Cases," *Annals of Emergency Medicine* 21 (1992): 782.

Comings, David E. *Tourette Syndrome and Human Behavior.* Duarte, Calif.: Hope Press, 1990.

Como, P. G. "Neuropsychological Function in Tourette Syndrome," *Advances in Neurology* 85 (2001): 103–111.

Culbertson, J. L., Newman, J. E., Willis, D. J. "Childhood and Adolescent Psychologic Development," *Pediatric Clinics of North America* 50, no. 4 (August 2003): 741–764.

Daly, E., MacDermott, E. J., Green, A. "Diagnostic Review of 66 Children with Learning Disability Attending a Single Center," *Irish Medical Journal* 94, no. 6 (June 2001): 184–185.

Darville, T. "Syphilis," *Pediatrics in Review* 20 (1999): 160.

David, R. B. *Child and Adolescent Neurology.* New York: Mosby, 1998.

Davis, Ronald D., and Braun, Eldon M. *The Gift of Dyslexia: Why Some of the Smartest People Can't Read and How They Can Learn.* New York: Perigee, 1997.

Davis, B., Krug, D., Dean, R. S. "Neuropsychological Clusters within Intelligence Levels for Learning Disabled Children," *International Journal of Neuroscience* 106, no. 3–4 (2001): 239–251.

Devlin, M. "Assessment and Treatment of Binge Eating Disorder," *Psychiatric Clinics of North America* 19 (1996): 761.

Dhigo, S. K. "New Strategies for the Treatment of Colic: Modifying the Parent-Infant Interaction," *Journal of Pediatrics Health Care* 12 (1998): 256.

Discolo, C. M., Darrow, D. H., Koltai, P. J. "Infectious Indications for Tonsillectomy," *Pediatric Clinics of North America* 50, no. 2 (April 2003): 445–458.

Dowel, S., et al. "Acute Otitis Media: Management and Surveillance in an Era of Pneumococcal Resistance: A Report from the Drug-resistant Streptococcus pneumoniae Working Group," *Pediatric Infectious Disease Journal* 18 (1999): 1.

Doyle, A. E., Faraone, S. V., DuPre, E. P., et al. "Separating Attention Deficit Hyperactivity Disorder and Learning Disabilities in Girls: a Familial Risk Analysis," *American Journal of Psychiatry* 158, no. 10 (Oct. 2001): 1,666–1,672.

Eichenfeld, L. F., et al., eds. *Textbook of Neonatal Dermatology.* Philadelphia: Saunders, 2001.

Eisenstein, E. M., and Amitai, Y. "Index of Suspicion: Organophosphate Intoxication," *Pediatrics in Review* 21 (2000): 205.

Emans, S. J., Laufer, M. R., and Goldstein, D. P. *Pediatric and Adolescent Gynecology.* 4th ed. Boston: Little, Brown, 1998.

Evans, G., Farberow, N., and Kennedy Associates. *The Encyclopedia of Suicide.* New York: Facts On File, 2003.

Ewing-Cobbs, L., Fletcher, J. M., and Levin, H. S. "Traumatic Brain Injury" in B. P. Rourke, ed. *Syndrome of Nonverbal Learning Disabilities: Neurodevelopmental Manifestations.* New York: Guilford Press, 1995.

Ferber, R. "Clinical Assessment of Child and Adolescent Sleep Disorder," *Child and Adolescent Psychiatric Clinic of North America* 5 (1996): 569.

Fernandes, J., Saudubray, J-M, Tada, K., eds. *Inborn Metabolic Diseases: Diagnosis and Treatment.* 3rd ed. New York: Springer-Verlag 2000.

Fireman, P. "Therapeutic Approaches to Allergic Rhinitis: Treating the Child," *Journal of Allergy and Clinical Immunology* 105 (2000): S616.

Fitzgerald, D. A., and Kilham, H. A. "Croup: Assessment and Evidence-Based Management," *Medical Journal of Australia* 179, no. 7 (October 2003): 372–377.

Flanagan, O., Nuallain, S. O. "A Study Looking at the Effectiveness of Developmental Screening in Identifying Learning Disabilities in Early

Childhood," *Irish Medical Journal* 94, no. 5 (May 2001): 148–150.

Fletcher, M. A. *Physical Diagnosis in Neonatalogy.* New York: Lippincott-Raven, 1998.

Foulon, W., et al. "Treatment of Toxoplasmosis During Pregnancy: A Multicenter Study of Impact on Fetal Transmission and Children's Sequelae at Age 1 Year," *American Journal of Obstetrics and Gynecology* 180 (1999): 410.

France, K. G., Henderson, J. M. T., and Hudson, S. M. "Fact, Act, and Tact: A Three-Stage Approach to Treating the Sleep Problems of Infants and Young Children," *Child and Adolescent Psychiatric Clinic North America* 5 (1996): 581.

Francis, H. W., and Niparko, J. K. "Cochlear Implantation Update," *Pediatric Clinics of North America* 50, no. 2 (April 2003): 341–361.

Frankenberg, W. K., et al. "The Denver II: A Major Revision and Restandardization of the Denver Developmental Screening Test," *Pediatrics* 89 (1991): 91.

Gaddes, William H., and Edgell, Dorothy. *Learning Disabilities and Brain Function: A Neuropsychological Approach.* New York: Springer-Verlag, 1994.

Garbutt, J., Jeffe, D. B., Shackelford, P. "Diagnosis and treatment of acute otitis media: an assessment," *Pediatrics* 112 (July 2003): 143–149.

Gardner, Howard. *Multiple Intelligences.* New York: Basic Books, 1993.

———. *Leading Minds: Anatomy of Success.* New York: Basic Books, 1995.

Gartner, L. M., and Lee, K-S. "Jaundice in the Breastfed Infant," *Clinical Perinatology* 26 (1999): 431.

Ghai, K., and Rosenfeld, R. L. "Disorders of Pubertal Development: Too Early, Too Much, Too Late, or Too Little." *Adolescent Medicine* 5 (1999): 19.

Gilberg, C., and Coleman, M., eds. *The Biology of the Autistic Syndromes.* London: Mackeith Press, 2000.

Glascoe, F. P. I., and Dworkin, P. H. "The Role of Parents in the Detection of Developmental and Behavioral Problems," *Pediatrics* 95 (1995): 829.

Goldsmith, A. J., and Rosenfeld, R. M. "Treatment of Pediatric Sinusitis," *Pediatric Clinics of North America* 50, no. 2 (April 2003): 413–426.

Gotoff, S. P., and Boyer, K. M. "Prevention of Early-Onset Neonatal Group B Strep Disease," *Pediatrics* 99 (1997): 866.

Green, W. H. *Child and Adolescent Psychopharmacology.* 3rd ed. Baltimore: Lippincott, Williams & Wilkins, 2001.

Greene, R. W. *The Explosive Child.* New York: Quill/HarperCollins, 2001.

Gross-Tsur, V., Landau, Y. E., Benarroch, F., et al. "Cognition, Attention, and Behavior in Prader-Willi Syndrome," *Journal of Child Neurology* 16, no. 4 (April 2001): 288–290.

Hagberg, B. A. "Rett Syndrome: Clinical Peculiarities, Diagnostic Approach, and Possible Cause," *Pediatric Neurology* 5, no. 2 (1989) 75–83.

Hagerman, R. J. *Fragile X Syndrome in Neurodevelopmental Disorders: Diagnosis and Treatment.* London: Oxford University Press, 1999.

Hall, C. B. "Respiratory Syncytial Virus and Parainfluenza Virus," *New England Journal of Medicine* 3444 (2001): 1917.

Harnadek, M. C. S., and Rourke, B. P. "Principal Identifying Features of the Syndrome of Nonverbal Learning Disabilities in Children," *Journal of Learning Disabilities* 27 (1994) 54.

Harris, J. *What Every Parent Needs to Know About Standardized Tests.* New York: McGraw Hill, 2002.

Haruda, F. D. "Meningitis—Viral Versus Bacterial," *Pediatrics* 112, no. 2 (August 2003): 447–448.

Hay, W. W., Hayward, A. R., Levin, M. J., et al. *Current Pediatric Diagnosis and Treatment.* New York: Lange Medical Books, 2003.

Herzog, D. B., et al. "Mortality in Eating Disorders: A Descriptive Study," *International Journal of Eating Disorders* 28, no. 1 (2000): 20.

Holmes, K. K., et al., eds. *Sexually Transmitted Diseases.* 2nd ed. New York: McGraw-Hill, 1999.

Holte, L. "Early Childhood Hearing Loss: A Frequently Overlooked Cause of Speech and Language Delay," *Pediatric Annals* 32, no. 7 (July 2003): 461–465.

Holtje, Katarina. *Start Them Off Right! A Parent's Guide to Getting the Most Out of Preschool.* New York: Alpha Books, 2002.

Hughes, E., and Lee, J. H. "Otitis Externa," *Pediatrics in Review* 22 (2001): 191.

Inglesby, T., et al. "Anthrax as a Biological Weapon," *Journal of the American Medical Association* 281 (1999): 2,127.

Iwamoto, M., Saari, T. N., McMahon, S. R., et. al. "A Survey of Pediatricians on the Reintroduction of a Rotavirus Vaccine," *Pediatrics* 112 (July 2003): e6–10.

Izard, C., Fine, S., Schultz, D, et al. "Emotion Knowledge as a Predictor of Social Behavior and Academic Competence in Children at Risk," *Psychological Science* 12, no. 1 (Jan. 2001): 18–23.

James, J. M. "Respiratory Manifestations of Food Allergy," *Pediatrics* 111 (June 2003): 1,625–1,630.

Jenkins, R. "Use of Psychotropic Medication in People with a Learning Disability," *British Journal of Nursing* 9, no. 13 (July 2000): 844–850.

Johnston, B. D., and Rivara, F. P. "Injury Control: New Challenges," *Pediatrics in Review* 24, no. 4 (April 2003): 111–118.

Johnston, L. D., O'Malley, P. M., Bachman, G. *Monitoring of the Future: National Survey Results on Adolescent Drug Use: Overview of Key Findings (NIH Pub. # 01-4923).* Bethesda, Md.: National Institute on Drug Abuse, 2001.

Journeycake, J. M., and Buchanan, G. R. "Coagulation Disorders," *Pediatrics in Review* 24, no. 3 (March 2003): 83–91.

Kann, L., Kinchen, S. A., Williams, B. I., et al. "Youth Risk Behavior Surveillance—United States, 1999," *Journal of School Health* 70, no. 7 (2000): 271–285.

Kaplowitz, P. B., Slora, E. J., Wasserman, R. C., et al. "Earlier Onset of Puberty in Girls: Relation to Increased Body Mass Index and Race," *Pediatrics* 108 (2001): 347–353.

Kaufman, F. R. "Type 1 Diabetes Mellitus," *Pediatrics in Review* 24, no. 9 (Sept. 2003): 291–300.

Kenna, M. A. "Neonatal Hearing Screening," *Pediatric Clinics of North America* 50, no. 2 (April 2003): 301–313.

Kimberlin, D. W., et al. "Natural History of Neonatal Herpes Simplex Virus Infections in the Acyclovir Era," *Pediatrics* 108 (2001): 223.

Knapp, J. F. "Updates in Wound Management for the Pediatrician," *Pediatric Clinics of North America* 46, no. 6 (1999): 1,201.

Kranowitz, Carol Stock. *The Out-Of-Sync Child: Recognizing and Coping with Sensory Integration Dysfunction.* New York: Perigee, 1998.

Kreipe, R. E., and Birndorf, S. A. "Eating Disorders in Adolescents and Young Adults," *Medical Clinics of North America* 84, no. 4 (July 2000): 1,027.

Labellarte, M. J., Walkup, J. T., and Riddle, M. A. "The New Antidepressants," Selective Serotonin Reuptake Inhibitors," *Pediatric Clinics of North America* 45 (1998): 1,137.

Lampe, K. F., and McCann, M. A. *AMA Handbook of Poisonous and Injurious Plants.* Chicago, Ill.: American Medical Association, 1985.

Lasley, M. V. "New Treatments for Asthma," *Pediatrics in Review* 24, no. 7 (July 2003): 222–232.

Lerner, Janet W. *Learning Disabilities: Theories, Diagnosis, and Teaching Strategies.* Boston: Houghton-Mifflin College, 2000.

Levelt, W. J. "Defining Dyslexia," *Science* 1. 292/5520 (May 18, 2001): 1,300–1,301.

Levine, M. D., Carey, W. B., and Crocker, A. C., eds. *Developmental-Behavioral Pediatrics.* 3rd ed. Philadelphia: Saunders, 1999.

Li, R., Zhao, Z., Mokdad, A., et al. "Prevalence of Breastfeeding in the United States: The 2001 National Immunization Survey," *Pediatrics* 111 (June 2003): 1,198–1,201.

Libby, A. M., Sills, M. R., Thurston, N. K., et al. "Costs of Childhood Physical Abuse: Comparing Inflicted and Unintentional Traumatic Brain Injuries," *Pediatrics* 112 (July 2003): 58–65.

Little, L. "Peer Victimization of Children with Asperger Spectrum Disorders," *Journal of the American Academy of Child and Adolescent Psychiatry* 40, no. 9 (Sept. 2001): 995–996.

Lovejoy, F. H., and Woolf, A. D. "Corrosive Ingestions," *Pediatrics in Review* 16 (1995): 473.

Lynfield, R., and Guerina, N. E. "Toxoplasmosis," *Pediatrics in Review* 18 (1997): 75.

Maffulli, N. "Lower Limb Injuries in Children in Sports," *Clinical Sports Medicine* 19 (2000): 637.

Maisonet, L. "Inguinal Hernia," *Pediatrics in Review* 24, no. 1 (January 2003): 34–35.

Mannucci, P. M., and Tuddenham, E. G. D. "The Hemophilias: From Royal Genes to Gene Therapy," *New England Journal of Medicine* 344 (2001): 1,773.

Massell, B. F. *Rheumatic Fever and Streptococcal Infection: Unraveling the Mysteries of a Dread Disease.* Cambridge, Mass.: Harvard University Press, 1997.

Matiz, A., and Roman, E. A. "Apnea," *Pediatrics in Review* 24, no. 1 (January 2003): 32–34.

McCarthy, C. A., and Hall, C. B. "Respiratory Syncytial Virus: Concerns and Control," *Pediatrics Review* 24, no. 9 (Sept. 2003): 301–309.

McGuigan, M. A. "Management of Acute Iron Overdose," *Pediatrics Annals* 25 (1996): 33.

McGuirt, W. F. Jr. "Gastroesophageal Reflux and the Upper Airway," *Pediatric Clinics of North America* 50, no. 2 (April 2003): 487–502.

Menkes, J. H., and Sarnat, H. B. *Textbook of Child Neurology.* 6th ed. Baltimore: Williams & Wilkins, 2000.

Milunsky, A. *Genetic Disorders and the Fetus: Diagnosis, Prevention and Treatment.* Baltimore: Johns Hopkins University Press, 1998.

Mittelman, D. "Amblyopia," *Pediatric Clinics of North America* 50, no. 1 (February 2003): 189–196.

Mosler, D. "The Association of Apgar Score with Subsequent Death and Cerebral Palsy: A Population-Based Study in Term Infants," *Journal of Pediatrics* 138 (2001): 798.

Mullins, M. E. "Measles-Mumps-Rubella Vaccine and Autism," *Pediatrics* 112 (July 2003): 206.

Mygind, N., et al. "The Common Cold and Asthma," *Allergy* 54 (1999): 146.

Needleman, R., and Zuckerman, Howard. "Temper Tantrums: When to Worry," *Contemporary Pediatrics* 6 (1989): 12.

Neumayr, L., Lennette, E., Kelly, D., et al. "Mycoplasma Disease and Acute Chest Syndrome in Sickle Cell Disease," *Pediatrics* 112 (July 2003): 87–95.

Norris, June, ed. *Handbook of Diseases.* Springhouse, Pa.: Springhouse Corp., 1996.

Nowak-Wegrzyn, A. "Future Approaches to Food Allergy," *Pediatrics* 111 (June 2003): 1,672–1,680.

Nyden, A., Billstedt, E., Hjelmquist, E., et al. "Neurocognitive Stability in Asperger Syndrome, ADHD, and Reading and Writing Disorder: A Pilot Study," *Developmental Medical Child Neurology* 43, no. 3 (March 2001): 165–171.

O'Keeffe, M. J., O'Callaghan, M., Williams, G. M., et al. "Learning, Cognitive, and Attentional Problems in Adolescents Born Small for Gestational Age," *Pediatrics* 12, no. 2 (August 2003): 301–307.

Olson, K. R., ed. *Poisoning and Drug Overdoses.* 3rd ed. New York: Appleton & Lange, 1999.

Parker, S., and Zuckerman, B., eds. *Behavioral and Developmental Pediatrics: A Handbook for Primary Care.* Boston: Little, Brown, 1995.

Parkinson, G. W., and Hike, K. E. "Bicycle Helmet Assessment During Well Visits Reveals Severe Shortcomings in Condition and Fit," *Pediatrics* 112, no. 2 (August 2003): 320–323.

Patel, N. J., and Sciubba, J. "Oral Lesions in Young Children," *Pediatric Clinics of North America* 50, no. 2 (April 2003): 469–486.

Payne, R. M., et al. "Toward a Molecular Understanding of Congenital Heart Disease," *Circulation* 91 (1995): 494.

Pellock, J. M., and Dodson, W. E. *Pediatric Epilepsy: Diagnosis and Therapy.* 2nd ed. New York: Demos, 2001.

Percy, A. K. "Research in Rett Syndrome: Past, Present, and Future," *Journal of Child Neurology* 3 (1988): S72–75.

Phipatanakul, W. "Environmental Indoor Allergens," *Pediatric Annals* 32, no. 1 (January 2003): 40–48.

Pruitt, D. B. *Your Child: What Every Parent Needs to Know About Child Development From Birth to Preadolescence.* New York: HarperCollins, 1998.

———. *Your Adolescent: Emotional, Behavioral, and Cognitive Development from Early Adolescence Through the Teen Years.* New York: HarperCollins, 1999.

O'Dwyer, M. E., and Druker, B. J. "Chronic Myelogenous Leukemia—New Therapeutic Principles," *Journal of Internal Medicine* 250 (2001): 3.

Ownby, D. R., Johnson, C. C., and Peterson, E. L. "Passive Cigarette Smoke Exposure in Infants," *Archives of Pediatric and Adolescent Medicine* 154 (2000): 1,237.

Rabban, J. T., Blair, J. A., Rosen, C. et al. "Mechanism of Pediatric Electrical Injury," *Archives of Pediatric and Adolescent Medicine* 151 (1997): 696.

Rajakumar K. "Vitamin D, Cod-Liver Oil, Sunlight, and Rickets: A Historical Perspective," *Pediatrics* 112, no. 2 (August 2003): e132–135.

Ramus, F. "Dyslexia. Talk of Two Theories,"*Nature* 412, no. 6845 (July 26, 2001): 393–395.

Randolph, C. "Latex Allergy in Pediatrics," *Current Problems in Pediatrics* 31 (2001): 131.

Remington, J. S., and Klein, J. O., eds. *Infectious Diseases of the Fetus and Newborn Infant.* 5th ed. Philadelphia: Saunders, 2001.

Rhee, D. J., et al., eds. *The Wills Eye Manual Office and Emergency Room Diagnosis and Treatment of Eye Disease.* 3rd ed. Baltimore: Lippincott, Williams & Wilkins, 1999.

Richek, M. A., Caldwell, J. S., Jennings, J. H., and Lerner, J. W. *Reading Problems: Assessment and Teaching Strategies.* Boston: Allyn & Bacon, 2001.

Rickards, H. "An International Perspective on Tourette Syndrome," *Developmental Medical Child Neurology* 43, no. 6 (June 2001): 428–429.

Riddle, M. A., Reeve, E. A., and Yaryura-Tobias, J. A. "Fluvoxamine for Children and Adolescents with OCD," *Journal of the American Academy of Child and Adolescent Psychiatry* 40, no. 2 (2001): 222.

Rockwood, C. A., Wilkins, K., and Beaty, J. H., eds. *Fractures in Children.* 4th ed. Baltimore: Lippincott, 1996.

Ross, R. N., et al. "Effectiveness of Specific Immunotherapy in the Treatment of Hymenoptera Venom Hypersensitivity," *Clinical Therapeutics* 22 (2000): 351.

Ross, H. E., and Ivis, F. "Binge Eating and Substance Use among Male and Female Adolescents," *International Journal of Eating Disorders* 26 (1999): 245.

Rotbart, H. A., and Hayden, F. G. "Picornaviruses Infections: A Primer for the Practitioner," *Archives of Family Medicine* 9 (2000): 921.

Rotbart, H. A. "Viral Meningitis," *Neurology* 20 (2000): 277.

Rotz, O. L., Khan, A., Lillibridge, S., et al. "Public Health Assessment of Potential Biological Terrorism Agents," *Emerging Infectious Diseases* (2002): 8.

Rovin, J. D., and Rodgers, B. M. "Pediatric Foreign Body Aspiration," *Pediatrics in Review* 21 (2000): 86.

Russell, J., and Hill, E. L. "Action-Monitoring and Intention Reporting in Children with Autism," *Journal of Child Psychology and Psychiatry* 42, no. 3 (March 2001): 317–328.

Sampayo, E. M. "Rotavirus Infections," *Pediatrics Review* 24, no. 9 (Sept. 2003): 322–323.

Sampson, H. A. "Food Allergy, Part 1: Immunopathogenesis and Clinical Disorders," *Journal of Allergy and Clinical Immunology* 103 (1999): 717.

———. "Food Allergy, Part 2: Diagnosis and Management," *Journal of Allergy and Clinical Immunology* 103 (1999): 981.

———. "Anaphylaxis and Emergency Treatment," *Pediatrics* 111, no. 6, part 3 (June 2003): 1,601–1,608.

Sams, H. H., et al. "Nineteen Documented Cases of Loxosceles reclusa Envenomation," *Journal of the American Academy of Dermatology* 44 (2001): 603.

Sawyer, M. H. "Enterovirus Infections: Diagnosis and Treatment," *Current Opinions in Pediatrics* 13 (2001): 65.

Schiff, D., and Shelov, S., eds. *Guide to Your Child's Symptoms, Birth Through Adolescence.* New York: Villard, 1997.

Schlaggar, B. L., and Mink, J. W. "Movement Disorders in Children," *Pediatrics in Review* 24, no. 2 (February 2003): 39–51.

Schutzman, S. A., and Greenes, D. S. "Pediatric Minor Head Trauma," *Annals of Emergency Medicine* 37 (2001): 65–74.

Scriver, C. R., et al. *The Molecular and Metabolic Bases of Inherited Disease*. 8th ed. New York: McGraw-Hill, 2001.

Sears, William, and Sears, Martha. *The Baby Book*. Boston: Little, Brown, 1993.

Shaeffer, J. L., and Ross, R. G. "Childhood Onset Schizophrenia: Premorbid and Prodromal Diagnostic and Treatment Histories," *Journal of the American Academy of Child and Adolescent Psychiatry* 41 (2002): 538.

Shelov, Steven P. *The American Academy of Pediatrics: Caring for Your Baby and Young Child*. New York: Bantam Books, 1998.

Shrier, L. A., Harris, S. K., Kurland, M., et al. "Substance Use Problems and Associated Psychiatric Symptoms among Adolescents in Primary Care," *Pediatrics* 111, no. 6, part 1 (June 2003): e699–705.

Sibbit, W. L., et al. "Neuropsychiatric Systemic Lupus Erythematosus," *Comprehensive Therapy* 25 (1999): 198.

Silverman, A., and Roy, C. C. *Pediatric Clinical Gastroenterology*. 4th ed. New York: Mosby, 1995.

Smith, Corrine, and Strick, Lisa. *Learning Disabilities: A to Z*. New York: Simon and Schuster, 1997.

Smith, G. A., Knapp, J. F., Barnett, T. M., et al. "The Rockets' Red Glare, the Bombs Bursting in Air: Fireworks-Related Injuries to Children," *Pediatrics* 98, no. 1 (1996): 1–9.

Smith, G. C., Pell, J. P., Dobbie, R. "Risk of Sudden Infant Death Syndrome and Week of Gestation of Term Birth," *Pediatrics* 111, no. 6, part 1 (June 2003): 1,367–1,371.

Smith, R. J., and Hone, S. "Genetic Screening for Deafness," *Pediatric Clinics of North America* 50, no. 2 (April 2003): 315–329.

Smyth, C. M., et al. "Klinefelter Syndrome," *Archives of Internal Medicine* 158 (1998): 1,309–1,314.

Snowling, M. J. "From Language to Reading and Dyslexia," *Dyslexia* 2001 January–March; 7(1): 37–46.

Sorensen, R. U., and Moore, C. "Antibody Deficiency Syndromes," *Pediatric Clinics of North America* 47 (2000): 1,225.

Spock, B., and Parker, S. *Dr. Spock's Baby and Child Care*. New York: Pocket Books, 1998.

Stein, David B. *Ritalin Is Not the Answer : A Drug-Free, Practical Program for Children Diagnosed With ADD or ADHD*. San Francisco: Jossey-Bass, 1999.

Stein, M. T., Zentall, S., Shaywitz, S. E., Shaywitz, B. A. "A School-aged Child with Delayed Reading Skills," *Journal of Developmental and Behavioral Pediatrics* 2001 April; 22 (2 Suppl): S111–115.

Sterni, L. M., Tunkel, D. E. "Obstructive sleep apnea in children: an update," *Pediatric Clinics of North America* 50, no. 2 (April 2003): 427–443.

Stevens, Laura J., and Crook, William G. *12 Effective Ways to Help Your ADD/ADHD Child: Drug-Free Alternatives for Attention-Deficit Disorders*. New York: Penguin Putnam, 2000.

Stoffman, Phyllis. *The Family Guide to Preventing and Treating 100 Infectious Illnesses*. New York: John Wiley & Sons, 1995.

Stratton, K., Gable, A., McCormick, M. C. *Immunization Safety Reviews: Thimerosal-Containing Vaccines and Neurodevelopment Disorders*. Washington, D.C.: Institute of Medicine, National Academy Press, 2001.

Stratton, K., Howe, C., Battaglia, F. *Fetal Alcohol Syndrome: Diagnosis, Epidemiology, Prevention, and Treatment*. New York: National Academy Press, 1996.

Suchy, F. J., ed. *Liver Disease in Children*. 2nd ed. New York: Mosby, 2000.

Sudderth, David, and Kandel, Joseph. *Adult ADD : The Complete Handbook: Everything You Need to Know About How to Cope and Live Well With ADD/ADHD*. Roseville, Calif.: Prima, 1997.

Swanson, H. L., and Sachse-Lee, C. "Mathematical Problem Solving and Working Memory in Children with Learning Disabilities: Both Executive and Phonological Processes Are Important," *Journal of Experimental Child Psychology* 79, no. 3 (July 2001): 294–321.

Swischuk, L. E. "Stiff and Sore Neck," *Pediatric Emergency Care* 19, no. 4 (August 2003): 282–284.

Teoh, D. L., and Reynolds, S. "Diagnosis and Management of Pediatric Conjunctivitis," *Pediatric Emergency Care* 19, no. 1 (February 2003): 48–55.

Ticho, B. H. "Strabismus," *Pediatric Clinics of North America* 50, no. 1 (February 2003): 173–188.

To, T. "Cohort Study on Circumcision of Newborn Boys and Subsequent Risk of Urinary-Tract Infections," *Lancet* 352 (1998): 1,813.

Toomey, S., and Bernstein, H. "Sudden Infant Death Syndrome," *Current Opinions in Pediatrics* 13 (2001): 207.

Townes, B. D. "Adult Outcome of Verbal Learning Disability: An Optimistic Note," *Seminars in Clinical Neuropsychiatry* 5, no. 3 (July 2000): 210–211.

Turkington, C. *The Poisons and Antidotes Sourcebook.* 2nd ed. New York: Facts On File, 1999.

———. *The Encyclopedia of the Brain and Brain Disorders.* 2nd ed. New York: Facts On File, 2002.

———. *Hepatitis C: The Silent Killer.* New York: Contemporary Books, 1998.

Turkington, C., and Ashby, B. L. *The Encyclopedia of Infectious Diseases.* 2nd ed. New York: Facts On File, 2003.

Turkington, C., and Dover, J. S. *The Encyclopedia of Skin and Skin Disorders.* 2nd ed. New York: Facts On File, 2002.

Turkington, C., and Harris, J. *Understanding Memory: The Sourcebook for Memory and Memory Disorders.* New York: Checkmark Books, 2001.

———. *Understanding Learning Disabilities: The Sourcebook for Causes, Disorders and Treatments.* New York: Facts On File, 2003.

Turkington, C., and Kaplan, E. F. *Making the Antidepressant Decision.* New York: Contemporary Books, 2001.

Turkington, C., and Sussman, A. *The Encyclopedia of Hearing and Hearing Disorders.* New York: Facts On File, 2000.

U.S. Consumer Product Safety Commission. 1999 Fireworks Annual Report: Fireworks-related deaths, emergency department treated injuries, and enforcement activities during 1999. (June 11, 2001) Online: www.cpsc.gov/library/1999fwreport6.PDF

Van Dyke, D. C. and Holte, L. "Communication Disorders in Children," *Pediatric Annals* 32, no. 7 (July 2003): 436–437.

Vazquez, M., Sparrow, S. S., Shapiro, E. D. "Long-Term Neuropsychologic and Health Outcomes of Children with Facial Nerve Palsy Attributable to Lyme Disease," *Pediatrics* 112, no. 2 (August 2003): e93–97

Vicari, S., Bellucci, S., Carlesimo, G. A. "Procedural Learning Deficit in Children with Williams Syndrome," *Neuropsychologia* 39, no. 7 (2001): 665–677.

Waasdorp, C. E. "Lessons Learned Following the Anthrax Experience," *Pediatric Annals* 32, no. 3 (March 2003): 193–194.

Waecker, N. J. Jr., and Hale, B. R. "Smallpox Vaccination. What the Pediatrician Needs to Know," *Pediatric Annals* 32, no. 3 (March 2003): 178–181.

Weber, S. M., and Grundfast, K. M. "Modern Management of Acute Otitis Media," *Pediatric Clinics of North America* 50, no. 2 (April 2003): 399–411.

Weir, E. "Raves: A Review of the Culture, the Drugs and the Prevention of Harm," *Canadian Medical Association Journal* 162 (2000): 1,843.

Wetmore, R. F. "Complications of Otitis Media," *Pediatric Annals* 29 (2000): 637.

Winner, B. J. "Disability and the ADA: Learning Impairment as a Disability," *Journal of Law and Medical Ethics* 28, no. 4 (2000): 410–411.

Wolf, L. E. "College Students with ADHD and Other Hidden Disabilities. Outcomes and Interventions," *Annals of the New York Academy of Science* 931 (June 2001): 385–395.

Woo, P., and Wedderburn, L. R. "Juvenile Chronic Arthritis," *Lancet* 351 (1998): 969.

Wood, R. A. "The Natural History of Food Allergy," *Pediatrics* 111 (June 2003): 1,631–1,637.

World Health Organization Department of Vaccines and Biologicals. "Safety of Mass Immunization Campaigns, 2002." http://www.

who.int/vaccines-documents/DocsPDF02/www669.pdf

Yorgin, P. D. "Renal Manifestations of Rheumatic Diseases Affecting Adolescents," *Adolescent Medicine* 9 (1998): 127.

Zaoutis, T., and Klein, J. D. "Enterovirus Infections," *Pediatrics in Review* 19 (1998): 183.

Zebrowski, P. M. "Developmental Stuttering," *Pediatric Annals* 32, no. 7 (July 2003): 453–458.

INDEX

Boldface page numbers indicate major treatment of a subject.